Readings in
Clinical Psychology
Today

Contributing editor, Barbara A. Henker

ASSISTANT PROFESSOR, DEPARTMENT OF PSYCHOLOGY,
UNIVERSITY OF CALIFORNIA, LOS ANGELES

Readings in
Clinical Psychology
Today

CRM BOOKS
Del Mar, California

Assistants to Dr. Henker:
Sue Ellen Holbrook, Maria Nemeth, Carol Whalen

Library of Congress Catalog Card Number: 73–91132
Standard Book Number: 87665–106–6

Manufactured in the United States of America
First Printing

Contents

Introduction

This collection of articles, selected from the pages of *Psychology Today*, presents the innovative concepts and recent research in the area of clinical psychology. No longer confined to the diagnosis and treatment of "mental disorder," modern clinical psychology is blending imperceptibly with personality theory, and with applied learning theory and social psychology as well. The articles chosen for inclusion reflect this breadth. Most of the selections are controversial; they are here either because they represent a challenge to our established ways of understanding and treating psychological problems or because they present a perspective not found in the usual textbook.

Today's clinical psychologists, like today's students, move in a time of ferment and urge to change. From the many changes taking place three main themes emerge. One is the trend, in the clinical study of personality, away from a preoccupation with pathology. Freud fostered the idea that ordinary, everyday behaviors such as memory lapses or slips of the tongue are indicators of hidden conflict. This diagnostic attitude of looking at behavior for clues to underlying problems or sickness no longer dominates clinical psychology—however popular it may be at cocktail parties. Instead, clinicians use much more than the single dimension of sickness versus health when they look at personality patterns. They are as interested in positive abnormalities as they are in negatively valued deviations. They employ a flexible array of concepts, and the approach is descriptive rather than evaluative. They focus as much on "what is going on" as on "what is wrong." Only a few of the readings here use the familiar labels associated with psychological "disorders"; more characteristic are rich, qualitative descriptions that imply no clear distinction between normal and abnormal psychological processes. Dreams, needs, social strategies, and even defenses are now assessed in terms of their adaptive value *for the individual.*

Just as clinical descriptions of personality are more than thermometerlike measures of sickness, psychotherapy is more than the treatment of mental disturbance. Therapy no longer implies a fixed set of techniques used only by highly trained experts. The cast, the staging, the script, and the props have all been expanded, in an almost limitless way. This thrust toward innovation represents a second theme in current clinical psychology.

A generation ago, Carl Rogers and the neo-Freudians altered the history of psychotherapy. The chair replaced the couch, and problems in living rather than fantasy and memory became the focus. Although different schools of therapy differed markedly in emphasis, there was general agreement on several issues: The goal was insight into one's problems, and the method was face-to-face interaction with a skilled therapist, either in dyads or groups. Almost every major therapist emphasized the *relationship* as the vehicle of therapy. Each school still had a set of procedures and conditions designed to guide the therapist, but rigid adherence to dogma and rules was beginning to disappear. Today, an even greater spirit of innovation pervades the entire field. Complacency and orthodoxy are rapidly being replaced by a self-critical, experimental attitude. Today's therapist tailors his treatment techniques to fit the problem rather than vice versa. The result is an abundance of new (but less dogmatic) schools of therapy, new personnel, and new techniques. Widely divergent approaches such as humanism and learning theory now coexist with only minimal friction; rosters of subprofessionals are now easing the shortage of trained psychotherapists; awareness training, encounter groups, and physiological conditioning are but a few examples of the new methodologies.

This innovative climate is part and parcel of the strong reaction against the medical model of personality change. *Therapists* still administer *treatment* to *patients* in clinical settings, but outside of medical environments we also have *behavioral* specialists or *human relations* counselors working with *participants* in centers, institutes, or even homes and offices. In some settings, even the word "therapy" is in disfavor because of its medical connotations. The pervasive influence the medical model has had is shown by the fact that one cannot discuss psychological problems without using medical terms. There are no adequate substitutes, as yet, for mental "illness," "psychopathology," or "treatment." There is no synonym for "clinical" psychology.

Current dissatisfaction stems mainly from the implications of the model. When a problem in living is seen as an illness, responsibility for cure tends to be vested in a specialist, and a passive role is assigned to the "sick" person. Few would claim the model is altogether inappropriate; rather, it has been overextended. Current research does indicate, however, that within limits the

traditional approach may still prove essential. One example is in the understanding of psychotic processes.
Another is in the application of learning principles to
therapy; if the behavior therapist is not seen as an
expert or if his instructions are disregarded, the technique is not productive.

A third trend is the growth of communication and
involvement between mental health professionals and
the community they serve. In the final section of the
book, it is obvious that the moral and clinical issues
surrounding "psychopathology" and "psychotherapy"
have now become public concerns. The broadened definitions of psychotherapy, the increasing numbers of
subprofessional therapists, and the advantages of group
techniques have made psychological methods of change
more available and more acceptable. In Everett Shostrom's view this enthusiasm and acceptance may have
come too fast. In our eagerness to abandon the medical
model and the "expert" figure of the therapist, we may
have thrown the baby out with the bathwater.

Ashley Montagu's paper raises another consequence
of discarding the medical model. We have long known
that some types of hallucinations and even maladaptive
behaviors have a biological base. Montagu forces us to
consider that criminal tendencies might also be biological in origin. If so, how should the criminal be treated
in our courts? When is a man to be held responsible for
his acts?

Taken together, these articles attest that the understanding of personal and interpersonal conflicts is one of
the most important frontiers in modern civilization.
The professions most concerned—psychology, psychiatry, and social work—are abandoning interdisciplinary
rivalries and outmoded theories to forge new approaches
and new insights. As these readings amply confirm,
today the questions far outbalance the answers.

I
Psychopathology and Personality Dynamics

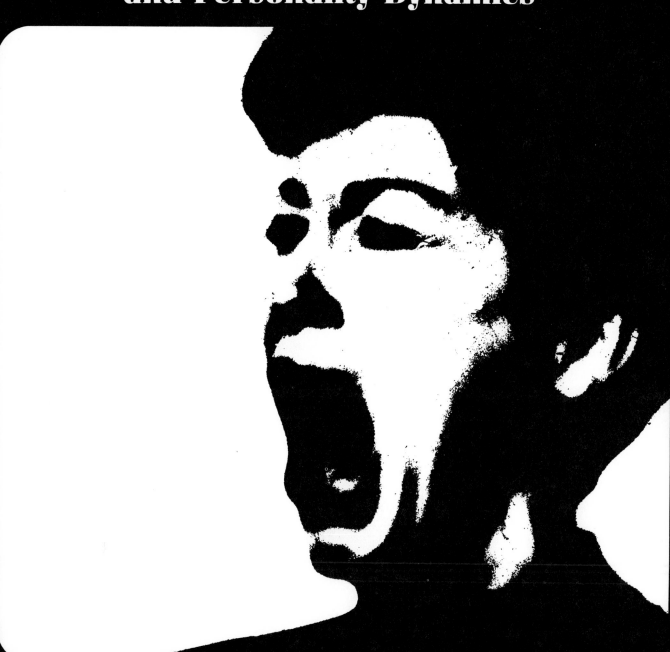

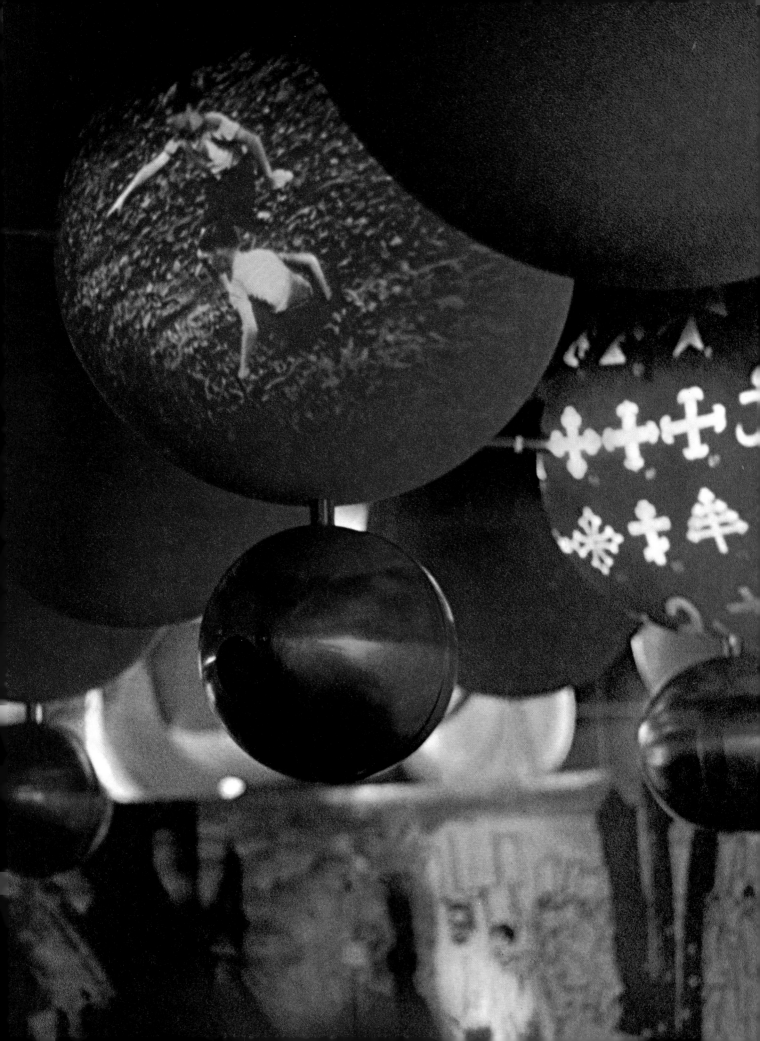

The Dreams of Freud and Jung
Calvin S. Hall and Bill Domhoff

Freud gave us a theory of mental life that has influenced virtually every discussion, formal and informal, of human motives held in the past fifty years. One of his most brilliant students, Carl Jung, shared Freud's interest in the workings of the unconscious, but the two disagreed on the importance of biological versus creative urges. Jung soon formulated his own theory and subsequently fathered what is today a small but vigorous school of therapists and writers.

Calvin Hall and Bill Domhoff provide an unusual perspective from which to view these two great thinkers. Their article has another value as well, in that it describes a systematic method of analyzing the content and structure of dreams. Dream analysis has usually been founded on the notion that dreams permit the expression, in disguised or symbolic form, of the dreamer's censored wishes. Hall and Domhoff point out that dream content often parallels waking thought and that dreams recapitulate actual experiences, feelings, and life styles. Though not forgoing intuitive interpretations, they have endeavored to systemize their analyses. For each reported dream, they tabulate numbers of people, classes of objects, types of interactions, and even lengths of lines. Such methods lend themselves to analyzing the Rorschach inkblot test and the Thematic Apperception Test (TAT), as well as dreams, personal letters, or even the productive fantasy of fiction.

When psychiatric research, normally content to draw on frailer men· for its material, approaches one who is among the greatest of the human race, it is not doing so for the reasons so frequently assigned to it by laymen. "To blacken the radiant and drag the sublime into the dust" is no part of its purpose, and there is no satisfaction for it in narrowing the gulf which separates the perfection of the great from the inadequacy of the objects that are its usual concern. But it cannot help finding worthy of understanding everything that can be recognized in these illustrious models, and it believes there is no one so great as to be disgraced by being subject to the laws which govern both normal and pathological activity with equal cogency. (From "Leonardo Da Vinci and a Memory of His Childhood," by Sigmund Freud.)

It is hard to imagine two more "illustrious models" in the matter of dream analysis than Freud and Jung. Both men analyzed their own dreams—and, at times, each other's—so it is fitting to demonstrate the usefulness of a new analytic method by applying it to *their* dreams.

What follows is a comparative and quantitative study of the dreams of Freud and Jung as they reported them in their writings. Its main purpose is to demonstrate the value of quantitative content analysis of dreams and to relate the information conveyed by the dreams to known facts about the character and behavior of the two men.

Freud reported twenty-eight dreams in two books, *The Interpretation of Dreams* and *On Dreams*. Jung reported thirty-one, in his autobiographical study, *Memories, Dreams, Reflections*. Although we would like to have had more dreams to work with, previous studies that we have conducted show that as few as twenty dreams reveal significant aspects of a dreamer's personality. Moreover, the two men's choice of dreams to report might be prejudiced. For example, Freud might have selected dreams favorable to *his* theory, and Jung might have selected dreams favorable to *his* theory. It does seem evident that the two men's reasons for relating their dreams in the first place were quite different. Freud used his own dreams to illustrate various aspects of his dream theory; Jung's purpose was the more personal one of illuminating the nature of his inner life and development. This difference in purpose is evidenced by the books in which the dreams appear. Freud's are published in scientific treatises; Jung's are reported in his autobiography.

In spite of differing purposes, we expected that objective methods of dream analysis would reveal differences between the two men that were congruent with differences in their biographies. We also expected to find many similarities in their dreams. There is, we think, a hard core of universality in the dreams of all human beings, no matter *when* they live, *where* they live, or *how* they live. Each dream was typed on a five by eight card. Freud's twenty-eight dreams and Jung's thirty-one dreams were shuffled together before they were scored. One of us (Dr. Hall) did all the scoring, using content scales described in *The Content Analysis of Dreams* by Calvin Hall and Robert Van de Castle. In order to achieve greater accuracy, each dream was scored twice. The dreams were scored for the following variables: length, characters, objects, aggressive and friendly interactions, success and failure, good fortune and misfortune, oral incorporation and oral emphasis, and castration anxiety, castration wish, and penis envy.

To find out what was typical about Freud's and Jung's dreams, their scores were compared with the scores obtained for 500 dreams reported by 100 young American men and, in some cases, with other norms. Although the exact age at which each of Freud's and Jung's dreams occurred is known in only a few cases, it is believed that, with one exception, they were all dreamed during adult life. The exception is a dream Jung reports having had when he was about four years old.

Here, then, are the results of our investigation into the dreams of Freud and Jung.

Length

The total number of lines in Freud's twenty-eight dream narratives is 286, just a shade more than ten lines per dream. His longest dream is thirty-four lines, his shortest is one line. The total number of lines in Jung's thirty-one dreams is 458, just shy of fifteen lines per dream. His longest dream is fifty-one lines, his shortest is four lines.

This fairly marked difference in average length of dream report is in keeping with the writing styles of the two men. Freud published as much if not more than Jung did, but Freud's style is compact and Jung's discursive. One cannot imagine Freud as the author of Jung's rambling *Memories, Dreams, Reflections*, nor Jung writing Freud's spare *Autobiographical Study*.

Characters

There are certain universal facts about the characters in all dreams. One of them, taken so much for granted that it is rarely commented upon, is that the dreamer is a character in virtually all his own dreams. Freud and Jung are no exceptions: they appear in all their own dreams. (In the Hall-Van de Castle system of content analysis, however, the dreamer is not counted as a character.)

Another universal is that men dream more about men than about women, but women dream about equally of the two sexes. Freud and Jung abide by this general rule. They have almost identical sex ratios. The ratio of men to women in Freud's dreams is 2.56 to 1, and in Jung's dreams it is 2.50 to 1. These ratios are somewhat higher than the average ratio for American college men, which is about 2 to 1. It is known, however, that the sex ratio increases with age.

Still another universal is the proportion of single and plural characters. (A plural character is an undifferentiated group or crowd.) The typical proportion is .70 single characters to .30 plural characters. Jung's dreams show exactly that proportion, and Freud's a proportion that is only slightly different, .73 single characters to .27 plurals.

Dreams reported by adults are always peopled by many more adult characters than adolescents, children, and babies. The proportion of adults in college men's dreams is .97. Freud's and Jung's proportions are .91 and .93, respectively, which are not significantly different from the norm.

Finally, there is a standard proportion of familiar and unfamiliar characters. A familiar character is a member of the dreamer's family, a relative, a friend or acquaintance, or a prominent person. An unfamiliar character is one who is not known to the dreamer in waking life. In typical dreams of men, .45 of the characters are familiar and .55 are unfamiliar. Freud's proportions are .53 for familiar characters and .47 for unfamiliar characters. Jung's proportions are .57 and .43. This difference between Freud and Jung is not significant, nor is the difference between their proportions and those of the normative group. Up to this point, the results of the analysis of dream characters merely demonstrate that both Freud and Jung belonged to the male half of the human race. But there are also differences in the dream characters of the two men.

Freud has more characters in his dreams than Jung does, 85 to Jung's 70, although Jung reports more dreams and longer ones. The number of lines per character is 3.4 for Freud and 6.5 for Jung. The density coefficient of people in Freud's dreams is much higher than it is for Jung. Jung's dreams are filled with scenery, architecture, and objects rather than with people.

This difference appears to be compatible with what is known about the two men. Freud was a sociable person. He had many close friends and disciples with whom he had very personal relationships. One imagines him surrounded by an entourage wherever he went. Jung was more solitary and kept would-be disciples at a distance. He spent much time in scholarly pursuits, poring over old manuscripts, and he was a lover of nature. Jung said of himself, "Today as then [in childhood] I am a solitary."

A difference in sociability between the two men is indicated by other evidence from their dreams and writings. Animals appear more frequently in Jung's dreams than in Freud's, which suggests that Jung identified more closely with the world of nature than with the world of men. He writes in *Memories, Dreams, Reflections*, "I loved all warm-blooded animals . . . Animals were dear and faithful, unchanging and trustworthy. People I now distrusted more than ever." Mystical, fictional, and historical figures turn up more often in Jung's dreams than in Freud's. This suggests that Jung lived more in the past whereas Freud lived more in the present. Indeed, Jung said that for years he felt more closely attuned to the past, especially to the Middle Ages and the eighteenth century, than to the present.

Jung dreams more about members of his family; Freud dreams more about friends and acquaintances. This implies that Jung's sociability expressed itself within his immediate family, and Freud's social life was centered more outside the family. It is interesting that although Jung was an only child for nine years and then had only one sister, and Freud grew up in the midst of a large family, both men raised large families of their own. Freud had six children, and Jung had five. Nonetheless, Freud seems to have looked persistently for intimate and even paternal relations outside his family.

A letter written by Freud to Jung is characteristic of his search for intimacy. Here is a passage from the letter, which is reproduced in *Memories, Dreams, Reflections*. "It is remarkable that on the same evening that I formally adopted you as an eldest son, anointing you as my successor and crown prince etc. . . . I therefore don once more my horn-rimmed paternal spectacles and warn my dear son to keep a cool head . . ." Given Jung's solitariness, his preference for nature and architecture, and his familial concerns, and also given his unsatisfactory relationship with his own father, it is not difficult to imagine how repelled Jung was by Freud's adhesiveness or to believe how quickly the two men went their separate ways.

Here, we think, lies the real secret of their break. After all, Swiss intellectuals such as Oscar Pfister, a Protestant minister, and Ludwig Binswanger, who introduced existentialism and phenomenology into psychiatry, remained personal friends with Freud despite considerable intellectual differences. But Freud did not try to make sons out of Pfister and Binswanger; and Pfister and Binswanger, unlike Jung, did not have depressive, moody fathers who lost their faith and spent time in mental institutions.

Objects

There are twelve classes of objects and a miscellaneous class in the Hall-Van de Castle system of content analysis. Three of the classes—architecture, implements, and body parts—have subclasses. There are

many more objects in Jung's dreams than in Freud's, 297 versus 196. This suggests, as does the larger number of human characters in Freud's dreams, that Jung was more object-oriented and Freud was more person-oriented.

Further support is given to this statement by the kinds of objects each man dreamed about. Jung dreamed more about houses, buildings, and architectural details—especially windows, doors, and walls—and more about nature and landscape than either Freud or the norm group did. Freud, on the other hand, dreamed much more about parts of the body, particularly parts of the head, than either Jung or the norm group did.

It is interesting to speculate on the symbolic meaning of these differences. If architecture and nature are female symbols, for the most part, and if body parts, especially the head, are displacements of the male genitals, then it could be inferred that Jung was more oriented toward the female and Freud was more oriented toward the male. This inference ties in with other data to be presented here.

Jung's dreams contain no references to money, whereas Freud dreams of money about as often as the norm group. Freud also refers more often than Jung to food, a fact that will be commented on later. Both men seldom mention implements, especially weapons and recreational equipment, which is probably not surprising considering that they were intellectuals and scholars.

Interaction

In Freud's dreams, there are sixteen aggressive and sixteen friendly interactions; in Jung's dreams, fourteen and eleven, respectively. When these figures are divided by the number of characters, the proportions are much the same for Freud and Jung. Moreover, they are in close accord with the proportions for male dreamers between the ages of thirty and eighty.

Other universal characteristics of Freud's and Jung's dreams are the large proportion of dreamer-involved aggression and friendliness as compared with witnessed aggression and friendliness, and the equal number of times that the dreamer is aggressor and victim.

With regard to the role of befriender and befriended, however, the two men are poles apart. Every time Jung is involved in a friendly interaction, he initiates the friendliness. Freud, on the other hand, is more often the recipient of friendliness (eight out of eleven times). The norm is midway between the figures for Freud and Jung. Does this signify that Freud wanted people to respond to him in a friendly manner and was sensitive about being rejected? It does seem that Freud was sensitive about being slighted: for example, his feelings were hurt that Jung did not make an effort to visit him when Freud made a trip to Switzerland. And Freud's biographer, Ernest Jones, says that Freud became quite annoyed when friends to whom he had written did not reply at once.

Another indication of Jung's greater social autonomy is that, when we consider only the dreams in which aggression or friendliness occurs (and not the total number of aggressive and friendly encounters in all the dreams), Freud has almost twice as many "interactional" dreams as Jung has. Freud's frequency agrees with the norm. In other words, Jung has fewer dreams in which he interacts in significant ways with other characters than does Freud.

By far the most interesting finding with respect to aggression and friendliness, however, is the striking difference in Freud's and Jung's aggressive and friendly encounters with male and female characters. The typical man has more aggressive interactions with men than with women, and more friendly interactions with women than with men. Jung's aggressive and friendly encounters with men and women are fairly typical. He has an aggressive interaction with about one out of four male characters in his dreams, and none at all with females. As for friendly encounters, Jung has about an equal number with men and women, which deviates slightly from the norm.

In Freud's dreams, the typical pattern is reversed. He has an aggressive encounter with one out of every four *female* characters, and almost none with males. On the other hand, he has many more friendly encounters with men than with women. These results suggest that Freud had an inverted Oedipus complex. The Oedipus complex is characterized by hostility toward other men and friendliness or love toward women. In an inverted Oedipus complex, the tables are turned. There is a friendly attitude toward men and a hostile one toward women. (Freud's pattern of aggression and friendliness with men and women is not like that of the typical woman, who is both more aggressive and friendlier toward men than toward women. Nor is it like the pattern of a group of male patients in a mental hospital, who showed more aggression than friendliness toward both men and women.)

Is there any evidence from his biography that Freud had an inverted Oedipus complex? Many people have concluded after reading Freud that he was hostile toward women. Ernest Jones says that Freud's attitude toward women was "old fashioned": Freud considered that their main function was to serve as "ministering angels to the needs and comforts of men." He thought women "enigmatic" ("What do they want?" he asked Marie Bonaparte); he was attracted to masculine women; he was "quite peculiarly monogamous." Jones says that "the more passionate side of married life subsided with him [Freud] earlier than it does with many men. We assume this means that Freud stopped having intercourse with his wife fairly early in their married life. That he was "quite peculiarly monogamous" suggests that he did not have affairs with other women.

As regards Freud's feelings for men, we know that he had a very intense relationship with Wilhelm Fliess. Freud spoke of overcoming his emotional homosexuality and admitted that alternations of love and hate affected his relationships with men. Jones also speaks of Freud's "mental bisexuality." By using the word "mental" as a qualifier, Jones implies that the bisexuality was never physically expressed. Freud wrote to his friend and colleague, Max Eitingon, "The affection of a group of courageous young men is the most precious gift that psychoanalysis has bestowed upon me." This remark is reminiscent of Michelangelo (whose art Freud greatly admired), who also found joy in being surrounded by young men.

It appears from his dreams, then, that Freud had an inverted Oedipus complex, and what biographical material is available supports this conclusion. Jung, on the other hand, seems to have had a fairly ordinary Oedipus complex, in the sense that hostility toward the father is inevitable. Nothing that is known of Jung's life changes the picture. He says in his autobiography that he felt much closer to his mother than he did to his father. When his father died, he immediately assumed the role of father in the household, even to the point of moving into his father's room. Small wonder that Jung did not want to become a son again, least of all the son of a father with an inverted Oedipus complex.

Success and failure in dreams are almost always experienced by the dreamer himself, and this holds true for Freud and Jung. Most men have an equal amount of success and failure in their dreams. So does Jung, but Freud has much more success than failure. In fact, he succeeds six times and only fails once. This suggests that Freud was more strongly motivated to succeed than Jung was. Jones' remark that fame meant very little to Freud does not square with the fairly obvious fact that Freud aspired to greatness.

Jung, on the other hand, though he may have had the same aspiration, did not do many of the things that would have helped him achieve fame. Unlike Freud, he did not found an international organization with its own journals and publishing house. He did not establish a chain of institutes throughout the world to promote his ideas. He did not encourage disciples. He preferred his stone tower to the bustle of the scientific marketplace. He did not seek worldly success, though he did not refuse it when it knocked at his door. Near the end of his life Jung wrote, "Today I can say it is truly astounding that I have had as much success as has been accorded me."

Good Fortune and Misfortune

Good fortune in dreams is rare; misfortune is commonplace. Freud and Jung, true to this universal pattern, have more misfortune than good fortune in their dreams. In fact, Freud has no good fortune at all. Jung, however, has more good fortune than is to be expected. Good fortune is defined as something favorable that happens to a person without any effort on his part, and without a friendly intent upon another character's part. Freud's lack of good fortune, taken together with his large amount of success relative to failure, suggests that he saw success as the result of his own efforts, and not as luck. Jung was more likely to view the world, at least in his dreams, as a cornucopia of benefits. The impression one gets from Jung's autobiography is that he was more fatalistic than Freud. He was inclined to let things happen to him, to let his life be lived rather than to live it. His life "developed naturally and by destiny"; he felt that it was ruled by forces over which he had no control, and that (though he spent much of his adult life trying) he did not completely understand. Freud was more rationalistic. By exercising reason, he felt that one could master the world.

It is customary in dreams for misfortune to befall the dreamer more often than other characters. This is the case in Jung's dreams, but the reverse is true for Freud. In his dreams, more misfortune comes to other characters than to himself. If misfortune to the dreamer is interpreted as an expression of self-punishment, then misfortune to others may be interpreted as a disguised expression of hostility. The dreamer intends harm to another person but he does not want to express it directly through an aggressive act. We have not been able to find any biographical substantiation for the high incidence of indirect hostility in Freud's dreams.

We do know from a previous study that having more misfortunes happen to characters other than the dreamer is less usual for men than for women. In this respect, then, Freud's dreams are more like those of women.

Oral Incorporation and Emphasis

Oral incorporation is scored whenever there is mention of food, eating, drinking, cooking, restaurants, and the like in the dream report. Oral emphasis consists of references to the mouth and to oral activities other than eating and drinking, as, for example, smoking, singing, and so forth. On both scales, Freud scores higher than Jung, whose scores agree with the norms. Freud probably had a lot of orality in his makeup. We know he smoked a large number of cigars. Jones informs us that Freud had a horror of ever having to be dependent upon others—a reaction formation against oral dependence. Freud's orality is also consistent with the fact that he received friendliness in his dreams more often than he initiated it. It is as if he wanted to be taken care of but fought this infantile wish. Orality is also consistent with the relatively high incidence of success and low incidence of good fortune in Freud's dreams. He wanted to achieve success through his own efforts partly in order to deny his underlying need to be dependent.

Orality does not appear to have played much of a role in Jung's life, nor does he seem to have had conflicts about being dependent upon others. On the contrary, Jung preferred to go it alone rather than be dependent on others.

Castration Anxiety and Penis Envy

The castration anxiety, castration wish, and penis envy scales reflect different aspects of the castration complex. Castration anxiety is shown in a dream by injury to part of the dreamer's body or damage to one of his possessions. Castration wish is shown when the same thing happens to another character in the dream. Penis envy reveals itself through the dreamer's acquisition of impressive phallic objects such as cars or guns. These three scales have been shown by Hall and Van de Castle to differentiate between male and female dreamers in a way consistent with Freudian theory.

There is little castration anxiety and no penis envy in either Freud's or Jung's dreams. Freud does express a wish to castrate others in a few of his dreams, but it does not exceed the norms. We may conclude that as far as their dreams tell us, neither of the men was unusually afflicted with this basic anxiety.

In Conclusion

This completes our survey of some of the scorable features of the dreams of Freud and Jung. The results show, as we thought they would, that the dreams have universal characteristics as well as individual ones. In this instance, the individual traits are the more interesting because the subjects are Freud and Jung.

Our findings suggest that "scores," that is, frequencies and proportions, obtained from counting various elements in reported dreams bear a meaningful relationship to the personality and behavior of the dreamer. This fact not only demonstrates the value of the system of content analysis devised by Hall and Van de Castle; it also shows that there are important continuities between dreams and waking life: our evidence from the dreams of Freud and Jung supports the idea that their dream behavior is congruent with their behavior in waking life. And the dreams shed considerable light on the breakup of their friendship.

These findings are really not very astonishing when one considers that dreaming is as much a form of behavior as anything a person does in waking life. It would be surprising if dreams failed to reflect the same basic wishes and fears that govern waking behavior, since behavior—all behavior, in our opinion—is to a large degree a product of the timeless unconscious. It is the timeless unconscious (Freud's term) that confers a pattern upon a personality and that grinds out the same forms of behavior over and over again, in dreams as in waking life. To the old question, "Am I a butterfly who dreams he is an awake person or a sleeping person who dreams he is a butterfly?" we reply, "It makes no difference." The dream state merely reveals more clearly the wishes and fears that guide our waking actions.

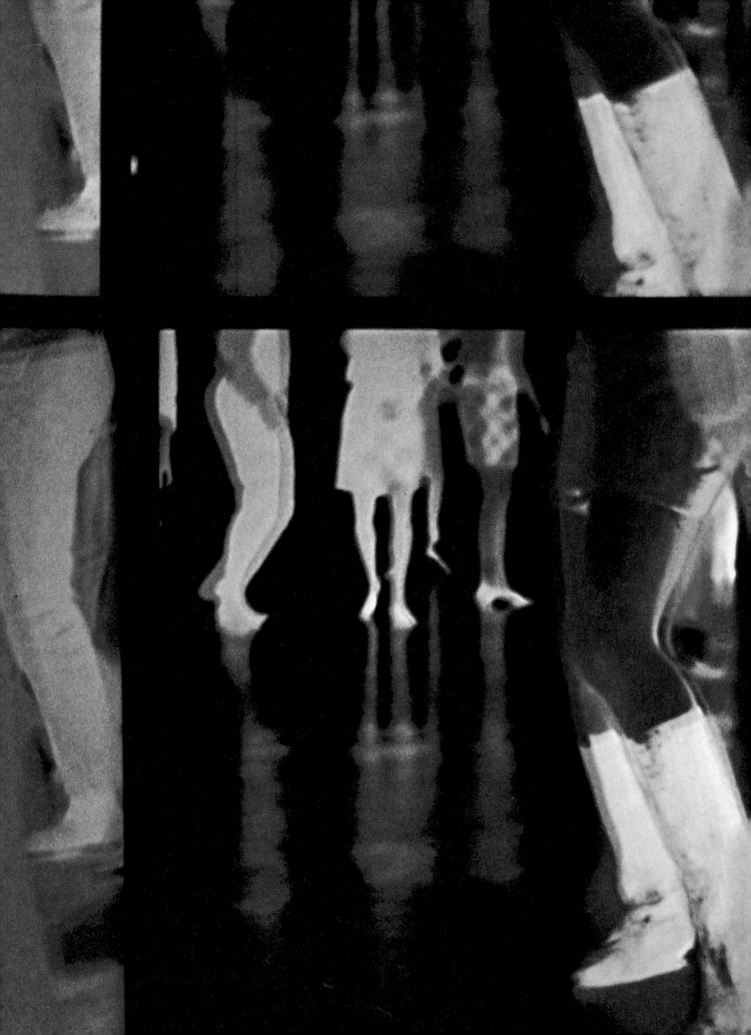

The Importance of Daydreaming
Jerome L. Singer

We've probably all heard a lecturer say, "Stop for a moment and imagine . . ." and in the next few sentences draw a fantasy picture or colorful analogy of something that is otherwise hard to describe. The image we form in our mind's eye helps us to understand the lecturer's message. Some of us will form better analogies than others because we are more skillful in objective daydreaming. The lecturer himself is probably a practiced daydreamer who uses fantasy in his creative and scholarly work as well as in planning his lectures.

Jerome Singer has spent many years studying the dreams of both children and adults. His research shows some support for the common notion that daydreaming is a retreat from stress or a substitute for overt action. According to Singer, however, these hypotheses about fantasies are far too simple. People can solve problems through fantasy as well as avoid them; daydreaming can arouse or reduce our anxieties and drives depending upon the situation.

Singer's attitude toward fantasy is similar to that described by Hall and Domhoff in the preceding article on the dreams of Freud and Jung. Dreams and daydreams are not so much a mysterious and unique aspect of consciousness as they are a part of the mainstream of ongoing behavior. The situations in which a man daydreams, the content of his fantasies, and the type of daydreaming he does form an integral part of his life style.

George, I've asked you three times to empty the garbage and you haven't moved."

"Sorry, Darling, I guess I didn't hear you. I must have been daydreaming."

"But you were looking straight at me!"

Mrs. Brown hears voices coming from five-year-old Timmy's bedroom. Momentarily startled, she soon realizes that Timmy merely is playing a game by himself, acting out the roles of the good guys and the bad guys.

The mother smiles proudly at Timmy's cleverness in shifting voices. Then she feels a pang of anxiety. Is something wrong with her son? Should he be talking to himself at his age? Isn't this a symptom of some emotional conflict?

These two cases illustrate a phenomenon most common to human experience. Daydreams intrude suddenly into the waking thoughts of almost everyone during a normal day and certainly surge into prominence in those quiet or solitary moments when we ride on trains, sit in waiting rooms, or prepare for bed.

The nocturnal dream, more vivid and dramatic, has been the focus of much attention in folklore, literature, and science from the days of Joseph in Pharaoh's court to the recent flurry of neurophysiological experimentation on sleep. Its paler cousin, the fleeting fantasy or distracting image we call the daydream, has always been of interest to creative artists but has been virtually ignored by scientific researchers.

These two hypothetical but typical cases point up some of the unknowns about daydreaming. Is George's reverie simply an escape from the unpleasant reality of taking out the garbage? Is his failure to hear his wife the sign of worthwhile, creative thinking, or is it a psychological defense against the humdrum character of his life?

And what is the nature of the fantasy play activity in which young Timmy is indulging? Is he abnormal? Is his taking of several roles the creation in effect of a world around Timmy that is not really there? Is it something that prepares him for skills in later life, or is it a passing characteristic of childhood? What kinds of cultural patterns foster such imaginative play or prevent its continuation?

Clearly, some systematic scientific understanding of the scope and function of daydreaming in children and in adults is called for. But how does one catch hold of so insubstantial a bit of fluff as a daydream for any kind of scientific study? Science usually requires objectivity, repeatability of the phenomenon, measurement, and experimental control. How to squeeze a daydream into that mold has so baffled psychologists that very little formal research on daydreaming has been done.

Well before the turn of the century, Sir Francis Galton proposed to study the range of human imagery, and William James called attention to the stream of thought as a significant human phenomenon. Psychoanalysts have, of course, made frequent use of their patients' daydreams in diagnosis and therapy. But behavioral scientists have devoted surprisingly little effort to examining daydreams or related types of self-generated internal stimulation experienced by the average person.

Indeed, in our action-oriented nation, the term "daydreaming" has assumed a negative connotation. But it does not seem likely that fantasizing is inherently pathological or even defensive. It seems more reasonable that daydreaming is a fundamental human characteristic, an autonomous ego function. Daydreaming is more than a readily available defense or escape; it is a valuable method we all use to explore a variety of perspectives.

My own interest in daydreaming evolved out of an earlier interest in the nature of imaginative behavior as shown clinically in such "projective techniques" as the Rorschach inkblots and the Thematic Apperception Test. Both of these techniques require a person to project his own feelings and ideas into an interpretation of ambiguous images—inkblots in the first case and nondescript drawings in the second. Presumably in doing so he reveals his general behavioral style and his dominant motivational pattern.

Especially interesting to me was Herman Rorschach's observation that people who look at inkblots and report seeing human beings in action—the so-called M determinant—are imaginative people, inclined to an original, rich inner life. The Rorschach M response has interesting implications for an understanding of imagination. Nevertheless, with the Rorschach data we still are dealing with an inferred measure of imagination based on reactions to inkblots—several steps removed from the underlying process which is of primary interest: the daydream itself.

Rather than attempting to explore daydreaming simply by making inferences from the Rorschach data, we decided to begin again and examine the phenomenon more directly. For some time now a program of research has been carried on under my direction at the City College of the City University of New York, with the close collaboration of various colleagues, in particular Professor John Antrobus.

Daydreaming Questionnaire

My first step was to devise a questionnaire, based on what I could learn from clinical literature and from the experiences of friends, relatives, and patients, as well as from my own introspections. This questionnaire consisted of a large number of actual daydreams; the person answered it by indicating how frequently he indulged in the various kinds of daydreams described. Over a period of time the questionnaire was improved and polished, and administered to almost 500 men and women, most of them college-educated. No data on persons of other socioeconomic levels are available at this time.

The questionnaire included such sample daydreams as these:

"I have my own yacht and plan a cruise of the Eastern seaboard."

"I suddenly find I can fly, to the amazement of passersby."

"I see myself in the arms of a warm and loving person who satisfies all my needs."

"I picture an atomic bombing of the town I live in."

"I see myself participating with wild abandon in a Roman orgy."

In analyzing the responses to the questionnaire, we saw at once that almost all adults engage in some form of daydreaming every day. Most of these daydreams take the form of fairly clear visual images. They occur chiefly during private moments, just before bedtime or during rides on buses or trains.

Most people report that they enjoy their daydreams. In content their fantasies stick fairly close to simple possibilities, although a very high proportion admit wildly improbable dreams such as inheriting a million dollars. A sizable minority report such fantasies as "being the Messiah," obtaining homosexual satisfactions, and murdering family members. Those individuals with a pronounced tendency to daydream seem to run the gamut of both realistic and bizarre fantasies. Apparently nothing human is alien to the imaginative realm of the accomplished daydreamer.

Men and women vary little in the frequency of their daydreams, but there is an understandable difference in the content of their fantasies. Women's daydreams clearly show their interest in fashions, while those of men display their enthusiasm for heroics and athletics. A recent independent study by Morton Wagman of the University of Illinois, using the same questionnaire, indicates that men report more explicitly sexual daydreams than women, while women have daydreams involving passivity, narcissism, affiliation (need for personal contact), and physical attractiveness.

Marriage precipitates no special pattern of daydreaming, but there are changes in the frequency of fantasy as people grow older. The peak of daydreaming seems to be in mid-adolescence, and then it falls off gradually, although fantasy persists well into old age. In later years daydreaming takes on a retrospective quality, for future possibilities are not only limited but rather frightening to the aged.

We compared the daydream responses of adults from several sociocultural groups—people from Italian, Irish, Jewish, Negro, Anglo-Saxon, and German subcultures. All of them were well-educated, middle-class Americans born of at least the second generation, but with both parents from the same national-origin background.

The order of daydreaming frequency reported was, from high to low, Negro, Italian, Jewish, Irish, German, and Anglo-Saxon. This order strikingly reflects the relative upward mobility, insecurity, and even the pattern of immigration of the various groups to the United States. The latter three groups represent subcultures that have pretty well "made it," socially and economically, in America (see Figure 1).

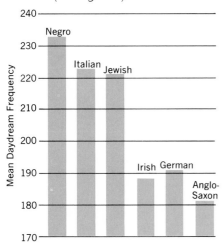

Figure 1. Daydreaming frequency of national-origin groups of Americans; note that the order of frequency strikingly reflects the relative upward mobility, and even the pattern of immigration, of these groups.

Interesting differences in the content of the fantasies also emerged. The Irish showed a tendency toward religious, extremely fantastic, or heroic daydreams. The Negroes fantasized about sensual satisfactions, eating well, comfort, fine clothes and cars.

What other personality characteristics, we asked, might be associated with the tendency toward frequent daydreaming? Psychoanalytic theory suggested one hypothesis: that relative closeness to one's mother might lead to greater inhibition and fantasy.

In order to examine this theory and to evaluate relevant personality factors, we gave the subjects a series of additional tests. All subjects answered a questionnaire designed to explore their attitudes about self, mother, father, and ideal self. They also filled out Cattell and Minnesota Multiphasic questionnaires, which provided

information on anxiety, repressive defenses, and self-awareness. They kept logs of their night dreams for a month, a technique developed by Rosalea Schonbar of Columbia University. In addition, they wrote Thematic Apperception Test stories or gave accounts of fantasies, which were scored by judges for imaginativeness and creativity.

In general, findings with the questionnaire and with projective measures support psychoanalytic theory. Men and women who report closeness to or identification with their mothers, or a rejection of their fathers' values, tend to daydream more frequently. They also remember more of their night dreams. On the projective tests, such individuals rate as more creative storytellers, are generally more self-aware and anxiously sensitive, and are less inclined to employ defense mechanisms such as repression.

Categories of Daydreaming

When we analyzed the results of some forty personality tests taken by college freshmen and matched them with the subjects' daydreaming patterns, we discovered that there were seven categories of daydreaming.

General daydreaming reflected a predisposition to fantasy with great variety in content and often showed curiosity about other people rather than about the natural world.

Self-recriminating daydreaming was characterized by a high frequency of somewhat obsessional, verbally expressive but negatively-toned emotional reactions such as guilt and depression.

Objective, controlled, thoughtful daydreaming displayed a reflective, rather scientific and philosophically inclined content, and was associated with masculinity, emotional stability, and curiosity about nature rather than about the human aspects of environment.

Poorly controlled, kaleidoscopic daydreaming reflected scattered thought and lack of systematic "story lines" in fantasy, as well as distractibility, boredom, and self-abasement.

Autistic daydreaming represented the breakthrough into consciousness of material associated with nocturnal dreaming. It reflected the kind of dreamy, poorly controlled quality of inner experience often reported clinically by schizoid individuals.

Neurotic, self-conscious daydreaming revealed one of the clearest patterns—the one most closely associated with measures of neuroticism and emotional instability. It involved repetitive, egocentric, and body-centered fantasies.

Enjoyment of daydreaming was characterized by a generally positive and healthy acceptance of daydreaming, an enjoyment of fantasy, and the active use of it for both pleasure and problem solving.

People who scored high on introversion showed a strong inclination to respond to internally generated material. Their daydreams were either fantastic and fanciful or controlled, orderly, and objective. This vividly calls to mind C. P. Snow's much discussed contrast of the literary-humanist scholar with the scientist-engineer. Both are given to inner activity, but they are very likely at opposite poles of the daydreaming dimension.

Daydreaming is not confined to adults; it also enters into the games of children. If we observe young children in a nursery or at a playground, those whose play is directly involved with physical reality can be separated from those who introduce make-believe characters, scenes, or times into their play.

Children's Daydreams

In one of our investigations, children between six and nine years of age were interviewed and observed in a series of situations. From their responses to questions about play habits, imaginary companions, and "pictures in your head," we classified them into high- and low-fantasy groups. We then told the children that we were looking for "astronauts of the future." We pointed out that astronauts have to sit quietly in a confined space for long periods of time and asked the children to remain seated in a simulated space capsule as long as possible.

The high-fantasy group were far better at sticking it out, presumably because they could create internal games to pass the time. These children also showed more creativity in storytelling and more achievement motivation. They were more likely to be firstborn or only children; they reported greater closeness to one parent, and they indicated that their parents played fantasy games with them and told them bedtime stories.

Clinically, the high-fantasy children were evaluated as more obsessional in character structure, with greater likelihood of Oedipal conflicts. The low-fantasy children more often were rated as hysterical personalities with pre-Oedipal conflicts—that is, problems with need satisfaction or aggression control, rather than problems relating specifically to parental figures.

Another study in this series, carried out by Bella Streiner and me, compared the dreams and fantasies of congenitally blind children with a matched group of sighted children. As could be anticipated, the variety and complexity of the dreams, daydreams, and imaginative play of the blind children were greatly limited. Their dreams, cast, of course, in verbal and kinesthetic imagery, stayed close to their own immediate life situations. The sighted children were off on rocket ships or flying carpets, but for the blind children a trip to the supermarket became a source of adventure in fantasy.

The contrast emerged when two children, one blind and one sighted, imagined an airplane flight. The blind child spoke of the fact that the boy in his fantasy did not know what an airplane was but that he had a pleasant trip and enjoyed traveling with his mother. The sighted child told of the plane hitting an air pocket, the pilot's unconsciousness, and the parents taking over controls of the ship.

Blind children, we discovered, were more likely to have imaginary companions, and to keep them to a later age than the sighted children. This is understandable when one remembers how dependent these children are on their parents or siblings for even simple maneuvers outside the home. Clearly, they develop make-believe companions, invariably sighted, as a comfort for the times when they are left alone.

Still another study, carried out under my direction by Sybil Gottlieb of the City University of New York, sought to determine whether children imitate adults in producing fantasy material. Several hundred children, who differed initially in fantasy predisposition, were divided into three groups. They were shown an experimental color movie involving a lot of activity by abstract figures. After they had seen the movie, an adult discussed the film with each group. One group was given a very *imaginative* interpretation of the film; the second group was provided with a *realistic* type of story, and the third was given merely a literal description of the "events" of the movie with a *neutral* content.

Then a second abstract film was shown and the children were instructed to write something about it. We were looking for answers to these questions: (1) In describing the second film, to what extent would the children imitate the adult interpretations of the first film? (2) What effect would their initial imaginative predisposition have on their response? and (3) Would the age of the children make a significant difference?

Results were rather clearcut. The elementary-school-age children showed a strong imitative effect. Direct mimicry was rare, but the story content that emerged showed that the adults' versions of the first film had a decided impact on the way the children responded to the second. Their fantasy predisposition was less influential than the content of the adults' stories.

The older children were less influenced by the adult models. Rather, their imaginative predisposition was the deciding factor in how they described the second movie. Regardless of which adult version they had heard, those junior-high-school children who were rated high in fantasy showed far more imagination in their stories.

These and other experiments lead us to believe that fantasy play is indeed a kind of cognitive skill, a fundamental potentiality of all children. Normal development seems to require some aspects of imaginative play. The child combines novel associations with scraps of adult behavior and weaves them into his limited repertory of concepts. Fantasy play is one way in which a child carries out his explorations, not only through interaction with his environment but also through playful combinations and reexaminations of new ideas.

As a child develops a game such as "house" or "knights attacking a castle," he acquires mastery over the elements of the game and thinks of better ways to play it. Whether alone and talking to himself or with a companion, he gains verbal feedback from the game and he may develop a more differentiated vocabulary and a wider repertory of images.

As he grows older and the pressure increases for socializing his play, the child gradually "internalizes" his fantasy. When parents accept his imaginative play, or when the child is not shamed away from such activity, he may continue his fantasy play into late puberty, becoming quite skillful at this form of self-entertainment.

Predictably, children in the middle of large families are less inclined toward fantasy play. They are caught up in direct imitation of other children. It takes time and solitude to develop a rich imaginative life. Indeed, the indications that slum children show less complex fantasy play than other children may be attributed to the facts that their lives are spent in crowded conditions and that they lack consistent adult models for imaginative activity.

Freud theorized that fantasy processes grew out of early hallucinatory experiences of children during periods of drive arousal when gratification was delayed. The child gradually would experience the fantasy of gratification, partially reducing the drive and enabling him to "hold out" until sustenance arrived.

Fantasy, Aggression, and Anxiety

Seymour Feshbach made some ingenious attempts to test Freud's theory that fantasy partially reduces an aroused aggressive drive. His subjects, having been angered by insults from the experimenters, showed less residual resentment after being given an opportunity to write aggressive Thematic Apperception Test stories or to view an aggressive prizefight film.

Richard Rowe and I applied this approach specifically to daydreaming rather than to projective fantasy. In our study we aroused anxiety instead of aggression. Our subjects were students who had to take surprise midterm examinations. Immediately after their test papers were collected, some of the students were allowed to engage in daydreaming. Others were assigned a distracting task. Results suggested that daydreaming did not reduce anxiety. If anything, daydreaming increased anxiety because the subjects could not avoid thinking about the situation in fantasy form.

But in other situations, daydreaming can reduce anxiety. In another study, Rowe placed subjects in a medical laboratory, taped electrical wires to them, and told them they shortly would receive an electric shock. Those subjects who daydreamed to divert themselves showed a reduction of the aroused heart rate caused by the threat of shock. But subjects who had no chance to daydream continued to show an accelerated heart rate. The subjects who were strongly predisposed to daydreaming, as measured by the daydream questionnaire, showed significantly less arousal in response to the

experimental situation than those with little inclination to fantasy.

An elaborate study by Ann Pytkowicz, Nathaniel Wagner, and Irwin Sarason of the University of Washington used subjects rated high and low in daydreaming. They were subjected to insults, then given a chance to daydream or to tell Thematic Apperception Test stories. The experimenters found that both TAT fantasy and daydreaming worked equally well in reducing anger, but they worked best for those persons already inclined toward daydreaming. Contrary to a simple drive-reduction hypothesis, the investigators noted that the amount of aggression was not reduced. As the subjects engaged in fantasy activities, they shifted their aggression from the experimenter to themselves.

It may be that practiced daydreamers can engage in distracting imagery in the fantasy realm, or work out resolutions of their fear or anger. Thus, fantasy changes their mood rather than reducing the amount of drive energy. Those not skilled in the use of fantasy, who are left to their own devices during a period of stress or anger, actually may become more uncomfortable.

The issue of the functional role of daydreaming in relation to motivational or emotional processes is far from resolved. Moreover, the problem has broader implications, such as the effects of violence or sex in literature, art, or movies. There is a general belief that sexual fantasy material is arousing and therefore ought to be limited to "mature audiences." But no restrictions are imposed on aggressive material presented to children. In effect, our folklore seems to argue that fantasy is drive-arousing in the sexual area but drive-reducing in the area of aggression.

The latter notion has been seriously questioned by the work of several researchers. But it is still not known whether predisposition to fantasy might be a critical factor. Perhaps the daydreaming child is less likely to be aroused to direct action after witnessing violence in life or in a movie than the child who has little experience in fantasy play.

Another series of studies in this program dealt with daydreams in relation to information processing. Let us assume that daydreaming represents a special case of "noise" produced by the unceasing activities of our active brains. Ordinarily we are forced to ignore these "signals" in order to steer our way through our physical and social environments. But when the flow of external information to be processed is markedly reduced, as when we prepare for sleep, there is a dramatic upsurge in awareness of one's interior monologues, self-generated imagery, or elaborate fantasy. Memories of the day's events flood into consciousness, touching off associations to earlier events or important unfinished business, leading to fantasies about what tomorrow will bring.

The results of a series of experiments designed to examine fantasy processes suggested distinct values in

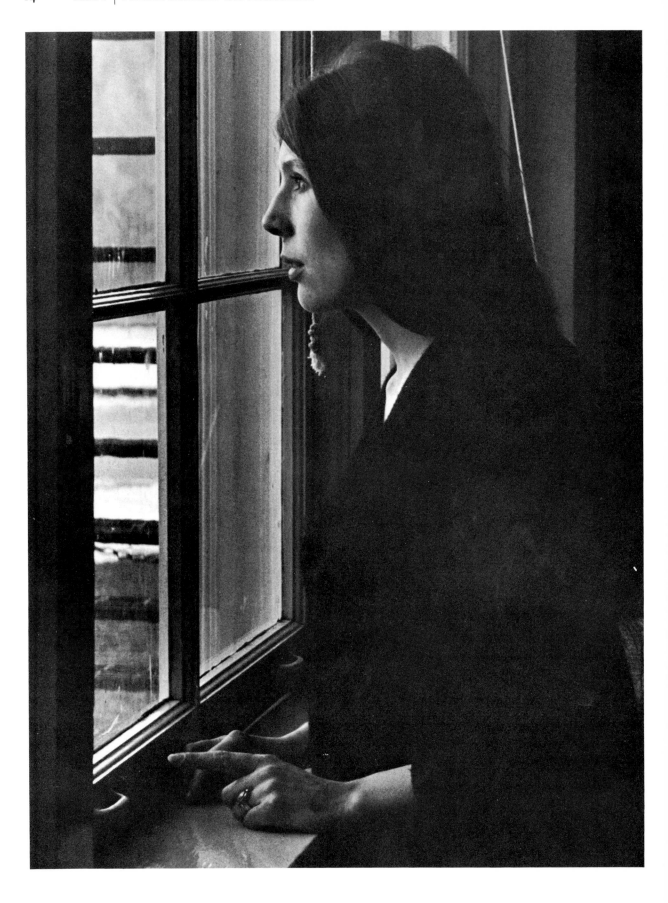

daydreaming and unearthed a wealth of materials about the process of fantasizing and free association. In one experiment subjects seated in a small, dark, sensory-restriction chamber reported their thought content every fifteen seconds. These signal-detection and vigilance studies gave us a sample of thought that was independent of any stimulus and unrelated to any task. Reports were filled with fantasylike content, following the predictions of information theory. In another experiment, the electroencephalograph was used to record the eye movement of subjects. Each person was left to think naturally, but whenever the polygraph showed periods of little or of considerable eye movement, he was interrupted and asked to report his thought content. Tests were also made during periods of instructed fantasy, when the subject was asked to imagine that his deepest secret wish was coming true, and during conscious suppression, when he was asked to suppress his secret wish as if he wanted no one to read his mind. The rapid-eye-movement studies made under the opposed conditions were compared. As a result of the study of these comparisons, we now can make a number of generalizations.

Daydreaming can keep us entertained or reasonably alert under dull, monotonous conditions, but at the cost of missing some of what is going on "outside." When extreme alertness is demanded in a complex environment, daydreaming is less useful and may even become dangerous. It is as if the individual makes rapid estimates of the degree to which he will have to pay attention to his environment, and then allows himself some appropriate margin of time or "channel space" to indulge in fantasies, interpretative glosses on the scenery or his situation, or some other form of self-stimulation.

The situation is analogous to that of a driver. On a road he knows well, with little traffic, he feels free to drift off into an extensive daydream. On an unfamiliar city street where external information is irregular and not readily anticipated, too much attention to his thought stream could be fatal.

To engage in a daydream, a person must withdraw part of his attention from his environment. When he is awake and in a normal environment, he somehow must screen out the material surrounding him. Perhaps he does this by fixing his gaze steadily at a spot in front of him, so that the image fades. With less external material to process, he can deal more effectively with internal material. This may account for the blank stare that tells us someone with whom we're conversing really isn't listening but is lost in thought.

One of the important conclusions drawn from our program of research is that the ephemeral fantasy need not be so elusive a phenomenon. The properties of man's inner experience can be systematically studied by formal methods as well as by clinical observation. While the scientist may never see the actual inner imagery any more than he can see an electron, it should be possible to employ certain physiological or reporting measures in a sufficiently systematic fashion to ensure that we are indeed zeroing in on private experience.

The early psychoanalytic view that daydreaming is compensatory, defensive, or drive-reducing does not seem either general enough or precise enough to become the basis of a model. Today it seems more reasonable to regard daydreaming as a consequence of the ongoing activity of the brain, and to apply models that relate to man's cognitive and affective environmental adaptation and his requirements for varied stimulation.

Very likely man's capacity to daydream is a fundamental characteristic of his constitution. Like other abilities—perceptual, motor, or cognitive—it is there to be developed depending on circumstances.

The practiced daydreamer has learned the art of pacing so that he can shift rapidly between inner and outer channels without bumping into too many obstacles. He has developed a resource that gives him some control over his future through elaborate planning, some ability to amuse himself during dull train rides or routine work, and some sources of stimulation to change his mood through fanciful inner play.

This heightened self-awareness also may bring to consciousness many things that persons who are less internally sensitive can avoid: awareness of faults, failures, or the omnipresent threat of global destruction. The daydreamer thus pays a price for his highly developed inner capacity. But perhaps it is well worth it.

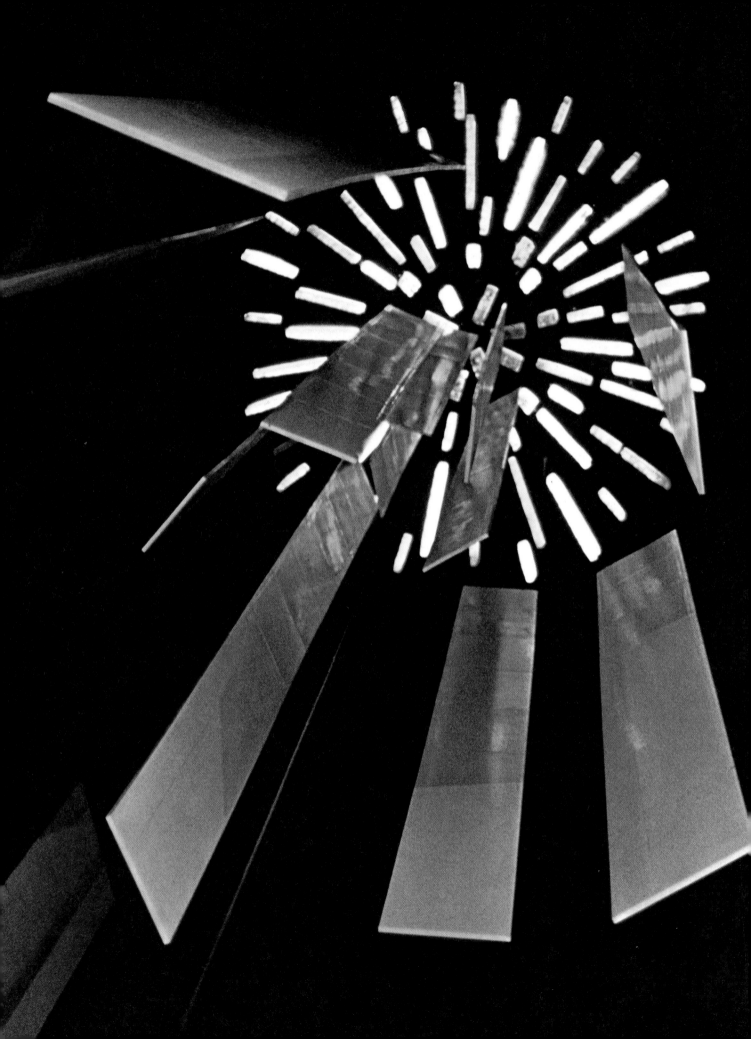

The Dream of Art and Poetry

Frank Barron

To the degree that creativity is an extraordinary process, it should be amenable to the researches of those studying abnormal psychology. Usually this field deals with negatively valued deviations and seldom inquires into positive abnormalities. Nietzsche, whose aphorism serves as motto for Frank Barron's essay, would today be diagnosed as a brilliant, creative, paranoid schizophrenic, and the paranoia and schizophrenia would interest many psychologists much more than the brilliance and creativity. However, some contemporary psychologists have recognized the imperative of studying both the negative and the positive valences of deviations from normality. Barron's investigations into the artistic sensibility are in this line.

Creative potential may be shown by an elevated IQ score, lots of intense and colorful dreams, or a particular pattern on the Rorschach, but the creative process is the unleashing of what these but pallidly indicate, and it involves a good deal more.

As Barron points out, not all creative individuals work in the fine arts. The artistic sensibility in greater or lesser degree exists in many persons whose creations are but fancy pies and elegant roofbeams. And it may exist though never surface in a good many more. Barron, among other writers, emphasizes the importance of nurturing whatever creative urges an individual harbors, for in our dehumanizing technological society such a sensibility is the strongest thrust toward self-identity we have.

Every man is a perfect artist in his dreams," wrote Friedrich Nietzsche a century ago.

Regretfully, I must say that I doubt it.

Of course, no one can say for sure what another man's dreams may be, considered as art, for only the dreamer may experience them; yet, I must doubt it. And regretfully, for there is an engagingly democratic appeal in this idea of a hidden realm of being in which at last all men are indeed created equal, and not only equal but equally perfect. It may seem ungracious to allow tedious research empiricism to encroach upon a vision of the ideal. Yet I am bound to report that I have interviewed hundreds of people about their dream life, and from hundreds more have collected written dream protocols. I have even studied variations in the symbolic richness of hypnotically implanted dream complexes. All the evidence points to variability and, alas, imperfection.

The evidence shows that people do differ widely in the frequency of remembered dreams, the vividness of dream imagery, the occurrence of color and color symbolism, the degree of reality or unreality in dream sequences, and the dramatic qualities of plot, characterization, and secondary elaboration. And in one of these studies, in which the written dream protocols were quite reliably rated for "originality," originality in dreaming proved to be significantly related to originality as measured by written tests of creativity.

My guess is that while every man is a sort of artist willy-nilly in his dreams as in his life, the esthetic quality of the product varies widely from person to person.

As usual, though, with Nietzsche, one must have second thoughts, for his aphorisms aim at the revelation through altered emphasis of an aspect of reality commonly unnoticed. In T. S. Eliot's words, "Between the conception/And the creation . . . Falls the Shadow" —even the great artist may fail on occasion to express his initial vision in the completed work of art. If we take Nietzsche's aphorism in this sense, it points to the need for talent and discipline in the exercise of the artist's craft, to make the perfect dream a perfect reality.

And there is still another shade of meaning in Nietzsche's statement. Though art may be conceded as the province of the artist, the kind of imagination that is essential to art may be very broadly distributed throughout the human species, coming to expression as art only under special conditions of individual and social motive and opportunity.

This interpretation would indeed jibe very well with the findings of empirical research by our psychological staff at the Institute of Personality Assessment and Research. We have studied highly creative men and women in the arts and sciences, and in creative professions, and we have studied also large numbers of individuals for whom the creative life seemed to exercise no special attraction. The characteristics of creative imagination, though not finding artistic expression, certainly appeared quite often in the groups of persons whose occupations were of the "practical" sort. And in such ordinary folk the motivational and personality correlates of measures of artistic aptitude were very similar to the characteristic motives and personal traits of artists themselves.

We can justifiably, therefore, speak of the poetic and artistic imagination as a quality of perception and thought that may be found in any man, artist or not. Whether it comes to expression in a socially recognized art form is a matter of choice, sometimes even of chance.

Perhaps it should not be so surprising to find artistic and poetical sensibility so prevalent, for the firmament in its furnishings and functioning invites us all to be poets and artists. In art, whether visual art or poetry and fiction, one finds repeated the same heart-grasping forms that follow upon the earliest perceptual discriminations. Think, for example, of the importance of circles and of orbs from the very beginning of individual life. There are, first of all, the eyes of the mother, upon which the infant characteristically will fix his gaze, for the movement of the mother's eyes provides the first assurance of a moving other self; then, the mother's breasts, which come to signify the earth itself, the source of abundance, and even in some kinds of adolescent poetic yearning the distant full moon. The moon is related in root language to words for womb, for mind, for month, for measurement; and the tides themselves go as the moon goes. The noticing of fingers and toes, the beginning of the enumeration of organs and the generic relation of the common numbers of systems of arithmetic, the bilateral symmetry of the body and the prevalence of symmetry in nature, the recognition of size, and of expansion and contraction, all set the stage for the emergence of natural philosophy. Thus the human form and the major constants of the external world, such as the moon, the stars, the turning of the

seasons, the sequence of day and night—these forms and rhythms are the early nonverbal beginnings of art and culture.

And once the phenomena of degrees of magnitude and of sequence are grasped, the central questions of classical philosophy soon state themselves in childish terms. I am thinking here not only of the great unanswerables ("Where do the stars come from, Daddy?"; "Who made God?"; "Why do we have to die?"; "Why did they kill the Baby Jesus?") but the questions of moral responsibility, justification for aggression, ownership, good and evil ("That was just an accident"; "He hit me first"; "That's mine and you can't play with it"; "Superman is good, he zaps the crooks; he's our friend"). The Roman Catholic Church requires that in order to sin one must have attained "the use of reason," and conventionally this is placed at about the age of six, but the particular three- and four-year-olds I have known best were all of them philosophers and moralists upon whose reasoning aged wisdom could hardly improve.

Most of the great mythic themes that repeat themselves throughout the world are capable of entering childish consciousness by age four. Freud has made us all too familiar with the clinical outcomes of the family romance, and the origins of the misfortunes of the house of Laius have been laid bare for all to see without leaving home. The unconscious crime of Oedipus the King, perceived by Tiresias through the clairvoyant wisdom given only to the blind, reminds us again of the coupling of day and night, now enacted in the psychic sphere as the conscious and the unconscious. Black is a frightening color—*die Schwarzmann*, the Bogeyman, Death, the big hole they put you in, the abyss. White is light, purity, elevation, innocence, completeness, heaven. All the colors have special symbolic meanings, as do the numbers. The colored, numbered, shaped world has been shaped to symbol, and the sequences of begetting, initiating, maturing, aging, and dying imbue all experience with an infinite nostalgia.

The artist is a person of acute sensibility who has recognized an opportunity to abet the growth of all human sensibility by communicating his private vision. In creating the work of art, he has built upon the childhood urge to self-initiated activity that will produce delight and has elevated his urge to the status of a mature and altruistic motive to communicate, testify, serve as a personal vehicle for the extension of the general consciousness. In a sense, he comes to remind us of the awesomeness of the world.

Adult artists and poets come in all shapes and sizes, and even sexes, just as children do, of course, and this variety characterizes their personalities as well. There is no single "artistic personality." In the course of the empirical research mentioned earlier, I have had occasion to scrutinize the personality test profiles of many famous contemporary writers and architects. I have been impressed by two facts: (1) that all sorts of different persons become writers or architects; and (2) that stare as we might at their personality profiles, we could never guess from the profiles alone what sort of work the persons would do in their chosen field—nor even what sort of field they would choose! This is not to say that no regularities may be discerned, however; it is merely to emphasize the great variety in personality that renders even more striking certain similarities in experiencing, in motivation, and in moral vision.

One might expect high intelligence to be one such common trait among persons of a high order of creative imagination. Indeed it is true that writers, architects, mathematicians, and scientists who are distinguished for creativity are also of quite high measured intelligence. The famous studies conducted by Terman and his associates, and particularly those collected by Catherine Cox in *The Early Mental Traits of 300 Geniuses*, showed that historically authenticated geniuses were greatly accelerated in their mental development as children, as well as being outstanding in intellectual attainments in their later years. Yet within her sample of intellectual geniuses the correlation of estimated IQ with eminence was low.

This finding is similar to the overall result obtained in our studies at the Institute of Personality Assessment and Research. However, it must be remembered that in all these studies researchers considered a highly restricted range of intelligence and of eminence or reputation for creativity. This extreme restriction of range on both counts would lead to a very considerable underestimation of the correlation of intelligence with creativity or eminence in the general population. Add to this restricted range a certain amount of inaccuracy, both in the measurement of intelligence and in the recognition of creativity, and it is not surprising that the relationships we have observed are small or insignificant.

Perhaps the more important fact is that the IQ among creative and eminent individuals is, on the average, quite high. This makes sense, of course, since a reputation for creativity usually rests upon the claim to success in the solution of difficult problems, in art as well as in science and the creative professions. For example, the theory of relativity was highly creative, and there is no doubt that only a person of genius-level intelligence, like Albert Einstein, could have produced it. Even to grasp the antecedent problems, much less to come forward with the original solution, required high intelligence.

In Catherine Cox's studies, eminent artists have an average estimated IQ of 135, which is very close to the measured average in our group of contemporary creative architects; "imaginative writers" in the Cox sample have an average IQ of 165, and scientists an average of 170. This estimate is somewhat higher than for contemporary writers and scientists in the IPAR studies, especially for scientists, but of course the degree of

eminence was also less in our samples of contemporaries. Overall, it is fair to say that the distinguished creative individuals in the IPAR studies have an average IQ in the neighborhood of 140.

Thus from our own recent findings, two statements that at first may seem mutually incompatible must be made:

1. Persons of a high order of creative ability are usually in the upper 10 percent, or perhaps upper 5 percent, of the general population in terms of IQ.
2. Within groups of such persons, even when highly creative persons are compared with merely representative persons in a profession that demands creative ability, there is usually no relationship between IQ and creativity.

In brief, for certain creative activities a specifiable minimum IQ probably is necessary in order to engage in the activity at all. But beyond that minimum, which may be rather low in certain nonverbal artistic activities, creativity is not a function of intelligence as measured by IQ tests. Of course, the most widely used IQ tests are heavily verbal in content and require a kind of thinking that stresses logic at the expense of imagination, unusual associations, and metaphor.

We must remember too that creativity can manifest itself in more modest but no less genuine form, and any one of us may be creative on our own terms, in our own way, doing our own thing: a housewife preparing a new dish or adding unexpected spice to an old one, a carpenter figuring out a new way to shape boards to one another, a clergyman making up a parable of his own, or even a confidence man thinking up a new way to bilk the unwary. But if in professions that are intrinsically creative in nature, neither intelligence nor personality makes the crucial difference, what does? As we have suggested, styles of experiencing, motives, and values or philosophy of life determine creative achievement.

We have found three distinct traits that mark the highly creative person. The first of these has to do with the relationships of complexity to simplicity, and of order to disorder. Creative individuals seem to be able to discern accurately more complexity in whatever it is they attend to. This results in part from the fact that they are attracted to complexity and find it more challenging, so that indeed there *is* more complexity for them to discern. They prefer phenomena and visual displays not readily ordered, or that present perplexing contradictions. When confronted with an ambiguous perceptual field, as in various inkblot tests, they seek the single synthesizing image that will unite many diverse elements.

This tendency has shown itself in a wide variety of the tests we use. One such test calls for metaphorical and poetic thinking. We present a stimulus image, such as *leaves being blown along in the wind*. Then we ask the respondent to create other images somehow equivalent to the stimulus. For example, leaves blown in the wind could be "clothes seen through the window of a Bendix dryer, being tossed up and down," or "a civilian population fleeing from advancing enemy armies" (scattered like untreed leaves before the winds of war). The stimulus images are varied in complexity. We can reliably appraise the degree to which their elements are reproduced in the respondent's suggested symbolic equivalence. The responses of creative individuals to this test are marked by a finely differentiated and apt symbolic equivalence.

Another relevant test is the Barron-Welsh Art Scale, in which line drawings of figures, systematically varied as to complexity, are presented, with instructions to choose the figures the respondent finds pleasing. The scale measures the similarity of one's preferences to those of artists. Artists prefer figures that are more challenging, more complex, less obviously balanced, dynamic rather than static, biomorphic rather than geometric. We have found that creative individuals in many different professional fields prefer the kinds of figures that artists prefer.

A second trait of creative people is perceptual openness, or resistance to premature closure. This is perhaps related to the first, since such an attitude provides more opportunity for complexity in the phenomenal field to develop. Our best measure of it derives from the theories of C. G. Jung, and opposes the perceptual attitude to the judgmental attitude. According to Jung, whenever a person uses his mind for any purpose, he performs either an act of perception (he becomes aware of something) or an act of judgment (he comes to a conclusion, often an evaluative conclusion, about something). If one of these attitudes is strong in a person, the other is correspondingly weak. The judging attitude is said to lead to an orderly, carefully planned life based on relatively closed principles and categories, whereas the perceptual attitude leads to more openness to experience, including experience of the inner world of self. The perceptual attitude facilitates spontaneity and flexibility.

In our studies, every group but scientists is predominantly perceptual rather than judgmental, and in every group, including scientists, the more creative individuals are more perceptually oriented, and the less creative are more judgmentally oriented.

The third characteristic of creative persons is reliance upon intuition, hunches, and inexplicable feelings. They trust the nonrational processes of their own mind. This too provides one of the bipolar oppositions in Jung's classification. The act of perception itself, according to Jung, may be of two kinds: sense-perceptive or intuitive. The sense-perceptive attitude emphasizes simple realism, and is a direct awareness of things as they most objectively are in terms of the evidence of the senses.

Intuition, by contrast, is an indirect awareness of deeper meanings and possibilities. Creative individuals are characteristically intuitive. Test results on the Myers-Briggs Jungian Type Indicator show that more than 90 percent of the creative individuals we have studied are predominantly intuitive. Experiments and interviews confirm the test scores.

One such interview was devoted especially to the fantasy life, ranging from daydreams to night dreams, and from hypnagogic experiences to transcendental experiences in full and acute consciousness. An unusually high percentage of creative persons claimed to have had experiences either of mystic communion with the universe or of feelings of utter desolation and horror. This statistic does not represent a checking of "yes" or "no" to a question such as, "Have you ever had a mystical experience?" They frequently described the prologues to these experiences with considerable vividness. Among other unusual experiences they described were being barraged by disconnected words as though one were caught in a hailstorm, with accompanying acute discomfort, or seeing the world suddenly take on a new brightness. These creative people also reported a high frequency of dreaming as well as a high frequency of dreaming in color, as compared with control groups we have studied.

The *motive to create* is of the greatest importance in actualizing creative potential. Our work with writers has led me to believe that there are many, many persons who have just as much technical potential as the creative writers who came to our attention, yet who do not write. In this as in other kinds of hard work, one must *want* to do it (or be compelled to, which at least for some artists does seem to be part of the story).

The motive to create has several aspects. One aspect, to which I have already referred, might be called "the cosmological motive." Such a tendency on the part of the creative individual to relate himself to nothing less than the universe and the meaning of human life has shown itself repeatedly and in many ways in our studies. In responses to the Symbol Equivalence Test, for example, there is a striking tendency for the artist to move from the commonplace stimulus image to the cosmic metaphor. And in projective tests, such as the Rorschach and the Thematic Apperception Test, the characteristic concern is with mythic themes, archetypal symbols, great inanimate forces, birth and death, and the symbolic rather than literal meaning of colors and shapes.

In creative writers, the classic existential problems of philosophy, such as the freedom-determinism problem, the problem of evil, solipsism, the mind-body problem, and the problem of induction, arise constantly both in their work and in their fantasies. The nature of man in his relationship to the cosmos is the general theme that engages and excites their imagination.

However, a difference must be noted here between

genuine artistic involvement and another kind of activity that is motivated primarily by a need for self-analysis or perhaps an attempt at self-therapy. Freud, I think, was not quite alert to this distinction in "The Poet and Daydreaming." Here I feel that he was not describing the genuine poet, who certainly does not moon about so pointlessly.

The creative writers we studied were distinguished for volume as well as quality of production. Dwelling upon death and the cosmos and the solitariness of the self can be an easy way of getting out of working. Sharpness of detail, sympathy and validity of characterization, discipline of form, tireless rewriting and shaping up of the outflowing material, and a touch of the old shoemaker's pride in craftsmanship and in keeping trade secrets are among the characteristics of creative writing and writers. Although their concern is with cosmic issues, these are brought to life in characterization and an unhackneyed use of language that invites the reader to experience through *his* own nature the reality that the writer perceives.

The motive to create need not be so lofty in origin or aims, of course. There is a simple pleasure in genuine self-expression that can be understood as a common good, something that is part of our nature as human beings. To sing, to dance, to paint, to play, to improvise, to dream a little in all sorts of ways that free us from the humdrum sort of realism, all these things we may do for the pure pleasure of expressing ourselves without our having an audience in mind or high art as a goal. Indeed, there is an ever-growing belief among educators that formal schooling itself should seek to develop the esthetic sentiment and to encourage the growth of artistic imagination. The late author and critic Sir Herbert Read had long argued that the development of artistic sensibility should be of central importance in education, particularly in the face of a society organized increasingly around machines and technology. In this view, esthetic education is a means for the realization of selfhood and for the preservation of human values in society. In a time when our society is beset by so many vexing problems, it is heartening to observe this increasing recognition of the value of art, imagination, and creativity.

Perhaps we could amend Nietzsche's remark to: "Let every man *become* a better artist in his dreams."

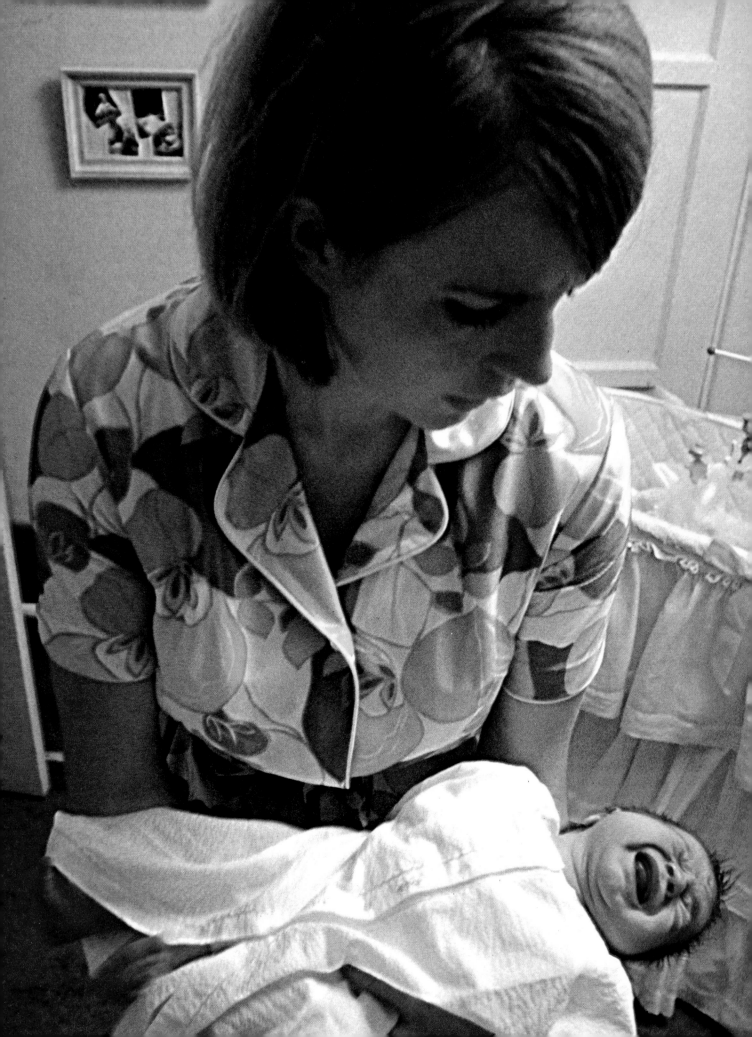

Mrs. Oedipus
Matthew Besdine

Matthew Besdine suggests that, as the myth of Oedipus is replayed on each analyst's couch, the analyst should peer more attentively at the role of Jocasta, the mother of Oedipus. A Jocasta-mother is a warm, intelligent, doting woman who binds her child to her, making herself his exclusive source for emotional nurturance. She and her son are inextricably tied in a conflicted, encompassing dependency on each other. In the pattern commonly called an unresolved Oedipus complex, the boy is hostile and fearful toward the father. He often adopts feminine emotional patterns and esthetic attitudes and values as a result of inadequate identification with the male role. Freud, Besdine points out, erred when he left the mother's place in this pattern in obscurity. For Besdine, the mother-child relationship appears to be the entity that generates true creativity in the child.

Besdine's essay is something of a rarity these days. In the current ambience of existentialism and mathematical models of man, few professional articles devote themselves to enriching the classical Freudian approach. Besdine here uses the historical perspective of the psychoanalyst and presents a remarkable illustration of the Freudian method of inquiry. His intense description of this mother-son configuration taps Freud's adaptation of the Oedipus myth and flows unhesitatingly into richly suggestive interpretation. Freud's original metaphor was more an evocative literary stroke than a clinical achievement; in amplifying the metaphor, the present essay does not mean to proffer treatment implications.

Let us call him Patient XY and consider him a composite of countless patients in analysis, or of a legion of troubled men. XY's father was dim, distant, or remote—either absent from the home physically, or absent as a paternal masculine force because of weakness, irresponsibility, or deep involvement in a successful career. XY's mother was a bright, warm, intelligent, forceful woman, but for one reason or another, these gifts of intellect and love were not laid at the feet of friends, society, or husband; they were poured out almost exclusively for her son, who was an only child, or the first child to survive, or a child born late, after earlier children had grown up and had left the home.

XY himself is intelligent and sensitive, but his relations with himself and with others are stormy, unhappy, or at least highly ambivalent. He craves a deep, binding, exclusive intimacy with others and yet continually jeopardizes such intimacy—when he doesn't repel it entirely —on the slightest of pretexts. Then he frantically seeks it once again, often succeeding once more in frightening away or exasperating the loved one.

He finds the possibility or fact of marriage almost nightmarish, and establishes close bonds only with women who are "safe"—with married women, known lesbians, or with women much older than he is. He is capable of lust only with women who can lay no claim to him as a permanent partner: whores, women of defective intelligence or much lower social position, or one-night stands of one kind or another.

He has a very strong homosexual streak, either overt or ferociously suppressed. All or most of his deep emotional and intellectual friendships occur with men. He tends to be paranoid, masochistic, and laden with a veritable crush of guilts. He often has some quasi-ruinous addiction—to gambling, to drink, to drugs, to crackpot schemes, or to wild extravagances of some kind. When this guilty activity has been indulged, he punishes or redeems himself by fantastic bouts of work, often equally ruinous in terms of health or temper.

XY is also capable of rich, childlike humor and fantasy; he often plays with words or ideas or the observed world as though with bright and very special toys. If you are walking down the street with him, he will often seem to perceive the environment quicker than you do. He may notice and call attention to a strange face, to a weird old tree, to a marvelously shaped rock or cloud. His attention seems to flit quickly, almost as though he were speed-reading the world. Yet he will retain a staggering amount of detail. Little bits and pieces of past experience continually pop up to be recombined in curious or witty ways. It is almost as though the whole of his experience must be kept in touch with, run through associatively like prayer beads.

XY tends to have a sharp tongue and is intolerant of people or things he dislikes. He tends to be—or appears to be—forceful, aloof, moody, cold, or snobbish among strangers, and sometimes even among friends. When he speaks of himself, he may often mention events or aspects of his childhood. And he will frequently mention his mother.

XY could be any number of analysands. He could be one of countless thirty-year-old decorators, architects, hairdressers, or musicians experiencing some typical homosexual panic or climacteric.

But XY could also be Christopher Marlowe, Goethe, Heinrich Heine, Leonardo Da Vinci, Michelangelo, André Gide, Balzac, Marcel Proust, Dostoevsky, Lytton Strachey, Oscar Wilde, Jean Paul Sartre, or Sigmund Freud.

Freud's Oedipus

Shortly after his father's death, Freud created and gave to the world his retelling or reinterpretation of the Oedipus myth. The result was a new emphasis on childhood sexuality, on the boychild's lust for his mother, on patricidal feelings, and on the role of the father as a second love object, threatening ogre, and crucial wedge separating the child from its all-enveloping maternal surround. Freud thus created a whole new focus not only for the "story" of man but for literary biography. In the light of his theories, many of the recorded lives of great men appeared lopsided, if not wholly inadequate; multivolume biographies were, in a sense, thick at the wrong end.

But it is not belaboring the obvious to point out that Freud was a late Victorian, that late-Victorian middle- and upper-class society had a strong patriarchal character, as well as deeply rooted myths and taboos about women, and that Sigmund Freud's Oedipus was just as much his own as Sophocles' was, or Michelangelo's "David" was. Like all great created "characters," Freud's Oedipus is both universalized and unique.

Partly as a result of his culture and partly as a result of his own character gestalt, Freud more or less edited out Jocasta, the mother of Oedipus. He allowed Jocasta to remain in plush obscurity, and this obscurity has become quite apparent in the altered lights of our own time and culture. Mid-twentieth century American society has quite consciously called attention to the altering, commingling roles of father and mother, husband and wife; it has watched with glee the spectacular death of the so-called paterfamilias.

In the orthodox Freudian view, Jocasta is merely the passive recipient of the oedipal lusts; her sexual, emotional, and intellectual life is almost wholly lacking in detail and dynamic. She merely subserves the larger, masculine plot. But the facts are there, both in the myth and in Sophocles' play. Jocasta's husband, warned by the Oracle that a manchild born to him would kill him, abstained from all sexual intercourse with his wife. However, a drunken orgy led to the birth of a child, Oedipus. Jocasta was then forced to abandon her child on the cruel mountain. In the play, she actually turned Oedipus over to a retainer for this purpose. She remained thereafter childless, then husbandless, until the grown Oedipus turned up, whereupon she bore him four children.

The bare bones of a character structure are there: a presumed craving for children, the absence of a normal sex life, grief for a child presumably dead and "half-murdered," as it were, and finally the complete removal of the husband.

Freud did not really apply his imagination to this set of facts; he did not consider sympathetically enough the fact that the Jocasta of Sophocles' play is a woman of considerable personal force and insight, and above all, that it is *she* who speaks the ripe words that all men dream of lying with their mothers.

What would happen if one placed the spotlight upon Jocasta as well as Oedipus and viewed them as an integral unity, as mother and child? This question came to mind as I studied the life of Michelangelo. The first ten years of Michelangelo's life had been almost unexplored, and a great deal of suppression and distortion continues to cloud the events of those years. It was known, however, that the infant Michelangelo was mysteriously expelled from the Buonarotti family and turned over to a stonecutter's wife, much as Oedipus of legend was found and raised by the childless queen of Corinth. Further investigations revealed similarities in the childhood and subsequent lives and works of many strikingly creative people. I have begun strongly to suspect that the mothering pattern typical of "Jocastas" may be in some ways essential to creative productivity, particularly in the field of the arts.

Jocasta-Mothering

We must clearly distinguish the complex configuration I call Jocasta-mothering from other kinds of mothering that have similar features. At one extreme, there is total rejection of the infant. Rejecting mothers may cling pathologically to a child, but they are aware only of their own needs; they are insensitive to cues and signals from the child. There is far more hate than love in such a relationship, and the child's intellectual development is retarded and distorted, often to the point of schizophrenia. That is certainly *not* Jocasta-mothering.

Somewhere in the middle of the mothering continuum is the mother who loves her infant tenderly but whose life is fulfilled in other loving relationships. She willingly allows her child to grow and to separate himself from her, and she consciously or unconsciously exposes him to appropriate masculine models. This is not Jocasta-mothering either.

Jocasta-mothering has had a number of not entirely satisfactory tags applied to it: overevaluating, overprotective, binding, overindulgent, doting, seductive, narcissistic, momistic. These terms, while accurate enough, do not seem to suggest strongly enough a peculiar but identifiable configuration having its own limitations, its own dynamics, and its own strange richness.

Jocasta-mothering presupposes a sensitive woman who is emotionally, sexually, and intellectually starved. It also presupposes or requires a bright, sensitive child, who can respond successfully to the subtly escalating demands of such a mother.

What happens, simply enough, is that the all-enveloping, intensely warm, intimate and tender mother-son interaction of symbiosis, so typical and necessary in the first year, is extended far beyond the normal cut-off point. It can continue through adolescence, even into manhood. The Jocasta mother becomes her child's companion, tutor, and principal emotional source. This exclusive mothering process nurtures and cultivates the fullest creative potential. Just as a gardener snips all but the central bud to secure prize flowers, the Jocasta mother devotes herself almost exclusively to her chosen child.

Quite often she introduces the child very early in life to her own delight in art, music, painting, or literature. The child become precocious, or intellectually mature and sensitive for his age, thus further reducing his chances at successful relations with his peers or with weak, dull, ineffectual, or harsh masculine models. As the child grows, both he and the mother become increasingly dependent upon one another for a satisfying life of the mind and emotions—and increasingly aware of this dependency.

The mother becomes frightened by this intimate dependency and periodically repulses the child; the child finds that vital intimacy cruelly shattered, then born again. He comes more and more to regard this marvelous blessing as two-faced, as half-suffocating or half-crippling. Yet it is the only close, tender, enriching relationship in his experience; he must constantly exceed himself to renew or recapture it. The prodigies of effort needed to do this seem to enlarge or train lifelong drives or capabilities; greater and greater effort is needed, more and more grandiose success is envisioned, and quite often accomplished.

Studies of the mothers of geniuses indicate that not only the intensity but also the *quality* of Jocasta-mothering is very high. These Jocasta mothers are often women whose originality, aliveness, and deep, wide-ranging interests make them outstanding people in their own right—as were the mothers of Goethe, Heine, Freud,

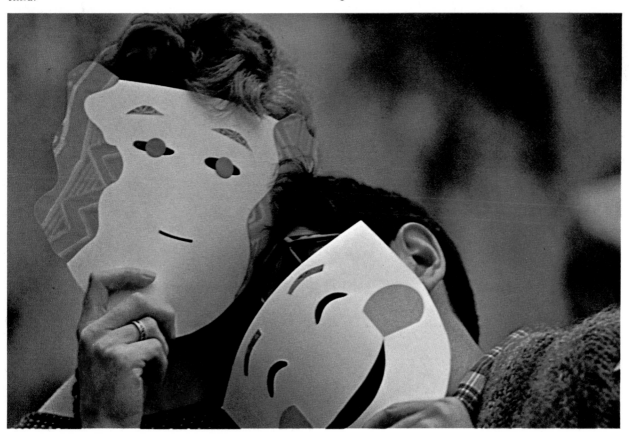

Proust, and Lytton Strachey, to name but a few.

Indeed, the character, gifts, and quickness of the mother, and her ability to interact with her gifted child in increasingly stimulating, complex, and imaginative ways during the first years of life, and her need and ability to continue that relationship well into adolescence and beyond, seem to furnish the soil in which the seeds of intelligence and creativity flourish most spectacularly.

The pattern of mothering I call Jocasta-mothering has frequently been cited as causing or contributing heavily to homosexuality. And we do indeed find among men of real creative originality that overt homosexuality, strong bisexuality, extreme marital difficulties, or an unusual incapacity to relate to women as peers occurs far too frequently to be coincidental or irrelevant.

My experience with analysands and with those who walk in from the pages of biography has led me to a number of tentative, more or less grudging, conclusions on this subject.

As the intense, tender, highly stimulating mother-son symbiosis extends into the oedipal period (five to seven years) and beyond, the son of a Jocasta finds himself increasingly looking at the world through the window of a room that is essentially and irreversibly *feminine*, in the good sense of that word. A love of fabric, color, form, scent, subtlety of design, indirection, suggestion —all the tangibles and intangibles of vibrant female life—form a cluster of sensations and stimuli that becomes home base for the child. (The domain of sheer intelligence, of powerful, acute, rational thought—to which the mother has usually introduced the child quite early—is, I believe, essentially sexless or neuter, though usually considered to have a male gender.) The vigorous masculine world becomes for the son of Jocasta increasingly a world seen from afar, in tantalizing or agonized glimpses. And as the absence of an undoubtedly masculine world becomes more and more acutely felt, male models or companions increasingly become the property of imagination, rather than of personal experience.

A search for idealized friends or companions begins usually in the world of imagination itself—in literature or art. This search becomes a lifelong impulse, often assuming the proportions not only of hero worship but of hero creation.

Since the one manifest impossibility of the Jocasta mother-son relationship is the satisfaction of physical lust, the sexual object must be found elsewhere, or else eschewed entirely.

In the *actual* experience of the Jocasta son, this object is often a woman who is quite unlike the mother in terms of sensibility, talent, or warmth. The sex object is often slovenly, or beneath notice as a human being. And it is often a man. The fact that lust may be more quickly and noncommittally satisfied by a homosexual partner can, however, only partially account for the choice of male love objects by so many sons of Jocasta.

It is the *imaginative* experience of Jocasta sons that seems to be crucial in explaining their actual love lives. Imagination is the realm of ideals, and for Jocasta sons the ideal tends to be a synthesis of what was lacking, and what was known. Such sons scramble through an often grubby sexual underworld looking for a companion or relationship that is or has all things: Apollonian maleness; physical beauty of a lithe, sensuous, graceful, or heroic sort; force of character and accomplishment; the kind of youthfulness or boyishness always lacking in children mature beyond their years; complete understanding, and, of course, an ego-dissolving love like the richly sensual intimacy characteristic of the first fused or symbiotic state.

Since life but imperfectly mimics art or imagination, such an impulse toward an ideal comrade or lover remains more or less unrealized in real life. In an environment that can be mastered and controlled—the artist's medium, in other words—such an ideal crops up again and again, sometimes disguised, sometimes not. This ideal hides in the absorbing metaphor, the ambiguous line, the Gioconda smile in all its ageless, infinite variety.

Michelangelo as a Jocasta Son

Michelangelo, for example, was much more at home with the heroes of his imagination, Jesus, David, Brutus, Hercules, and Moses, than with the father figures or the lovers of his "real" life. As a boy of twelve, or younger, he sought out the older artist, Granacci; as a teen-ager, the luminaries of the Plato Academy; and later, Pope Julius II, who employed him to do his Tomb (containing the "Moses") and the ceiling of the Sistine Chapel.

As Michelangelo grew older, he was attracted to a series of young men, usually in their teens. Not till his sixty-third year could he establish even a platonic friendship with a woman. Though he died just short of ninety, he never married.

The pendulumlike "agony and ecstasy" of all his relationships is best documented in the letters, sonnets, painting, drawings, and marbles inspired by Thomasso Cavalieri, a teen-ager whom Michelangelo fell in love with at the age of fifty-seven. Snapping out of a suicidal depression, the artist wrote: "You are . . . matchless and unequaled, light of our century—paragon of the world . . ." He revealed in a poem, beginning "The horseman always riding in the night," that Cavalieri was his dream lover. In a letter to Cavalieri, he shows his symbiotic attachment and dependence, and confesses: ". . . the boundless love I bear you . . . Your name nourishes body and soul filling both with such delight that I am insensible to sorrow or fear of death. . . ." To a friend, he wrote ". . . if he were to fade from my memory, I think I should instantly fall dead."

The patterns of love are presented even more pointedly in the Cavalieri sonnets and drawings. The "Phaeton," the "Tityos," and the "Rape of Ganymede" are quite open. In the last of the drawings, Michelangelo portrays young Cavalieri as the godlike, all-powerful lover who sweeps down, overwhelms and seizes him, taking him off to heaven to be his lover. It is quite similar to rape fantasies found in certain female patients. The awesome, all-powerful, godlike Cavalieri was an idealized, imaginative creation of the artist with which, in the flesh, he was bound to be frustrated, disappointed, and furious.

The way in which Michelangelo saw and felt mother figures is characteristically grim, aloof, and distant. They never look lovingly at the infant in their arms. The glowing ecstatic mother in adoration, a theme so common to his contemporaries, is never attempted. Most of his life women were for him distant Madonnas untouched with eroticism. On the other hand, his male nudes on the Sistine ceiling, in the "Doni Madonna," the "Bacchus," the "David," and the "Battle of Centaurs," have that nuance and erotic quality men usually find in women. One has only to compare the hairless adolescent Adam and the newly created Eve of the Sistine vault, for they tell their own story of the psychosexual reality of Michelangelo. At no point in his life did he create a female adolescent the equivalent of the "David" or the "Ignudi."

Michelangelo's sense of guilt showed constantly in his life and work. In a self-portrait, he sits upon a horse, a Roman soldier crucifying St. Peter. In the statue of the "Victory," he is a vanquished old man, crushed by his love of Cavalieri and other adolescents. Obsessed with his sinfulness, he cries out in agony, "So near to death and yet so far from God." He shudders in terror at his expectancy of doom, fearing "the double death" of his body and immortal soul.

In expiation he seeks a saintly life, portraying himself as the martyred Saint Bartholomew in the "Last Judgment." In another self-portrait, he is St. Nicodemus in the service of the martyred Jesus. In real life, he devoted himself for his last seventeen years in saintly service as chief architect of St. Peter's, accepting no earthly reward; a labor of love to please the Popes and the Father in heaven for the "good of his soul." His deepest agonies compelled him to create his most beautiful masterpieces, hopefully expecting to be accepted and loved rather than repulsed and punished.

Art from Torment

For the Jocasta son, be he a Michelangelo or not, the real world is unstable, ambivalent, and extreme in a primitive, emotionally regressed way. He is constantly seeking to bind it up, to make it one. Hence you tend to get from him the kind of comprehensive, synthesizing, metaphoric thought represented not only by Plato (or Freud for that matter) but also by the major religions of the world.

Indeed, it could be argued that the life of the historical Nazarene, as we know it from the Gospels, bears the clear imprint of Jocasta-mothered genius. There is, for instance, the ineffectual, older father; the astonishing intellectual precocity; the rebellious parting from the mother; the absence of any sexual relations with women yet the intense sympathy for the prostitute; the vanity, the egocentricity, and fig-blasting temper; the exclusively male band of disciples and companions; the beautiful, profound, lovingly simple stories; the emphasis on childlikeness; the search for an all-loving, all-wise, and powerful father; the guilt, the atonement, the courting of and achievement of personal destruction. And finally, the staggering accomplishment: the creation of a complex picture or image in which men for two thousand years have read the death of the body on the cross or pinwheel of the world, and the entrance into a proper spiritual home through that necessary death.

It is all very curious. It would seem that Jocasta-mothering represents a deviation or pathology in terms of the mothering process. Nevertheless, it seems to create drives or force fields of personality that, though producing mostly misery and torment in real life, express themselves in the realms of art and thought as extraordinarily potent, comprehensive, or beautiful things.

Jocasta sons cannot wholly trust and yield to intimacy because they get caught in it in the same consuming, ego-dissolving way in which they first experienced love. They are inordinately demanding; when the loved one cannot meet these demands, they withdraw, deeply hurt and angry. The defenses go mile-high—from paranoid fury to complete dissociation of all emotional states— and soon enough come crashing down again. Their actual world is constantly receding from them, or shattering into bits. Therefore they must, *somehow*, create an unambiguous, comprehensive world or resting place that will hold and heal their experience, and they *must* work for and win that lover, who is somewhere. Such a world is built of canvas and paint, or Carrara marble, or wood, or words; more often than not, so is the lover.

As a practicing analyst, I would be the last to deny that most people who have the character structure *so* typical of homosexuality are lonely, miserable, unrealized people, sadly and trivially withered on the vine of human potentiality. Yet far too many truly creative people have to some degree the same personal dynamic or gestalt, a dynamic whose genesis I prefer to locate in the kind of mothering I attribute to Jocasta.

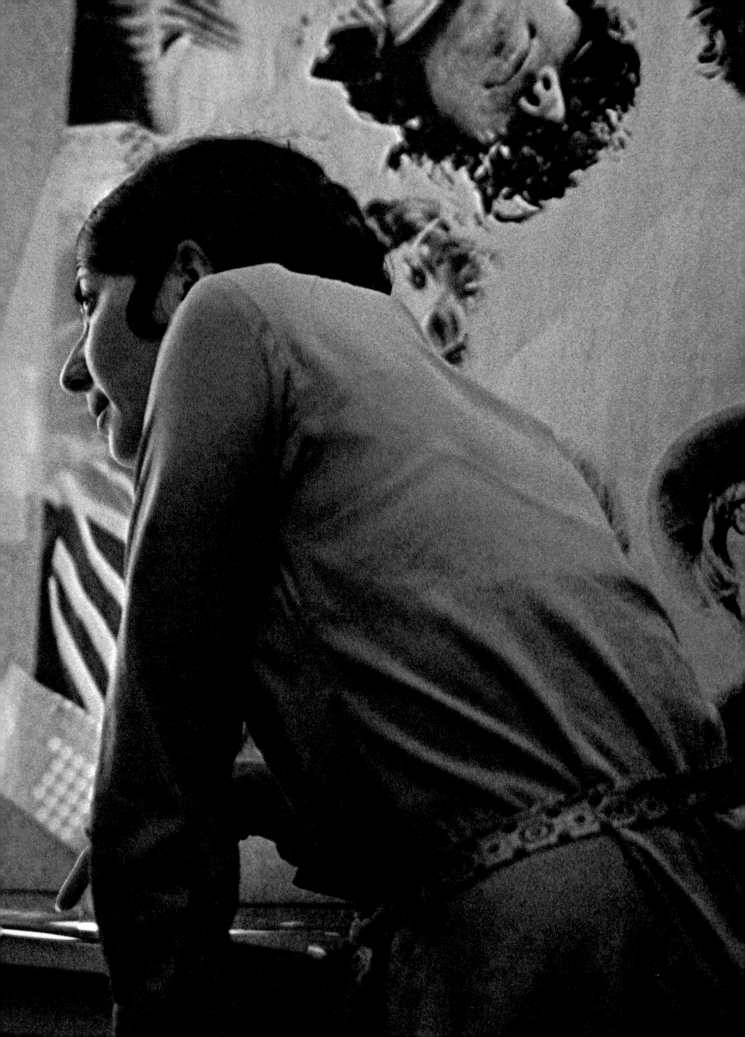

The Grim Generation

Robert E. Kavanaugh

A recurrent theme in this book is that looking within the individual for the source of his difficulties is at best a partial solution. Another theme is that the old distinctions between normal and pathological simply don't fit most psychological problems. Through the evaluative glasses of the middle-aged adult, this entire generation of college students is "maladjusted." Through the students' own eyes, each of them experiences a whole set of existential neuroses or identity crises.

If one wants to apply clinical or psychiatric terms to the "now" generation, there are ample symptoms to diagnose. There are the interpersonal manipulations and socialization failures of the personality (character) disorder; or the inner frustrations and anxious confusion of the classic neurotic; or even the suspicions of the paranoid and the hallucinations or loss of reality contact—albeit mainly drug-induced—of the temporary psychosis. Yet these clinical terms seem uniquely ill suited to understanding this generation and the difficulties they experience.

Like most college counselors, Robert Kavanaugh is more interested in helping solve the problems of the grim generation than he is in applying psychodynamic and clinical diagnoses. He sees six major patterns among today's students, ranging from the benevolent dreamers to the malevolent militants. In writing to an audience of university faculty and administrators, Kavanaugh asks that they honestly listen to the needs and demands voiced by these troubled students. Solutions will not be found in clinics and classifications. A partial answer will come when authorities and educators willingly join today's anguished youth in a committed search for realistic, constructive alternatives to our society's present dissatisfactory way of life.

What are the changes in today's college student? The public is conditioned to see the student in terms of revolt, dope, sex, or the image transmitted by the mass media. But I am a college counselor. I see unsmiling faces, peer into dreamless eyes, hear indictments of parents and country, am frightened by threats of anarchy, listen to pleas for instant friendship, react to demands for student power, and cringe at the nakedness of youth without hope.

There are drastic changes in the students, and they are more than passing whims of a few.

I dare write about the changing student only in light of the adage: "In the land of the blind, the one-eyed man is king." But I write after seventeen years as university lecturer, administrator, campus pastor, and counselor.

There is an absence of mirth on today's campus, a lack of humor. Long before the new student uprisings, even before the recent assassinations, life on campus had become intensely grim. Gone are the sick jokes, gone is the practical joke and the belly filled with goldfish. Humor magazines, planned buffoonery, and silly laughter—long typical of college youth—are as rare as popularity for administrators. A Rowan and Martin "Laugh-In" can trigger giggly smiles, but the self-generated humor of the inner man, which normally helps the self gain perspective, is decidedly rare.

Perhaps the cause lies in the grimness of contemporary life or in the uncertainty of tomorrow. Perhaps it lies in the pressure for grades or in the frustration experienced as values crumble. No matter what the cause, life without laughter is pained and out of focus. Despite an alleged increase in sexual license and party atmosphere on campus, the cared-for student of today is not the carefree student of other years.

Our era of instant communication means instant feedback to the campus of mass media reports about student action. The scene is one of comic tragedy. Selective reporting provides easily memorized stage directions, and students—in search of an identity—seem to become what the commentators on our culture "direct" them to be.

The *malevolent dreamers* are the only students who drive me to say the prayer I read in the eyes of many administrators: "Oh, God, restore to us the apathy of the 1950s." No matter what their label—activists, leftists, radicals, or anarchists—their cause is the overthrow of all authority and every institution, with little regard for means and almost no regard for consequences. Their motivation ranges from philosophical theories of revolution to inner pain and frustrated hurt. A few choose gradualism and nonviolent change, but I see them in astonishing numbers almost psychopathically wed to violence—now. Campus administrators still hopefully advocate dialogue, liberal professors still believe rational debate can direct this admirable energy along nonviolent channels; this stand is being tested hard and many academicians are retreating to the safe ground of the more precise *rule of law*.

Radical students debate mostly with each other or with faculty members of similar philosophy, and administrators get little hearing. Radicals have deep respect for rational debate, but few activists venture to "fly without a flight plan" gained by prior group agreement. And the popular view that unkempt appearance is characteristic of an angry mob pushes the radical groups further away from all outsiders. And even further.

Other students protect the activists, for they share the activist concern for social and political betterment while lacking the activist daring to be heard. They also lack the ability to come up with alternate solutions. The continued stability of campus activism lies in this body of quiet sympathizers.

Black activists seem ambivalent. Sometimes they want to go it alone, sometimes they want the support of white brothers. They walk, speak, and give orders with new confidence; they know that administrators are scurrying to put both more time and more money into minority-student recruitment and support. They know too that faculty planners are desperately arranging curricula in Afro-American studies, that professional schools will admit minority students who are "almost" qualified, and that all academe blushes with shame.

The largest and least often identified type on campus can be called the *kept generation*. The dominant characteristics here are good reputation and moderation. Preoccupation with grades, noninvolvement in extracurricular affairs of a serious nature, and an overriding tone of cynicism are other characteristics. They make mock of the hippy, debunk the activist, berate administrators, con the faculty, and associate only with one another.

Their morality stems from habit and fear, not from internalized conviction. They are adept at the dual standard, attending church only at home, writing letters as family peace and finances dictate, and cribbing on exams. They *ran* the family home and still *command* by phone or letter. In a sense they are what their parents designed.

If members of the kept generation accept an office, it is for personal benefit; if they take dope, it is out of

curiosity or conformity; if they make love, contraceptives are more important than passion. They hate war because they must go. They abhor violence because it blights their plans. Though they loudly mock the student left, they fail to articulate the political right. Cynicism marks their typical humor: "Every time I eat a Hershey bar, I project a death wish." Their identity crisis is deferred, their umbilical cord strained but not severed.

The mark of the kept generation is on enough brows to determine the fate of this generation of students. Anarchists warn that if they sleepwalk back to suburbia, they will find it in ruins. And should they awaken to involvement in social problems, it is these kept kids who will tilt the balance of campus upheaval.

There are other students who are monastically hidden in the cells of their own personal concerns and who join the community only for the common prayer of the classroom. They are a taxpayer's delight because they use no campus services other than the academic. Their number is legion; they go uncounted because they are seldom noticed. The *monastic generation* includes the married student who works nights, the shy commuter, the virginal fat girl, and the 4.0 student who studies incessantly. The monks have little to say on campus radicals, answer no polls, and seldom see a psychiatrist. Their views rarely are tinged with cynicism and only infrequently with self-pity. They are the potential dropouts who refuse to drop out.

Benevolent dreamers are the young men and women who have passed through their identity crisis. They have "lost" their parents or "found" them in a new adult relationship. You see them tutoring in the inner city, raising funds to educate minority youth, leading campus governments, editing newspapers, and forming ad hoc committees. They are prominent in every legal and vital facet of campus or community life. They are willing to be measured. With high ideals and dreams for a better world, accompanied by the drive and ambition to make them effective, these students work mightily to avoid the basely utilitarian overtones they despise in their society. Especially is this true of the benevolent dreamers in the ranks of the nonviolent New Left.

They feel threatened and wounded by draft demands, prospects of urban violence, and the "immoral" approval of war, by racism, poverty, and overpopulation. They feel strapped, stifled, and betrayed by their elders. Such students are not unduly fearful of revolution but they opt for peaceful reform of American institutions. They are abrupt with tradition, suspicious of advice, impatient with authority, and disdainful of duplicity.

Because their cause is seldom sensational and their tactics rarely flamboyant, they are not newsworthy. Some of them try drugs in their desperation for answers, but if so they do not continue, for—even if drugs help—they prefer the fight for legality to illegal involvement. They oversimplify life's complexities, switch heroes easily, and, beneath their confident exterior, they are depressed, anxious, and confused.

Small in number but important to the total picture are the *hippies*. Imitated by other students and often confused with nonacademic hippies, the authentic campus hippy is more than a court jester or a whipping boy. He frightens or disgusts those who measure men by garb, and he confounds those who listen patiently to the rationale for his life style. He is trying, albeit naively, to downgrade material concerns.

The hippy hopes to find himself, to discover meaning and sanity in life. His experience with American life has been brief but distasteful. Usually from a home that is broken or breaking, the campus hippy resembles a soft-spoken Isaiah, decrying middle-class foibles. He preaches human love and worth in the face of campus scoffing and community snickers. Though he probably loves others no more than most of us, love is his shibboleth.

The campus hippy provides few answers. He prefers to raise questions. Unable to visualize life in any but simplistic terms of love and community, the hippy regularly locks in to the dream world of his inner self, where felonies, personal inadequacies, selective service, economics, and social shallowness cannot touch him. Most hippies are somewhat paranoid about police and community harassment. They are a joy to counsel if handled respectfully in the framework of their own world.

Interestingly, though the hippy student professes little concern for grades, his marks tend to be above average.

And yet few campus hippies survive a full four years of college pressure. They drop out. But those who successfully negotiate the narrow path to graduation are potentially great people. They are willing to live in poverty, ready to share puff and pad, and they are able to follow their own convictions in the face of ridicule and scorn.

Campus hippies offer interesting predictions about their own future. Precious few forecast their own return to the Establishment when "their thing" is finished. The majority foresee the possibility of a permanent subculture, though they lack the concept of marriage or family that would allow such a continuance.

The saddest group on campus is one I see as the *graveyard generation*: the hippy who is on his way out and no longer can meet academic demands; the overextended student who holds on despite lack of talent or motivation until rescued by a face-saving transfer, by mononucleosis, or by wise counseling; the disillusioned youth, crushed by home problems, ineffective love affairs, or financial duress; the late bloomer in his budding days of failure; the student who punishes overanxious parents by his academic reluctance; and the one who is psychologically ill.

For this group, the gravestone always can be rolled away from the tomb by a meaningful love affair, by counseling, therapy, or even by survival through development.

I see today's students move with sudden fluidity from group to group, or even reflect several strains at once. I see them belonging to one group while masking affiliation to another.

Many of the changes I see in today's students can be traced to our changed family structure. Crashed or crashing marriages at home intensify the student identity crisis. The failure of the home, the school, and the church to transmit a sound and solid value system further heightens the expected crisis. Today's student lacks a strong parental figure or a deeply indoctrinated sense of values to polarize his identity crisis. Yesterday's authoritarian father and overworked mother, community-backed teacher and "heaven-hell" church generated clearer paths for rebellion or acceptance. Polarization is hardly possible when family authority is vested in "daddy-son" or "mommy-daughter," when teachers are overly accepting, when churches impart vague platitudes. The student is torn between acceptance and rejection and confused by a diffusion of goals and values.

Because of its altered structure and increased mobility, the family creates personal isolation and insulation. At best, today's family offers only limited opportunities for intimate relationships. When these are bungled by conflict or parental incapacity, the laboratory for friendship becomes the large high school, the shifting neighborhood, the dwindling extended family, or a church.

The results show in the demise or changing structure of the fraternity-sorority system, faculty-student aloofness, the grasping and groping for instant friendship, and the solidification of monogamous dating practices. Rare is the student who can cope simultaneously with several close relationships.

A new vision of the family is in the making. Rarely does the campus male animal fight for his woman. Children play an ever decreasing part in the college view of marriage. By admission—and even the reluctant permission—of the male, the wife dominates the married campus couple. And parental benefactors control the campus marriage with financial aid more often than the mendicant lovers realize.

Traditionally, youth uses the future for dreaming, the past for bragging, and the now for living. Yesterday there was little reluctance to permit the present to flow into the future. There was always the promise of a pleasant tomorrow. Some of today's students still enjoy the American dream: the ranch in suburbia, the niche in megapolis, the bench in St. Petersburg, the eternity box at the end. But a growing number believe they have tasted the "capitalistic dream" only to find it embittered by the prospect of war, jail, or emigration. Activists lash out to increase their alternatives. Most students lock in to the present and struggle to manufacture articulate dreams. They have no experience with the world they desire in their tomorrow.

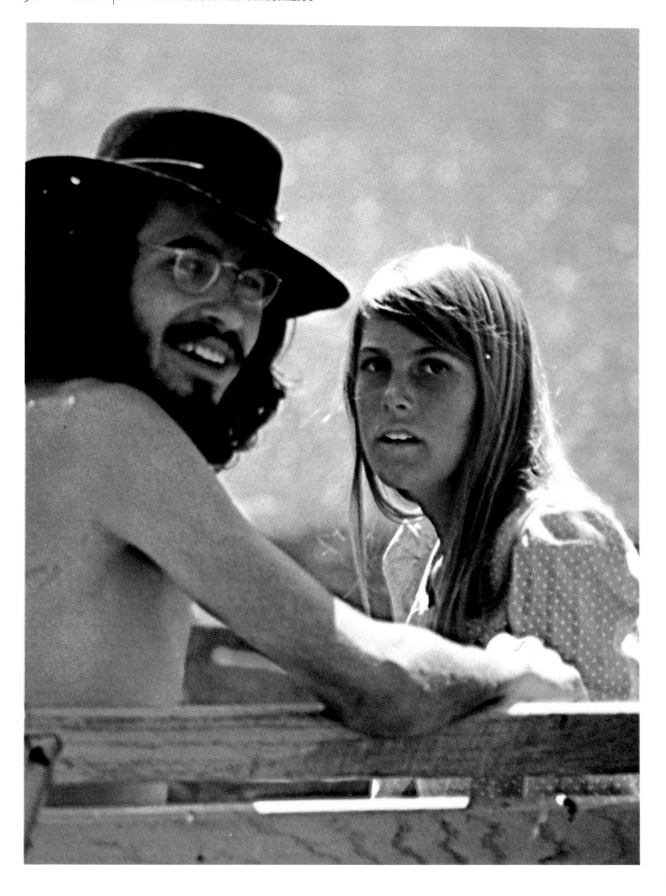

Adoration of the present pervades the campus. The drug user readily admits his need to zero in on the present. Drugs add an intensity and reality to his dreams and fantasies that reality denies. The maximum decibel roar of the stereo provides the hard rock fan with a lesser lock-in. So do the total preoccupation with theoretical math, the endless hours in a lonesome lab, isolated hetero- and homosexual love affairs, attempts at oriental meditation, devotion to alcohol, addiction to cars, and insulated aloofness. Even concern for distant injustices, like the war in Vietnam and poverty in the inner city, makes the present tolerable.

This mania to make the present bearable results in an increased preoccupation with death, both in contemplated suicide and in folk music or other art forms. Violence that does not disturb the present (such as that depicted on movies or TV) is groovy, but fist fights (part of the entertainment on yesterday's campus) are strangely absent.

The search for meaning and values *is* a major factor in student unrest. And the central campus value is this search for values. The framework for the search is one of mutual acceptance: each man has his own bag; don't interfere. (The unpracticed observer can read this non-intervention as a modern version of Cain and Abel, but it is more likely a stand against indoctrination and for individual freedom.) And the search intensifies as the excellence of the campus ascends from junior-college caliber to university level.

Organized religion plays a decreasing role on campus and possibly is saved from extinction only by the superior clergy assigned to most campuses. Scientific humanism attracts numerous students and continues as the "bag" for most faculty members. Political activism and expanding social concern provide new life for the departments of philosophy, political science, sociology, and religion. Oriental cults attract fewer than the press, radio, and TV imply.

Verbalized values are more negative than positive. Students speak out in terms of rights and rarely in terms of duties. There is almost no evidence of a right-wing viewpoint in social, political, or moral matters, even though the confused students seem ripe for simplistic, solid answers.

The much-publicized growing sexual promiscuity is not general practice on the campus. Shyness, introversion, vestigial guilt, self-doubt, and the fear of rejection keep students from the practice of their preaching, even

with pills and intrauterine devices to reduce their fear of pregnancy. Actually, premarital pregnancies are on the wane, "sleeping around" is not admired, and premarital sex is practiced most often in a semiresponsible and monogamous relationship.

Besides the vertical gap between this generation and the last there is a horizontal gap between students of the far left and their middle-of-the-road peers, between the science major and the artist, the engineer and the social scientist. As campus departments insulate themselves in their own concerns and jargon, upper division students share the isolation. A music student put it this way: "Dante could re-create the *Inferno* by putting me in eternity with two engineers."

Students are strangely willing—for the present—to grant the faculty immunity from the rebellious anti-authoritarianism they focus on the administration. This in spite of countless unintelligible or ill-prepared lectures, archaic and haphazard teaching methods, unjust and unscientific grading systems, and sharply limited faculty office hours. *There are signals that this divine right is ending.*

The student of today studies much harder than any college student before him, even that post World War II generation of veterans. The standard of achievement is higher today and today's student worries more.

The 1968 college student already has conquered the American home, exchanging roles with his parents. He has been victorious over his high school, where he found boredom instead of challenge. Now he is poised to lay siege to the American university.

The survival of the university seems to depend on whether faculty and administrators can provide a dream, a hope for tomorrow. Students want—they demand—that their dream include an end to injustice and to the suppression of truth and reality. They no longer want duplicity in morals. They demand a relevant curriculum and a concerned faculty. They want leaders who will take a stand on issues, who can provide meaning, a flame for their apathy, a respect for their right. They want leaders whose lives embody their dreams, leaders who listen. They want leaders who will work with them in the face of the nihilistic anguish of their hopeless present.

Academic arrogance will get us nowhere. These student demands are going to be hard to meet. I am just a counselor who listens. But I know the threat to every tree in the groves of academe if there is no change.

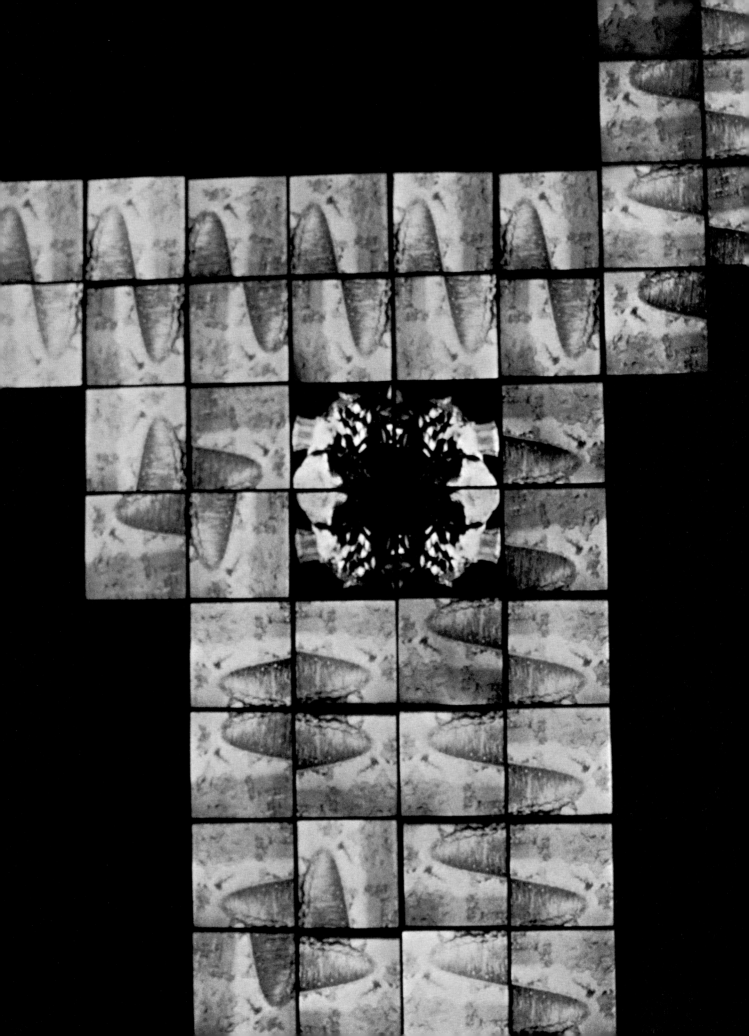

The Psychology of Religious Experience

Walter Houston Clark

Clinical psychologists have often touched the edges of the study of religion. Some have used religious faith as an index of personal stability. Others have seen religious beliefs, particularly when stated concretely, as indications of either uncritical intelligence or delusional states. Few psychologists have pursued the study of religious experience in and of itself, in spite of the fact that religious commitments can rival or exceed psychotherapeutic changes in a person's basic life style.

Walter Clark works with a very broad definition of religious experience. Not only does he include conversions to formalized faiths but he also allows transformations generated by drugs or during acute psychotic episodes. He considers as a true religious or mystical experience one that effects pronounced changes in both thought processes and actions. In some cases, the change is for the better, as when criminals are rehabilitated after taking LSD or when depressed persons gain, through a mystical experience, a reason and purpose for living. At other times, however, a religious experience has deleterious effects. A psychotic retreats further into delusions or a contrite parishioner is consumed with guilt.

Given the potency of religious experience, scientific psychology is interested not only in the phenomenon itself but in the reasons for its positive and negative effects on the individual personality.

A few years ago an inconspicuous member of one of my classes sought me out. The mother of a family, she told me about a religious experience of a mystical nature, a story she had confided to no other living person. Not understanding it, except in its general nature, I listened sympathetically but gave no advice. But the incident seemed to set in motion a psychological and religious process of surprising proportions. Shortly afterward she became more active in her church. Now others seek her out to take leadership in discussion groups, and, to her embarrassment, church members refer problems to her that, more appropriately, should go to the pastor. Besides being much more forceful, she is more attractive, and she herself is amazed to find that she is becoming a positive force for good in the community and in her family instead of just another aging housewife.

This is an illustration in a commonplace, contemporary person of the influence that religion may have in the transformation of personality. I have seen and studied such phenomena in ordinary men and women, and in many persons undergoing a religious experience under psychedelic drugs. The psychological study of religion is as fascinating as man himself, and as compelling as his fascination with God.

We have records of something happening in the personalities of eminent men and women of history— Socrates, Moses, the Buddha, St. Paul, St. Francis, Teresa of Avila, the French mathematician Pascal, John Wesley, and Jesus. In large part, it was to seek the source of this power in scores of intense souls that William James wrote his great treatise, *The Varieties of Religious Experience*, certainly the most notable of all books in the field of the psychology of religion and probably destined to be the most influential book written on religion in the twentieth century.

It is a paradox that, in view of such evidence, modern psychologists should be so incurious about the dynamics involved and so neglectful of a force in human nature with such influence for both good and evil in human personality and human history. Since the time of William James, the psychological study of religion has fallen on dull days. In our day, its prestige has gradually begun to revive, but the conventional psychologist still tends to observe it warily as a subject that he is not quite sure belongs in his field.

And this is not hard to understand. In the 1920s, behaviorism was obtaining a firm grip on psychology. The aim of shaping psychology into another natural science still seemed to be within reach if all psychologists would only agree to neglect the mind and to confine themselves to a study of environmental stimuli and resulting behavior.

But religion, particularly if one wishes to probe its depths and make sense of it, requires the study of the inner life more than almost any other human activity. With its close associations to theology and philosophy (more universally acknowledged in William James' day, incidentally), considering the psychology of religion as a natural science seems far from ideal.

Mystical Experience

By far the most interesting, instructive, and yet puzzling phenomenon of religious experience is the mystical one. I would agree with William James that "personal religious experience has its root and center in mystical states of consciousness." This characteristic seems to me to separate religious consciousness from other forms of consciousness. All other aspects of the religious life have their counterparts in man's secular life. A mystical state alone is *sui generis* and is so different from any other psychological state that subjectively it is seldom mistaken for anything other than religion. A mystical state produces a particular kind of perception involving what is probably the most intense positive psychological experience known to man. It may be compared to romantic love. Yet mystics, in order to serve God, have been known to desert their possessions, their previous ways of life, and those whom they love. It is the very differentness of mysticism that causes trouble for the mystic. He finds no words to explain exactly what he has experienced unless he is talking to other mystics. Thus the mystic is often a lonely person, keeping within himself the expression of his pearl of great price, the thing that gives meaning to his life.

The psychologist, unless he is a mystic himself (which he seldom is), is forced to rely on the words of the mystic to describe the experience, though he also notes the sharp changes in behavior that frequently accompany mystical states. The feature most often reported and that seems to be at the core of the experience is a perception of unity, accompanied also by a sense of timelessness, of holiness, and by the feeling that one has directly encountered ultimate reality, accompanied by a sense of great peace. It would be easy for the psychologist to pass off this strange state of ecstasy as just another aberration, were it not for the wholesome changes of personality that often follow it. Certainly, even if such transformations do not occur every day, one might suppose that a thorough study of them would at least throw some light on the nature of personality change and human creativity.

| THE ROLE OF DRUGS | In the study of religious experience and personality change, I will venture to mention a controversial but incomparable tool for the study of this elusive area—psychedelic drugs. Formerly I was extremely critical of the religious value of the drugs. However, I have experimented on myself and have had an opportunity to participate with others in research. My conclusions were not unlike those of William James after he had tried nitrous oxide, the psychedelic of his day. He said:

One conclusion . . . is that our normal waking consciousness, rational consciousness as we call it, is but one special type of consciousness, whilst all about it, parted by the filmiest of screens, there lie potential forms of consciousness entirely different. . . . We may go through life without suspecting their existence; but . . . no account of the universe in its totality can be final which leaves these other forms of consciousness quite disregarded. . . . My own experiences . . . all converge towards a kind of insight to which I cannot help ascribing some metaphysical significance.

Certainly if the psychedelics do not release genuine religious experiences, then the differences are so subtle that even religious experts cannot tell the difference, apart from knowing that a drug has been involved. The experiment that did the most to convince me that the psychedelics triggered mysticism was the following: Dr. Walter N. Pahnke, in a Harvard doctoral study, set up nine criteria of mystical experience using principally those of Princeton's expert, W. T. Stace, and William James. He then gave 30 milligrams of psilocybin to ten theological students, and to ten others he gave a placebo. None of the twenty were informed which they had received. All of them then attended the same Good Friday service. In their descriptions after the service, nine of the ten who had been given the drug reported unmistakable characteristics of mystical phenomena, while only one who had taken the placebo did, and his reaction was very mild.

What further supports many psychedelic experiences as being religious is that, when the subject reports a religious experience, therapeutic results are often more marked. This was the case with pioneer experiments in which massive doses of LSD were given to hopeless alcoholics in Saskatchewan by Humphrey Osmond and Abram Hoffer. After five years, half of the sample of sixty cases were still found to be nonalcoholic. "As a general rule," Hoffer reported, "those who have not had the transcendental experience are not changed; they continue to drink. However, the large proportion of those who have had it are changed."

There also has been experimentation with criminals in Europe and the United States. In order to find out for myself what the results had been, I studied several convicts to whom Dr. Timothy Leary had given psilocybin and who, according to his report, had encountered religious experiences of a life-changing nature. Some of these convicts definitely had fallen by the wayside—through lack of follow-up after the controversial Leary project collapsed.

But I discovered a rather remarkable phenomenon. Those who had remained in jail had started what they called the "Self-Development Group," a very successful AA type of self-rehabilitation that continued on a nondrug basis. One middle-aged armed robber, serving a twenty-year term, in a drug session had seen a vision of Christ. Shortly afterward, he said, "All my life came before my eyes, and I said, 'What a waste!' " Now, five years later, this man, a group leader, is considered by the authorities to be completely rehabilitated.

The point of these experiments is that not only do subjects, after psychedelic therapy, talk like religious people, but religion for them has had the effect of radically changing their values and attitudes. The drugs seem to do what the churches frequently only *say* they do in their talk of salvation, redemption, and rebirth. All this is not to minimize the real dangers and problems of the drugs but to call attention to certain facts that have not appeared often in the news media and to point out the connection of the drugs with religion.

The psychologist of religion faces some formidable problems. Even the definition of religion is a matter of great dispute. Several years ago I asked a number of experts in the field of the scientific study of religion to define what they meant by the word *religion*. Of sixty-eight replies, no two were exactly alike, and even when replies were grouped, the categories differed. This is hardly a happy situation for a discipline making any pretense to being a science.

History of the Study

Yet the psychology of religion is beginning to emerge from its long period of exile. Strangely enough, this discipline of psychology owes its emergence in no small measure to another genius who held religion in much lower esteem than did James. That man was Sigmund Freud, who was able to seduce large numbers of modern scientific psychologists through his own scientific background and through his insistence, which at least in his early days seemed completely sincere, that he was strictly a scientist and nothing more.

Actually, to an extent that Freud himself did not realize, he was an artist of the human soul. While his observations involved close study of the lives of his patients, his intuitions and speculations went far beyond pedestrian reports of stimuli and responses to them—the responses, of course, and some of the stimuli as well, being merely the products of his patients' inner lives. Aided by a clarity of style hardly matched in such a complex field, Freud opened the doors to the study of man's subjectivity for many behaviorists, whose studies and writing were thereby enriched. As examples I might mention the followers of the Yale behaviorist Clark Hull—men like John Dollard, Neal Miller, and O. Hobart Mowrer.

More directly, Freud set an example through his own writings on religion—through books like *Totem and Taboo*, *The Future of an Illusion*, and *Moses and Monotheism*. He dealt with religion as merely the search for a father image and as "the universal neurosis of mankind." But he wrote more about religion than any other single subject except sex. That this interest may have had its roots in the connection of his forebears with Jewish mysticism is suggested in a volume by David Bakan. Then Freud occasionally alarmed some of his close followers after conversations lasting into the early hours when he said he had times when he could almost bring himself to believe in many things, even

"der liebe Gott!" Certainly this interest has led many Freudians and neo-Freudians to think and write of religion.

One of the most influential of the latter was the Swiss psychiatrist Carl G. Jung, whom Freud at one time had designated as his successor. Though a more obscure writer than Freud, Jung was more positively and openly religious. It was he who declared that, among his patients over the age of thirty-five, there were none whose problems did not have their roots in religion. Like Freud, he found the principal roots of religion in the unconscious, especially in what he called the racial unconscious, by which he explained the universal aspects of much religious symbolism.

Somewhat nearer to the orthodox academic psychological tradition in America have been several scholars, all presidents of the American Psychological Association in their day, who have written on the subject, though none has worked in the psychology of religion as his major field. The list includes Gardner Murphy, the late Gordon Allport, O. Hobart Mowrer, and Abraham H. Maslow. Of these, perhaps Allport did most toward making the subject academically respectable, through his volume of lectures, *The Individual and His Religion*. Maslow includes religion among the "peak experiences" that are the fruits of what he calls B-cognition, the source of human creativity.

A somewhat different influence on the psychology of religion, one especially strong in theological schools and churches, has been exerted by clinical pastoral psychology. This movement in the United States has had an interesting history.

In the early 1920s a middle-aged clergyman, considering his life a failure, was hospitalized with the diagnosis of catatonic schizophrenia. Through his stay in the hospital, he became convinced of the need of many mental patients for adequate pastoral care. On his recovery, after some difficulty with conventional administrative ideas as to the value of religion for mental patients, he persuaded Dr. James A. Bryan, Superintendent of Worcester State Hospital in Massachusetts, to appoint him the first chaplain at a mental hospital in this country. Shortly after his appointment, the chaplain persuaded several theological students to study ministry to the mentally ill under his direction.

Thus started the clinical pastoral counseling movement in the theological schools, a training now required in at least one-third of the Protestant theological schools and in some form optional with most other seminaries, including many of the Catholic and Jewish seminaries. The clergyman who started it all was Anton T. Boisen, who died a few years ago at the Elgin State Hospital in Illinois, where he was Chaplain Emeritus, honored and lamented by thousands of students and patients.

About the time that Boisen began his ministry to the mentally ill, one of the first of a long line of volumes in the field of religion and mental health appeared—*Pas-*

toral Psychiatry and Mental Health, by James Rathbone Oliver, both a psychiatrist and a clergyman. One of the most articulate contemporary writers in this field is Seward Hiltner of Princeton Theological Seminary. However, recently authors in religion have multiplied themselves in so many volumes that they have become increasingly repetitive and even boring.

There has been a fringe benefit, however, in enrichment for clinical psychology. Theologians usually not noted for their attention to the practical or empirical have been forced to take some notice of mental health and of the fact that the clinician may often lead his patient to consider matters of "ultimate concern." The best-known theologian to encourage dialogue with therapists was the late Paul Tillich, particularly in his book *The Courage to Be.* And the greats in psychology all have responded to his dialogue. There are recordings of conversations with Carl Rogers, Hobart Mowrer, Erich Fromm, and with the man who perhaps was Tillich's closest friend, Rollo May.

But let us look again at Anton Boisen in another way. One of the striking facts in the lives of many great religious leaders has been abnormality, which sometimes has grown into full-blown psychosis. Ezekiel's visions of complicated flying beasts and "wheels within wheels" are only darkly understandable, while some of Jeremiah's words and actions mark him as, at the very least, a peculiar fellow. At one time Jesus' family and friends spoke of him as "beside himself," while George Fox, founder of the Society of Friends, probably would have been hospitalized in this day and age. William James discusses this subject in the first chapter of his *Varieties.* Of Boisen's psychic instability there is no doubt. He acknowledged it himself, and the records of the diagnosis and his stay still remain at Worcester State Hospital in Massachusetts.

His sickness gave him an incomparable opportunity to observe a psychosis from the inside. In addition to this, having a scholarly cast of mind, as he recovered he had an opportunity to observe his fellow sufferers and to reflect on his observations. The result was his *Exploration of the Inner World,* a contemporary minor classic filled with original observations on the nature of schizophrenia and on the value of religion as a dynamic aspect of many cures. He regarded catatonic schizophrenia, from which he suffered, as the presentation to the patient of a crisis in his life so profound as to drive him into a panic. The very profundity of the problem offered religious dimensions to be coped with only by a radical religious decision.

Thus, the crisis tended to "make or break" the individual, leading either to rapid cure or to continued deterioration. For this reason Boisen saw religion as an essential therapeutic tool for many patients, one that might make the difference between sickness and health, and out of which strength might come. In this way he explained the power of George Fox and other unstable religious leaders. Psychologists have acknowledged the originality of Boisen's theories, and while they would not for the most part generalize them to the extent that he did, most would grant that at least they fit his own case very aptly.

| TWO OPPOSING APPROACHES | The relationship between religion and mental illness suggests a paradox with respect to religion and mental health, and thus leads to two schools of thought. On the one hand are those who see religion as a positive force leading to a sense of well-being and optimism, tending to reduce morbid human attitudes and to maximize healthy-mindedness. On the other hand are those who make much of the association between religion and mental illness. Psychiatrists in the latter camp frequently stress the fact that there are some patients in whom the very consideration of religion will touch off a psychosis, and the fact that almost any mental hospital can display a varied assortment of self-styled messiahs and Jesus Christs. An interesting example of three such personalities is found in Rokeach's *Three Christs of Ypsilanti.*

Actually, the situation is much too complex for either of these views to be the whole truth. It is worth mentioning William James' two famous types of religion, the "religion of healthy-mindedness" and that of the "sick soul." James sees them simply as two differing expressions of religion usually associated with differing types of temperament or life style, though these may alternate within a single personality. The healthy-minded person expresses his religion in a context of exuberance and joy. He minimizes the tragedies of life and may even systematically deny the existence of sickness and evil, as in Christian Science, according to James. James points out that this way of dealing with life works well for some people and thus empirically demonstrates its core of truth.

But there are others who cannot turn away from life's tragic elements, its sicknesses, strife, injustices, and its suffering. Men are not born equal, with an equal chance in life, and death is the only leveler. An honest facing of such facts leads to a much deeper probing of the meaning of life than "the religion of healthy-mindedness," even though it may not produce cheery apostles. The title of one of Kierkegaard's books is *The Sickness Unto Death,* and one must acknowledge that this particular gloomy Dane produced some of the most searching religious observations of the last century. James, at least when he wrote *The Varieties,* looked on the sick soul as one who recognized a truer dimension of religion and life.

If one looks at these two religious styles, they may be seen not as mutually exclusive but as two roads to religious growth. There are none of the great religious faiths that do not provide for the expression of both. The greatest literary production of the Hebrew Bible—and indeed one of the great pieces of world literature—is the Book of Job, a consideration of suffering and its relation to evil. But the same Bible is filled with an account of the triumphs as well as of the disasters of the

Children of Israel. The theme of death and resurrection is a universal one in religion, derived from the depths of human nature. It is significant that the Passion of Christ's Crucifixion is followed by His Resurrection. Good Friday is linked with Easter. This symbolizes that alternation in human destiny, that dialogue of opposites through which religious development takes place.

This search for understanding of the process of religious growth will bring any religious psychologist worth his salt to the delicate and fascinating field of religious experience. I say *delicate*, for the churches have widely differing but nevertheless very positive convictions in the area. One runs the risk of offending some people no matter what one says or how carefully one phrases one's research and thought. This is one reason that psychology is somewhat gun-shy about religion. But such subjects as conversion, mysticism, possession, and prophecy need to be dealt with not only by the psychologist of religion but by any psychologist who pretends awareness of the total man.

It is an oversimplification, of course, but we can see religious life as containing two interrelated but very different psychological functions. Rudolf Otto, in *The Idea of the Holy*, has termed them the *rational* and the *nonrational*. If we liken the religious pilgrim to a ship in voyage, we might designate as the rudder the critical, directive, rational, and reasonable parts of the pilgrim's nature; the ship's propulsion then would be the nonrational, the feeling and intuitive elements, providing energy, liveliness, and movement. Perhaps in this respect religion is simply a special case of all of life. But we might note that a boat, no matter how strong its rudder, would get nowhere without an engine, while a rudderless ship with a powerful engine would be a hazard to itself and to all navigation. Thus religion through the ages has needed the prophet, the convert, the seer, the martyr, and the saint as well as the theologian and the priest.

This well may be why the more dynamic forms of religion often deprecate the scholar and the rationalist. It also helps explain why churches so often have been afraid of religion in its livelier forms. The church develops the conservatism typical of any institution, and it prefers saints to be dead before it begins to worship them.

Partly because the churches at about the turn of the century made more of the phenomenon of conversion, James (and E. D. Starbuck, his predecessor in the field of the psychology of religion) devoted many pages to this phenomenon. The bad name that conversion has acquired among scholars is due partly to the fact that some churches have forced on their members a highly emotional experience of unsettling shallowness, which has obscured the significance of many a sudden conversion of life-saving proportions. The founders of Alcoholics Anonymous are an outstanding example. Against a background of brainwashing and Pavlovian theory, William Sargant gives some reasons for the power of sudden conversion, both for good and for ill, in *Battle for the Mind*.

It seems to me that religion at its best can be illustrated well by contrasting the two great psychologists, Gordon Allport and William James. In *The Individual and His Religion*, Allport speaks of "mature religion" as self-critical and as possessing its own motivational force; as consistent in its moral consequences; as comprehensive and integrative; and, finally, as eternally questing.

James tries to define what he sees as religion at its best in the chapter "Saintliness," in *The Varieties*. He defines the best thus:

A feeling of being in a wider life than that of this world's selfish little interests; and a conviction, not merely intellectual, of the existence of an Ideal Power . . . A sense of the friendly continuity of the ideal power with our own life, and a willing self-surrender to its control . . . An immense elation and freedom as the outlines of the confining selfhood melt down . . . A shifting of the emotional center towards loving and harmonious affections, towards "yes, yes," and away from "no" where the claims of the nonego are concerned.

James is not uncritical of some of the excesses of saintliness. Yet, when we compare his view of high religion with Allport's, we sense a wide gap. Allport is the rationalist.

Most college students take to Allport—the rudder. But some prefer James. These tend to be the more sensitive, more emotional ones, those who may have experienced the aesthetic and the mystical in their own lives, and who may be scorned a bit by their more rational classmates. Perhaps this is reminiscent of the situation on the Harvard campus in James' day, when his colleagues shook their heads at the vagaries of their attractive colleague.

We can trace this difference in emphasis to roots in James' own nature—half artistic and half intellectual, with mystical sensitivities of a profound nature, heightened through his experience with nitrous oxide and other experiences of which he spoke only to his intimates. Thus, we can bring these two students of religion into dialogue and take from each his characteristic contribution to theory as we derive from them the rational and nonrational components in religion at its best.

But, taken as a whole, the psychologist's contribution to religion is mainly a rational one. The psychologist is like the music critic, who can analyze and therefore help the hearer to appreciate. And so, as a psychologist of religion, I work to understand when I can. But ultimately I must stand in awe before what, as a psychologist, I cannot match—the authentic religious life. This is the subtlest, most profound, yet puzzling and paradoxical, of the achievements of the human spirit. It is religion *par excellence*, which has the power to transform human life and so give it meaning, and it is for these reasons that the religious consciousness is the most fascinating object of study of all human phenomena. At least, that is how one psychologist of religion sees it.

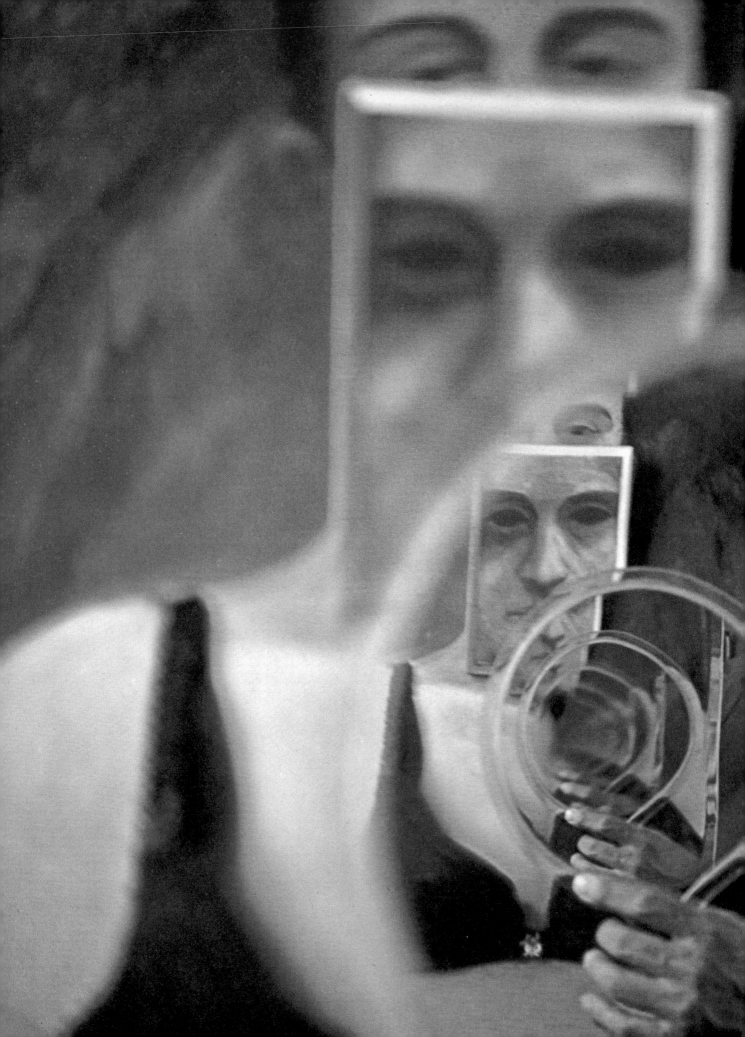

Homosexuality and Social Evil

Martin Hoffman

This article, like Kavanaugh's and others, underlines the need for both professionals and the public to reconsider our definition of mental illness. Should we continue to regard as "mentally ill" a person whose behavior patterns deviate from society's codes of conduct? Many people engage in some type of homosexual behavior or relationship at least once during their lives. Others do so more often or over a period of time and yet lead fairly normal lives. Only a small minority become homosexually oriented to the extent described here by Martin Hoffman and, according to him, still fewer show evidence of other aberrations.

Hoffman would have us suspend the assumption that homosexuals are, by their nature, seriously disturbed. In his view, the fundamental problem for the homosexual lies not in his relationships with his lovers and cohorts but in his relationships with the nongay world. It is one's self-definition, perhaps, that sets the stage for psychological conflict. In the homosexual's case, he has, in accepting the role of homosexual, assumed a self-identity and set of behavior patterns that ensure alienation from the rest of society. To the degree that he realizes that he is unacceptable in a society whose ethics he nonetheless values, he experiences conflict. He learns to devalue himself and those like him. It is, thus, more a sensitivity to social standards than a negation of them that leads to his lonely, troubled existence.

Every occupation has its hazards. One hazard of theoretical work in psychology and psychiatry is psychologism: overemphasis on psychological factors in explaining puzzling phenomena. Psychologism plagues the study of homosexuality. All the phenomena of this complex sexual orientation have been explained by the psychoanalytic theory of homosexuality—a brilliant but nevertheless incomplete analysis.

This theory is set forth clearly and economically in Otto Fenichel's classic work, *The Psychoanalytic Theory of Neurosis*, which dazzles with its profound insights into what most of us regard as a very mysterious kind of behavior. Unfortunately, we link his study with another idea: the disease concept of homosexuality. This concept holds that homosexuality, by its very nature, is always either a mental illness or a symptom of such an illness. I immediately reject this idea as too sweeping a generalization. Emotional disturbance causes many men and women to become homosexual. But a number of studies now show that there are many homosexual men who are not emotionally disturbed.

Because my own research and clinical practice has been almost entirely with male homosexuals, I am not going to discuss female homosexuality, except to mention a few differences between the two groups in order to make a theoretical point. This article is on male homosexuality; I even use the term homosexuality to refer to male homosexuality alone.

The Hooker Study

Evelyn Hooker, psychologist at the University of California at Los Angeles, made the classic study that refuted the disease concept of homosexuality. She found thirty homosexuals, not in treatment, whom she felt to be reasonably well adjusted. She then matched thirty heterosexual men with the homosexuals for age, education, and IQ. Hooker then gave these sixty men a battery of psychological tests and obtained considerable information on their life histories. Several of her most skilled clinical colleagues then analyzed the material. They did not know which of the tests had been given to the homosexual men and which to the heterosexuals; they analyzed the tests blind. Hooker concluded from their analyses that there is no inherent connection between homosexual orientation and clinical symptoms of mental illness. She stated: "Homosexuality as a clinical entity does not exist. Its forms are as varied as are those of heterosexuality. Homosexuality may be a deviation in sexual pattern that is in the normal range, psychologically." This conclusion is based on the fact that the clinicians were unable to distinguish between the two groups. Nor was there any evidence that the homosexual group had a higher degree of pathology than the heterosexual group.

A number of more impressionistic studies, based on psychiatric interviewing, support Dr. Hooker's conclusions. Two London psychiatrists, Desmond Curran and Denis Parr, reported in the *British Medical Journal* in 1957 that of 100 homosexual men seen in psychiatric consultation, only 49 percent had any significant psychiatric abnormalities. In late 1966, the Homosexual Law Reform Society, based in Philadelphia, wrote to a number of distinguished behavioral scientists, asking their opinions on the relation of homosexuality to psychopathology. The responses to the society from some of the country's most eminent scientists supported the position that Dr. Hooker and I hold: that homosexuals are not necessarily mentally ill.

Let me quote a few of the responses.

Paul H. Gebhard, Ph.D., director, Institute of Sex Research, Indiana University (founded by the late Alfred C. Kinsey): "the collective opinion of the members of the Institute for Sex Research . . . based on extensive interviewing and other data is as follows . . . homosexuality is not a pathology in itself nor necessarily a symptom of some other pathology."

Norman Reider, M.D., training analyst, San Francisco Psychoanalytic Institute, and recently visiting professor of psychiatry at the Albert Einstein College of Medicine in New York: "Homosexuality per se is no evidence of psychopathology."

John L. Hampson, M.D., associate professor of psychiatry, University of Washington: "In most instances the homosexual life-style is the product of certain complex early learning influences and should not be thought of as a 'mental illness' or 'psychopathology' . . ."

Fallacies in the Disease Concept

One could go on with further quotations refuting the fallacy that homosexuality is necessarily connected with mental or behavioral disorder. There is, to be sure, opinion on both sides. It seems to me, however, that the opposing view—that homosexuals are all sick—arises from two main sources. First, since the concept of sin is no longer in fashion in Western thought, we do not know how to label behavior when we disapprove of it on moral grounds. Second, psychiatrists who assert that homosexuality is an illness generally know homosexuals only as patients. Since psychiatric patients are disturbed, therapists conclude that they represent the general homosexual population when, in fact, they are

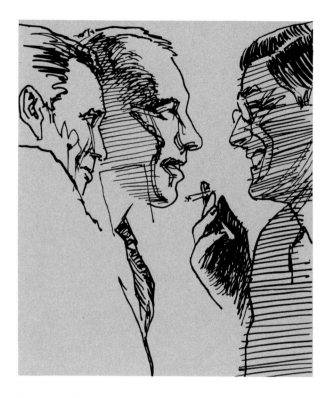

but a small fraction of it. As Dr. Judd Marmor, analyst and editor of the book *Sexual Inversion* wrote: "If the judgments of psychoanalysts about heterosexuals were based only on those they see as patients, would they not have the same skewed impression of heterosexuals as a group?"

This issue made me want to conduct a nonclinical, ethnographic field study of the male homosexual population in the San Francisco Bay area. I reported on this study in my book, *The Gay World: Male Homosexuality and the Social Creation of Evil*. As a clinical psychiatrist, I was seeing only disturbed homosexuals, and I wanted to find out what kinds of lives other members of that group were living. So, I interviewed many homosexual men to learn whether they suffered from mental disorder. I examined them as psychiatrists usually do, asking about their doubts, anxieties, possible phobias, depressions, and the like. Large numbers of them showed no clinical signs of mental disturbance. I am convinced, after talking to these men, most of whom had never sought psychiatric treatment, that one of the most important causes of the currently fashionable disease concept of homosexuality is that clinicians do not see a representative sample of homosexuals. If they did, they would be hard put to maintain their dogmatism about *all* homosexuals.

An example of the dogmatism is a magazine article called "A Way Out for Homosexuals," by Philadelphia psychiatrist Samuel B. Hadden. (Group therapy is the "way out.") Hadden says, "In my observation, homosexuals are deeply troubled people" (again the cliniçian's fallacy), "their numbers are increasing" (he gives no evidence for this, and there is none), homosexuality is "a grave social problem" (yes it is, but hardly in the manner Hadden thinks it to be), "from earliest childhood none of the homosexuals I have known have been truly psychologically healthy individuals" (one would hardly expect this from a psychiatric patient population!).

Hadden implies that homosexuals are abnormally prone to violence. This is utterly fallacious. In the most recent Institute for Sex Research report, which deals specifically with sex offenders, no categories were needed to describe homosexual acts that might involve force. In contrast, categories involving force (for example, rape) were needed to analyze the data on heterosexual acts. As the report states, "the use of force is rare in homosexual activity."

Finally, consider this statement by Hadden: "In my view, we should treat homosexuality as a handicapping disorder. *And I further believe that society has a right to expect those afflicted to seek treatment . . .*" (my italics). He clearly implies that those homosexuals—the vast majority—who do not wish to become heterosexual should be forced into psychiatric treatment. Let us be quite aware that Hadden's pronouncement borders on frank totalitarianism. Should all individuals who deviate from current social norms be forced to conform, whether or not their behavior harms others? Is psychotherapy to operate in an atmosphere in which the patient has the ultimate right to make up his own mind about what he will do with his private life, or is psychotherapy to become an agent of social control?

In the light of Hadden's remarks, we may do well to note the attitude of Communist China toward deviants. Some Chinese prisons for brainwashing are called "hospitals for ideological reform." And Mao Tse-tung has said, "our object in exposing errors and criticizing shortcomings is like that of a doctor in curing a disease. . . ." Robert Jay Lifton, who quotes this line in *Thought Reform and the Psychology of Totalism,* goes on to say, "In all of this it is most important to realize that what we see as a set of *coercive maneuvers, the Chinese Communists view as a morally uplifting, harmonizing, and scientifically therapeutic experience.*"

Assuming, then, that the disease concept of homosexuality is a gross oversimplification that carries dangerous implications, are there, nonetheless, any connections at all between homosexuality and psychopathology? Yes, there are a number that we can group into two general categories: psychological and sociological.

Psychodynamic Explanations

The psychological factors are well covered in the psychoanalytic theory of homosexuality. Reaction-formation, or the defensive substitution of one feeling for another that is unbearable, can lead to homosexuality. For example, a boy may hate his father or brother

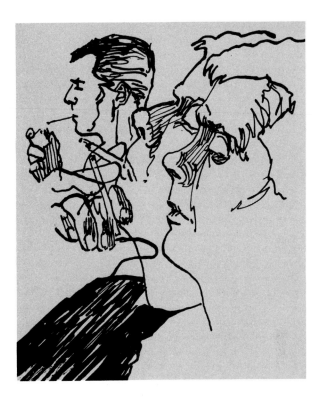

and also may be unable to express his hostility. So he changes hate into love by that substitutive magic that is the hallmark of defense mechanisms. If the love becomes sexualized, it may lead to a homosexual object-choice. Another explanation for homosexuality involves incorporative wishes toward the male, the penis, or masculinity. The homosexual may feel chronic emasculation. He may be able to achieve some sense of reparation only by taking the penis of his partner into his own body. In this way he thinks he has incorporated some of the imputed masculinity of the other man into his own deficient organism.

These psychodynamic explanations are very striking and highly appealing. I am sure they are true for a number of homosexual men. There exists no good evidence that they or any other psychoanalytic constructs explain all homosexual behavior. In fact, we do not know very much about the relation between sexual arousal and the symbolic triggers that act on the central nervous system, leading to the complex sets of behaviors that form the various stages or types of sexual arousal. Until we know about the mechanisms of sexual arousal in the central nervous system and how learning factors can set the triggering devices for these mechanisms, we cannot have a satisfactory theory of homosexual behavior.

We must point out that *heterosexual* behavior is as much of a scientific puzzle as homosexual behavior. Why, for example, is a particular man aroused by a large-bosomed brunette on a movie screen? Reflection reveals that we really do not have a satisfactory answer, and until we do we cannot answer analogous questions about homosexual arousal. We assume that heterosexual arousal is somehow natural and needs no explanation. I suggest that to call it natural and thereby to dismiss it is to evade the whole issue; it is as if we said it is natural for the sun to come up in the morning and left it at that. Is it possible that we know less about human sexuality than the medieval astrologers knew about the stars?

Psychoanalytic theories postulate that if an individual's sexuality is formed as described above, it must run a pathological course throughout his life, inasmuch as his sexual behavior is merely the acting out of unresolved childhood conflicts and problems. Such a viewpoint is attractive, for it seems to explain some very problematic homosexual behavior.

Promiscuity

One of the characteristics of homosexual interaction in the public places of the gay world—bars, beaches, parks, streets, and steam baths—is that sex is anonymous and promiscuous, not typically associated with affection or even, often, with identifiable individuals. John Rechy's novel *City of Night* describes such pick-up places and their way of life, as does my own book. Very often, in these places, one man is simply meeting or having sex with another of a certain physical type and does not want to know anything about his partner. Superficial acquaintanceships do spring from these meetings, and not infrequently the men repeat the sexual encounter. What is striking about these acquaintanceships, and even about many of the love affairs that last for several weeks to several months, is their shallowness. These people use each other in an instrumental, narcissistic way to gratify their own fantasies. Their partner is not really a lover, though he is often called by that label, but rather a necessary aid to acting out of the sexual (and nonsexual) fantasies that analysts believe originate in childhood. The man with a compulsion to fellate one individual after another until his conquests run into the hundreds may simply be vainly trying to replenish his masculinity. The two lovers who had had a stormy, tempestuous six-month relationship before one finally moves out may be acting out a sadomasochistic game in which the reaction-formation against hostility toward other males can be functional for only a time. During periods when it does not repress that hostility, there may be terribly long bouts of friction, punctuated by episodes of sexual activity.

Of course, such descriptions could easily fit many heterosexual couples; homosexuals have no monopoly on problematic relationships. But what is so striking about male homosexual alliances, in contrast to both heterosexual and female homosexual alliances, is their fragility, their tendency to be transitory, and the all-pervading promiscuity that characterizes the public places of gay life. Lesbians, who would perhaps be expected from a psychoanalytic point of view to have the same instability in their relationships, actually have much longer-lasting ones and do not in any way use public places for anonymous sexual contact, as homosexual men do. They do not cruise streets or parks and do not use lesbian bars—which are much less numerous—the way males use their gay bars. Lesbian bars are more like social clubs, where they go with their lovers to meet friends. Homosexual men also make some such use of bars, but cruising for an anonymous partner is specific to the male and not to the female homosexual.

Which ought to lead one to ask the so often unasked question: Just how much of male homosexual behavior can be explained by the fact—and this fact alone—that such relationships involve two *males*? The question at first sounds like a tautology, but I hope it will be seen that it is far from that. For I think it can be said that much of what seems to the observer as pathologic in male homosexual behavior is merely the result of having two men in a sexual situation. Most of what has been said, only partly in jest, about males being promiscuous by nature and females being the stable member of the heterosexual pair is true. Without the stabilizing female the dyad tends to break up. When two females interact, as in lesbian relationships, the dyad tends to be more stable.

Psychological Effects of Social Condemnation

I have saved for last what I regard as the most significant cause of unhappiness and psychopathology in the

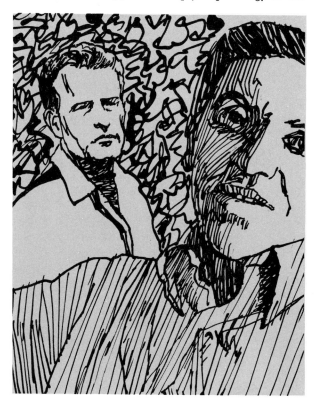

gay world: society's attitude toward homosexuality. I regard this as so significant both because social attitudes have been so little discussed in psychological writings on the subject and because they are, at least in theory, the most correctable and therefore the most pertinent for our immediate consideration.

Society has not only regarded the homosexual with the most abusive scorn; it has also preferred to think (until very recently) that homosexuality does not even exist, that is, is *unthinkable*—in spite of the fact that there are literally millions of Americans who are exclusively or predominantly homosexual. The ramifications of this attitude on the life of the homosexual are subtle and far reaching. A great deal of the anonymous promiscuity in the gay world can be understood only if we consider that the homosexual *cannot* be open about himself and his identity. His anonymity is forced upon him by the very society that, partly by means of the disease concept of homosexuality, condemns him for its consequences. His promiscuity results, in part, from the social attitudes that prevent him from living with another man in dignity and openness.

One of the critical ways that this pressure operates is by means of the social sanctions that would be visited upon the homosexual if his sexual orientation were known. The treatment accorded homosexuals by their employers, their acquaintances, their families, and by government agencies—especially the military—constitutes a continuing hidden scandal in the moral life of our nation. In a more subtle and terrible way, social condemnation acts directly on the homosexual's conception of himself. A well-known fact in the study of oppressed minorities is that they, tragically, adopt toward themselves the degrading view that the larger society has of them. The homosexual accepts this stigma. He views himself as queer, bad, dirty, something a little less than human. And he views his partner in the same way. Paul Goodman, describing some of his own homosexual encounters, says of some of his partners, "since they disapprove of what they are doing, they are not supposed to like the partner in it." How, then, can we expect them to have any kind of stable, meaningful relationship after the initial sexual thrill is over? (James Baldwin's novel *Giovanni's Room* describes what happens to a homosexual relationship as a result of such self-definitions.)

Self-condemnation pervades the homosexual world and, in concert with the psychodynamic and biological factors that lead toward promiscuity, makes stable relationships a terrible problem. In spite of the fact that so many homosexual men are lonely and alone, they cannot seem to find someone with whom to share even part of their lives. This dilemma is the core problem of the gay world and stems in large measure from the adverse self-definitions that society imprints on the homosexual mind. Until we can change these ancient attitudes, many men—including some of our own brothers, sons, friends, colleagues, and children yet unborn—will live out their lives in the quiet desperation of the sad gay world.

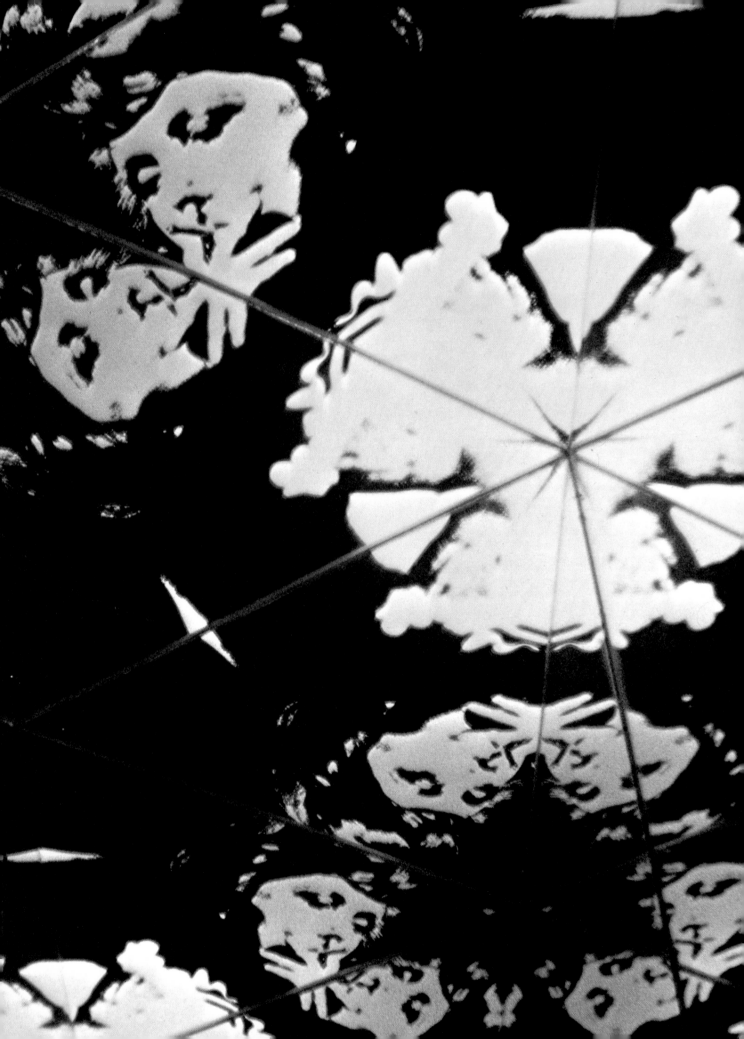

The Shattered Language of Schizophrenia

Brendan Maher

Definitional models of psychopathology are constantly and rapidly changing. Does a college student who doesn't know what to do with his life have an "existential neurosis"? Is it helpful to say that a juvenile offender has a "character disorder"? Is aggression a symptom or an action? Experts themselves may disagree sharply over whether to label a given behavior pattern "pathological."

In one area of psychopathology, however, the experts do usually reach unanimity, and that is in deciding whether someone should be called "schizophrenic." What does a schizophrenic person do that makes him so obviously different from any other person? He communicates oddly. His language, spoken or written, is so different that even untrained college students can detect the schizophrenic quality.

What precisely is this quality? And why are schizophrenic individuals unable to communicate in the ordinary way? Brendan Maher reviews the historical explanations for this bizarre use of language and bases his own account on the schizophrenic's difficulty in inhibiting associations and in maintaining attention. He offers the hypothesis that these difficulties are physiological in origin. In doing so, Maher reanimates the old question: Is there a relationship between genius and madness? Here the tentative answer is "yes."

Somewhere in a hospital ward a patient writes:

"The subterfuge and the mistaken planned substitutions for that demanded American action can produce nothing but the general results of negative contention and the impractical results of careless applications, the natural results of misplacement, of mistaken purpose and unrighteous position, the impractical serviceabilities of unnecessary contradictions. For answers to this dilemma, consult Webster."

The document is never sent to anyone; it is addressed to no one: and perhaps intended for no reader.

Another patient, miles away, writes:

"I am of I-Building in B . . State Hospital. With my nostrils clogged and Winter here, I chanced to be reading the magazine that Mentholatum advertised from. Kindly send it to me at the hospital. Send it to me Joseph Nemo in care of Joseph Nemo and me who answers by the name of Joseph Nemo and will care for it myself. Thanks everlasting and Merry New Year to Mentholatum Company for my nose for my nose for my nose for my nose for my nose."

A British patient writes:

"I hope to be home soon, very soon. I fancy chocolate eclairs, chocolate eclairs, Doenuts. I want some doenuts, I do want some golden syrup, a tin of golden syrup or treacle, jam . . . See the Committee about me coming home for Easter my twenty-fourth birthday. I hope all is well at home, how is Father getting on. Never mind there is hope, heaven will come, time heals all wounds, Rise again Glorious Greece and come to Hindoo Heavens, the Indian Heavens, The Dear old times will come back. We shall see Heaven and Glory yet, come everlasting life. I want a new writing pad of note paper . . ."

Yet another writes:

"Now to eat if one cannot the other can—and if we cant the girseau Q.C. Washpots prizebloom capacities—turning out—replaced by the head patterns my own capacities—I was not very kind to them. Q.C. Washpots under-patterned against—bred to pattern. Animal sequestration capacities and animal sequestired capacities under leash—and animal secretions . . ."

Experienced clinicians, when called upon to diagnose the writers of language like this, agree closely with each other (80 percent of the time or more). The diagnosis: schizophrenia. Nearly every textbook on psychopathology presents similar examples, and nobody seems to have much difficulty in finding appropriate samples. It would seem obvious that there must be a well-established and explicit definition of what characteristics language must possess to be called schizophrenic. But when we ask clinicians to tell us exactly what specific features of an individual language sample led them to decide that the writer was schizophrenic, it turns out that they aren't exactly sure. Instead of explicit description, the expert comment is likely to be: "It has that schizophrenic flavor," or "It is the confusion of thought that convinces me."

Impressionistic descriptions abound. The language is described as *circumlocutious, repetitive, incoherent,* suffering from an *interpenetration of ideas, excessively concrete, regressed,* and the like. Doubtless, all of these descriptions have merit as clinical characterizations of the language. Unfortunately, they are quite imprecise, and they give us no adequate basis for developing theoretical accounts of the origin of schizophrenic language. This is, of course, hardly surprising. Quantitative studies of language have been notoriously laborious to undertake. However, two recent developments in behavioral sciences have combined to change the situation quite significantly. The first of these is the development of language-analysis programs for computer use, and the second is the increasing sophistication of psycholinguistics as a framework for the study of applied problems in the psychology of language.

The Cipher Hypothesis

Before turning to look at the consequences of these developments, we should glance at the kinds of hypotheses that have already been advanced to account for schizophrenic language. The first of these might be termed the *cipher hypothesis.* In its simplest form this says that the patient is trying to communicate something to a listener (actual or potential) but is afraid to say what he means in plain language. He is somewhat in the same straits as the normal individual faced with the problem of conveying, let us say, some very bad news to a listener. Rather than come right out and tell someone directly that a family member is dying, the informant may become circumlocutious and perhaps so oblique that his message simply does not make sense at all.

In the case of the schizophrenic patient, however, it is assumed that the motives that drive him to disguise his message may be largely unconscious—that he could not put the message into plain language if he tried. Where the normal person is trying to spare the feelings of the listener by his distortions and evasions, the patient purportedly is sparing his own feelings by the use of similar techniques. This analogy can be stretched

a little further. Just as the normal speaker is caught in a dilemma—the necessity to convey the message and the pressure to avoid conveying it too roughly—so the patient is caught in a conflict between the necessity of expressing himself on important personal topics and the imperative need to avoid being aware of his own real meanings. Thus, so the cipher hypothesis maintains, it is possible in principle to decipher the patient's message —provided one can crack the code. This hypothesis assumes, of course, that there really is a message.

Obviously, the cipher hypothesis owes its genesis to psychoanalytic theory. In essence, it is identical with Freud's interpretation of the relationship between manifest and latent dream content. Unfortunately, from a research point of view, this hypothesis suffers from the weakness of being very hard to disprove. No two patients are assumed to have the same code, and so the translation of schizophrenic language into a normal communication requires a detailed analysis of the case history of the individual writer. As the code that is discovered for any one case cannot be validated against any other case, the hypothesis rests its claim to acceptance upon its intrinsic plausibility vis-à-vis the facts of the life history of the patient. But plausible interpretations of a patient's language may reflect the creative (or empathetic) imagination of the clinician rather than a valid discovery of an underlying process governing the patient's utterances.

One more or less necessary deduction from the cipher hypothesis is that language should become most disorganized when the topic under discussion is one of personal significance and less disorganized when the topic is neutral. To date, no adequate test of this deduction has been reported. In the absence of this or other independent tests of the cipher hypothesis, it must be regarded for the time being as, at best, an interesting speculation.

The Avoidance Hypothesis

A second explanation has been that the patient's communications are confusing and garbled precisely because he wishes to *avoid* communicating with other people. This hypothesis, which we shall call the *avoidance hypothesis,* interprets the disordered language as a response that is maintained and strengthened by its effectiveness in keeping other people away. Presumably, the normal listener becomes frustrated or bored with such a speaker and simply goes away, leaving the schizophrenic in the solitude he seeks. This theory rests, in turn, upon the assumption that the patient finds personal interactions threatening. We might expect that casual interactions—such as chatting about the weather—are relatively unthreatening and do not provoke avoidant disorder in language. The language disturbance should become more evident when the threat of personal involvement arises.

At this level, the avoidance hypothesis cannot be distinguished from the cipher hypothesis. The main difference between the two is that the avoidance hypothesis is concerned with a *dimension* of incomprehensibility and does not imply that the incomprehensible can be unscrambled. Both of these hypotheses have their attractions.

"For answers to this dilemma, consult Webster," wrote the first patient we have quoted. Is he just playing a word game with an imaginary reader or is there a meaning to his message? We might remark on the similarity of the prefix in many of the words he uses: *subterfuge, substitution; unrighteous, unnecessary; mistaken, misplacement; contention, contradiction.* His message might, indeed, sound like a random sampling from a dictionary.

Or did the dictionarylike nature of the "message" only occur to the patient himself toward the end—and hence the closing remark? In any event, the sample seems to fit plausibly into the notion that some kind of enciphering was going on between the patient's basic "message" and the language that he wrote.

Our fourth sample of schizophrenic language, on the other hand, seems to be absolutely incomprehensible. Fragments of phrases, neologisms (*girseau*) and repetitions—*sequestration* and *sequestired*—combine into a jumble that seems to defy understanding. It is hard to believe that there might be a message in disguise here, or even that the language was uttered with any wish to communicate.

Although both hypotheses can be made to seem plausible, they are intrinsically unsatisfying to the psychopathologist. They do not deal with the most fascinating problem of schizophrenic language: why does a particular patient utter the particular words that he does rather than some other jumbled-up sequence?

Interfering Associations

Some beginnings of an answer to this question have begun to emerge. Years ago, Eugen Bleuler commented on the presence of *interfering associations* in schizophrenic language. He suggested that the difficulty for the patient was that ideas associated with the content of his message somehow intruded into the message and thus distorted it. A patient of his, whom he had seen walking around the hospital grounds with her father and son, was asked who her visitors were. "The father, son, and Holy Ghost," she replied. These words have a strong mutual association as a single phrase, and although the last item, "Holy Ghost," was probably not meant as part of her message, it intruded because of its strong associative links with other units in the message.

Bleuler also noticed the difficulty that patients seemed to have in *understanding* a pun, despite their tendency to talk in punning fashion. A patient asked about her relationships with people at home says, "I have many ties with my home! My father wears them

around his collar." The pun on the word *tie* was unintentional, hence humorless.

Against the background of this general hypothesis of interfering associations, my students and I began investigations of schizophrenic language some years ago in Harvard's Laboratory of Social Relations. Our first concern was with the original question of definition. What must language contain to be labeled schizophrenic? Our work began with a plea to over 200 hospitals for examples of patients' writings—whether the patients were schizophrenic or not. Colleague response was rather overwhelming, and we amassed a very large number of letters, documents, diaries, and simple messages written in almost every state of the Union. (Many of these were inappropriate to our purposes. A carton of documents in Spanish from a Texas hospital, some brief obscenities scribbled on matchcovers and dropped daily onto the desk of a colleague in a St. Louis hospital, and other similar items were eliminated, of course.)

From this mass, we selected a set of documents that were legible, long enough to include several consecutive sentences—and written in English. These texts were then read by a panel of clinicians. Each text was judged independently and then was classified as *schizophrenic language* or *normal language*. (We obtained typical interjudge agreements of around 80 percent.) At this juncture we did not know whether the writers of the letters had been diagnosed as schizophrenic or not. Our concern was with the characteristics of the language—and with the clinicians' reactions to it.

Our two sets of texts then were submitted for computer analysis with the aid of the *General Inquirer* program. This program codes and categorizes language in terms of content and also provides a summary of grammatical features of the language. Out of this analysis, we developed some empirical rules (or a guide on how to write a document that a clinician will judge schizophrenic). Two of the most reliable rules were:

1. Write about politics, religion, or science. Letters dealing with global social issues of this kind are highly likely to be regarded as schizophrenic by clinicians.
2. Write more *objects* than *subjects* in sentences. Typical sentences consist of enumerations of classes of objects in a form illustrated in our second and third examples above: "Send it to me, Joseph Nemo, in care of Joseph Nemo and me who answers by the name of Joseph Nemo"; or "I fancy chocolate eclairs, chocolate eclairs, doenuts." Or in chains of associations at the end of a sentence. When, for example, a woman patient writes: "I like coffee, cream, cows, Elizabeth Taylor," the associational links between each word and the one following seem obvious.

This kind of associative chaining already had been described clinically by Bleuler; hence it was hardly surprising that the computer should find it to be a reliable discriminator in our document samples. What began to interest us, however, was the fact that these associations interfere most readily at the end of a sentence. Why not chains of subjects or chains of verbs, and why not at the beginning or middle of a sentence? Furthermore, why is this kind of interference found clearly in some schizophrenic patients and yet never occurs at all in others?

Disruption of Attention

For some time it has become increasingly apparent that, in schizophrenia, *attention* is greatly disrupted. It is hard for a patient to remain focused on any one stimulus for any length of time. He is unable to "tune out" or ignore other surrounding stimuli. These distract him; they enter consciousness at full strength and not in an attenuated fashion as they do with the normal person. Reports by the patients themselves make the point dramatically:

"Things are coming in too fast. I lose my grip of it and get lost. I am attending to everything at once and as a result I do not really attend to anything."

"Everything seems to grip my attention, although I am not particularly interested in anything. I am speaking to you just now but I can hear noises going on next door and in the corridor. I find it difficult to concentrate on what I am saying to you."

"I cannot seem to think or even put any plans together. I cannot see the picture. I get the book out and read the story but the activities and the story all just do not jar me into action."

Experimental tasks that require close attention, tasks that call for fast reactions to sudden stimuli, or any continuous monitoring of a changing stimulus field are almost invariably done poorly by schizophrenics. Sorting tasks, where the subject must organize objects or words into conceptual groups, are progressively more difficult for the schizophrenic if irrelevant or puzzling factors appear in the material.

We may regard the focusing of attention as a process whereby we effectively inhibit attention to everything but certain relevant stimuli in the environment. As attention lapses, we find ourselves being aware of various irrelevant stimuli—the inhibitory mechanism has failed temporarily.

It is possible that an analogous set of events takes place when we produce a complex sequence of language. Attention may be greater or lesser at some points in a language sequence than at others. The end of a sentence—the period point—may be particularly vulnerable to momentary attentional lapses: one thought has been successfully completed, but the next one may not yet have been formed into utterable shape. Within a single sentence itself, there may be other points of comparative vulnerability, though not perhaps as marked as at the sentence ending.

Uttering a sentence without disruption is an extremely skilled performance but one that most of us acquire so early in life that we are unaware of its remarkable complexity. (However, we become more aware of how difficult it is to "make sense" when we are extremely tired, or ripped out of sleep by the telephone, or distraught, or drunk.)

Single words have strong associational bonds with other words—as the classic technique of word association indicates. We know that the word "black" will elicit the response "white" almost instantaneously from the majority of people. The associational bond between black and white is clearly very strong. Strong as it is, it will not be allowed to dominate consciousness when one is uttering a sentence such as "I am thinking about buying a black car." Our successful sentences come from the successful, sequential inhibition of all interfering associations that individual words in the sentence might generate. Just as successful visual attention involves tuning out irrelevant visual material, so successful utterance may involve tuning out irrelevant verbal static.

By the same token, disordered attention should lead to an increasing likelihood that this kind of interference will not be inhibited but will actually intrude into language utterance. Its most probable point of intrusion is wherever attention is normally lowest.

| PUNS | "Portmanteau" words or puns provide unusually good occasions for disruptive intrusions. Consider, for example, the word "stock." This word has several possible meanings, each of them with its own set of associations. Financial associations might be *Wall Street, bonds, dividend,* and the like. Agricultural associations might include *cattle, barn,* and *farm;* theatrical associations might be *summer, company,* and the like. Webster's Third International Dictionary gives forty-two different definitions of the word *stock,* many of them archaic or unusual but many of them common. If one set of meanings intrudes into a sentence that is clearly built around another set of meanings, the effect is a pun, and an accompanying digression or cross-current in surface content. The sentences—"I have many ties with my home. My father wears them around his collar"—seem to skip, like a stone on a lake, from *ties* (bonds) to *home* to *father* to *ties* (neckties). On the surface, this is a witty statement, but the speaker had no idea of what was really going on inside or underneath the form of words. The statement was therefore unwitting and hence unwitty.

Loren Chapman and his associates, in work at Southern Illinois University, demonstrated that schizophrenics as a group are more open to interference from the most common meaning of a punning word. When we use a word like *stock* as a stimulus for word association, we discover that most normal respondents give financial associations first and may find it difficult to respond when asked to "give associations to another meaning." Associations to the other meaning are weaker or less prepotent and only emerge under special instructional sets. Chapman's work suggests that if the plan of a sentence calls for the use of a weaker meaning, the schizophrenic runs some risk that associational intrusions will interfere and actually produce a punning effect.

On the other hand, if the plan of a sentence involves the stronger meaning, then there may be no intrusion of associations. And if associations do intrude, these intrusions will appear relevant to the sentence and will not strike the listener as strange. Which meanings will be strong or weak will depend to some extent upon the culture from which the patient comes. (Personal experience may, of course, produce uniquely strong or weak associations in individual cases.) However, Chapman was able to predict correctly the direction of errors for schizophrenic patients as a group on the basis of estimates of strength obtained from normal respondents. Thus, some patients may have personal idiosyncrasies, but the associations that interrupt the schizophrenic are generally the same as those that are strong for the population at large.

A parallel investigation I conducted at the University of Copenhagen included a study of the language of Danish schizophrenics. I observed the same general effect: patients were liable to interference from strong meanings of double-meaning words. English is a language that is unusually rich in puns, homonyms, cognates, and indeed a whole lexicon of verbal trickery. But it seems plausible to suppose that in any language in which double-meaning words are to be found, this kind of schizophrenic disturbance may be found.

From these observations we can begin to piece together a picture of what happens when schizophrenic intrusions occur in a sentence that started out more or less normally. Where a punning word occurs at a vulnerable point, the sequence becomes disrupted and rapidly disintegrates into associative chaining until it terminates (see Figure 1).

We may look at schizophrenic utterances as the end result of a combination of two factors: the vulnerability of sentence structure to attentional lapses and the inability of patients to inhibit associational intrusions, particularly at these lapse points. From this point of view, the problem of language is directly related to the other attentional difficulties that the schizophrenic has; he is handicapped in making language work clearly, just as he is at any other task that requires sustained attention. The emotional significance of what the schizophrenic plans to say may have little or no bearing on when an intrusion occurs, or what it seems to mean. Any sentence with vulnerable points in its syntactic or semantic structure may result in confusion, whether the topic is of great psychological importance or has to do with a patient's harmless liking for chocolate eclairs and doughnuts.

Serious and sustained difficulties in the maintenance of attention suggest a biological defect. Peter Venables at the University of London has suggested swimming or unfocusable attention in schizophrenia may be connected with low thresholds of physiological arousal—stimuli can be very weak and yet trigger strong physiological reactions. This low arousal threshold is found mostly in acute, rather than chronic, schizophrenia.

Evidence from studies of a variety of attentional tasks supports this interpretation. Additional and intriguing evidence was obtained by one of my students, Dr. Joy Rice at the University of Wisconsin. Using electrochemical (galvanic) changes in the skin as a measure, she found that schizophrenic patients who were most responsive to noise stimulation were also the patients who showed the most difficulty in dealing with the meaning of punning sentences. The magnitude of galvanic skin response to external stimulation is presumably greatest in patients with low initial arousal levels (and hence the most receptivity to external stimulation). Rice's data may therefore support the notion that verbal associational interference is part and parcel of a total syndrome, of which biological control of attention is a crucial central focus.

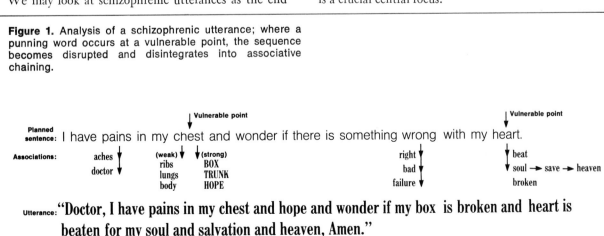

Figure 1. Analysis of a schizophrenic utterance; where a punning word occurs at a vulnerable point, the sequence becomes disrupted and disintegrates into associative chaining.

Planned sentence: I have pains in my chest and wonder if there is something wrong with my heart.

Associations:

aches	(weak)	(strong)	right	beat
doctor	ribs	BOX	bad	soul → save → heaven
	lungs	TRUNK	failure	broken
	body	HOPE		

Utterance: "Doctor, I have pains in my chest and hope and wonder if my box is broken and heart is beaten for my soul and salvation and heaven, Amen."

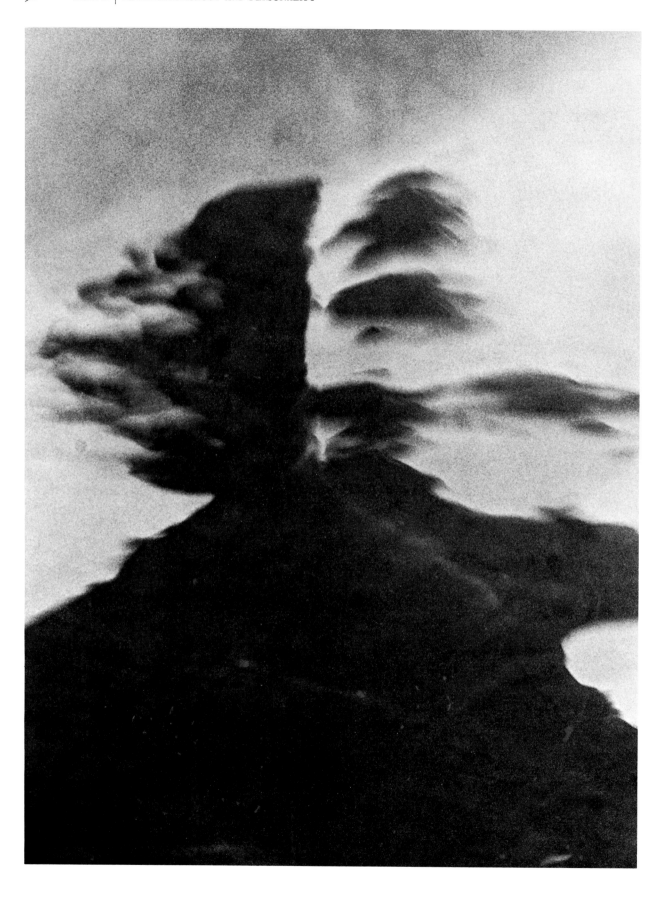

Art and Madness

Recent research into the effects of LSD has shown that it is people with low initial arousal systems who have the "good trips"; the most cursory glance at literary biography will reveal an extraordinary number of poets and writers who were "sensitive," "neurasthenic," and so on. Which leads me to a sort of Parthian speculation.

Look again at the four samples quoted in the beginning of this article. What you see there, I think, is the literary imagination gone mad, if I may use so unclinical a term here. The first sample, had it come from the pen of someone whose brain we trusted, might almost be a crude parody of ponderous political tracts of socio-economo-political gobbledygook of one sort or another. In the second, the fragment, "With my nostrils clogged and Winter here," is really not bad, and one wouldn't be terribly surprised to find it occurring in, say, the *Cantos* of Ezra Pound. In the third quotation, there are unmistakable echoes from the New Testament, Lord Byron, and Ralph Waldo Emerson, or rather echoes from an entire chamber of the literary heritage. The kind of wordplay indulged in throughout the fourth quote is not essentially different technically from that employed by the later James Joyce, or by the John Lennon of *In his own write*.

What is lacking from these samples, so far as we can tell, is context and control and the critical, or pattern-imposing, intelligence. It would seem, therefore, that the mental substrata in which certain kinds of poetry are born probably are associative in a more or less schizophrenic way. (In the case of poets like Dylan Thomas or Hart Crane, of course, these substrata had to be blasted open by liquor.) The intelligence that shapes, cuts, edits, revises, and erases is fed by many conscious sources, most of them cultural; but the wellsprings seem to be, as poets have been telling us for centuries, sort of divine and sort of mad.

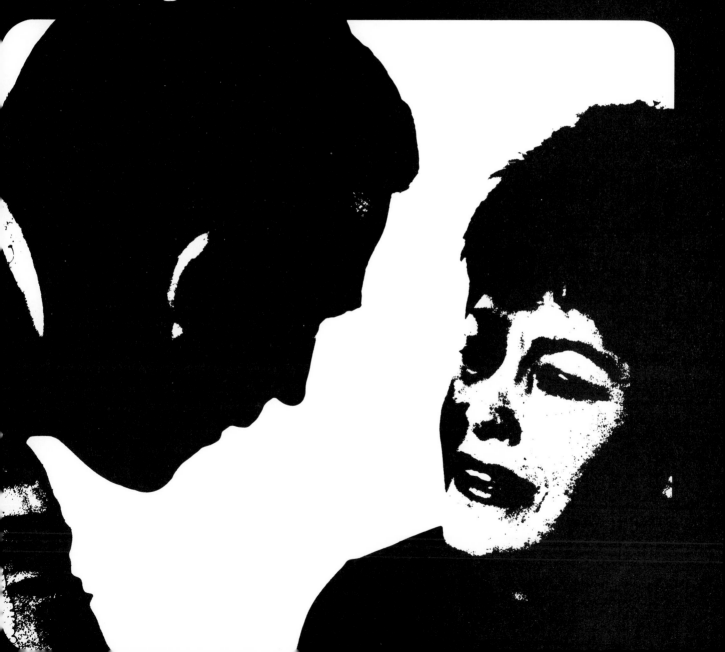

II
Psychotherapy and Behavioral Change–Research and Theories

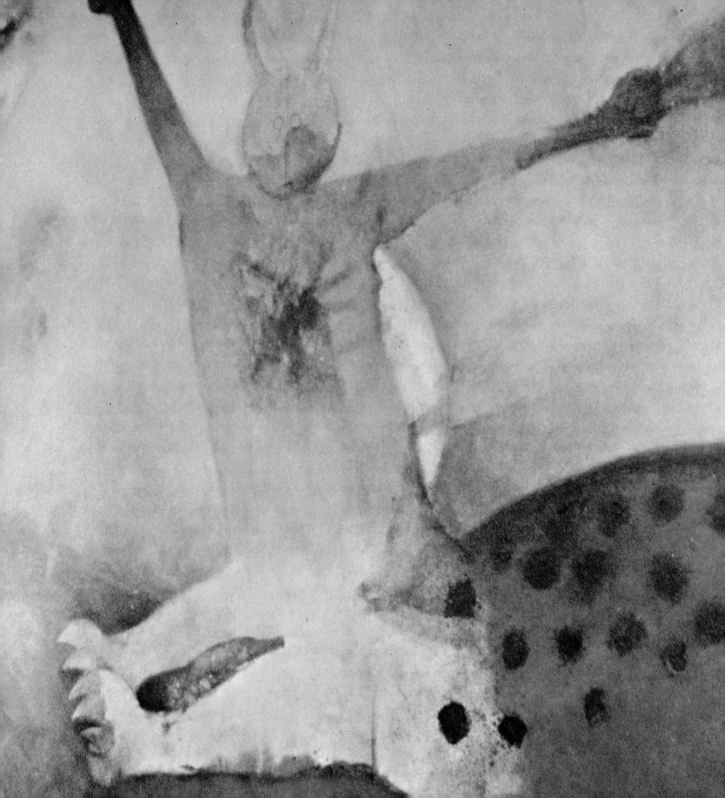

From Freud to Fromm

Jerome Brams

Freud is the founding architect of psychotherapy, and psychoanalysis is its anlage. Since Freud, subsequent systems of psychotherapy have formed themselves in one of two ways, either by directly repudiating or by selectively incorporating Freudian doctrines and techniques. The former is the way of behavior modification, advocated by Hans Eysenck in the following article, and of encounter group therapy, described by Frederick Stoller in a later selection. The latter includes those therapeutic approaches retaining remnants of classical psychoanalytical theory to the degree that they are often called neo-Freudian.

Erich Fromm is one of the most important and best known psychoanalysts in the neo-Freudian line. A dominant influence in the history of psychology for several decades, Fromm's ideas now form a viable school of psychotherapy. Jerome Brams here compares Fromm's theories and techniques with those of Freud. Fromm's views, he finds, are much less pessimistic. Fromm widens Freud's focus on sex and aggression into analyses of anxiety, alienation, and narcissism. The Frommian therapist is less historical, less enigmatic, and less passive than the Freudian.

For reasons varying from economic to theoretical, the psychoanalytic orientation is becoming more and more disfavored. The rapid proliferation of new treatment forms is a sign of this trend. Whether modifications such as Fromm's can revive Freudian psychotherapy remains to be seen.

Psychoanalysis. Say the word. Ask for a name, and the most usual response—after one names one's own analyst—is Freud. And then? Names like Jung, Adler, Sullivan, Horney, and Fromm come quickly to mind.

The genius and insights of Sigmund Freud into the nature of man have been recognized many times over and remain without parallel. His contributions in advancing an understanding into the unconscious forces that he viewed as the wellspring for all human motivation are the cornerstone on which all later psychoanalytic theories are based.

Since the 1940s, Erich Fromm has become more and more prominent on the lists of those with major influence in psychoanalysis, perhaps because his basic theme and penetrating study correspond closely to the mid-twentieth-century *Zeitgeist*: the alienated man. The theme is an existential one, and though Fromm himself would not approve being labeled as an existential psychoanalyst, his descriptions of man's dilemma and

modes of relating to the world have been borrowed and used by many who do describe themselves in this fashion.

Although also frequently classified as one leading proponent of the neo-Freudian school—along with Horney, Sullivan, and Kardiner—Fromm objects to this label as well, for he sees his work as an attempt to broaden the base of Freud's discoveries, not to change them, and as an effort to interpret them in terms of contemporary philosophical and sociological concepts.

Fromm is better described as the outstanding advocate of a humanistic approach in psychoanalysis and currently is writing a systematic presentation of his views.

The Psychology of Personality

When asked to compare the views of Freud and Fromm, many people see only a contrast between biological and cultural determinism. Freud is labeled a biological determinist, one who sees the motivated behavior of man as springing from his innate biological equipment, while Fromm is referred to as a cultural determinist, one who views man's motivation as determined by cultural influences.

Such an easy differentiation does both men an injustice. It ignores those areas in which there is more implied agreement than disagreement. Freud did not deny the importance of cultural influence on behavior, especially as a shaping and controlling agent over the aggressive and sexual instinctual drives that he saw as the two primary sources of human motivation. Nor has Fromm, more especially in his later writings, neglected the importance of constitutional factors in motivation and in the strength and intensity of the characteristic ways by which one orients one's self to the world.

However, Freud's observations on the unconscious motivating forces behind man's behavior lend themselves to a more pessimistic view of what it means to be human than Fromm's views do. (The orthodox Freudian psychoanalyst would sooner describe this as *realistic* than as *pessimistic*.) Freud saw man as driven by an unconscious pleasure principle to seek the reduction of tensions that emanate from the two basic instinctual drives, sexuality and aggression, which he classified more broadly as life instincts and death instincts. In his view, society is constructed on the renunciation of direct and immediate instinctual gratification, which results in inner conflict and neurotic behavior. Thus, the more repression demanded by society, the greater the incidence of neuroses among the populace. The motivational strength of these irrational instinctual forces, the development of inner controls against their breakthrough into conscious awareness, and the understanding of their role in the development of personality and neurosis are constant themes in Freud's work.

The idea of such motives as self-actualization, a will to meaning, and transcendence of the human condition—concepts that today find expression in the more humanistic and existential views of man—are not to be found in the writings of Freud. He was exceptionally impatient with such philosophical speculation. Freud saw all values, morality, love of any kind, art, justice, religion, indeed all that is part of the structure of civilization, as coming from the two basic drives. Yet in spite of his pessimism about the relative strength of man's rational and irrational qualities, Freud still held out the possibility that at some distant time, reason would play a more significant role in man's behavior.

Fromm does not disagree with Freud on the strength of unconscious irrational passions that can drive man to the brink of catastrophe, but he emphasizes the presence of human needs that spring from the existential conditions of man. He insists that man carries within himself potentialities for growth and for productiveness. Given the proper conditions in a culture and society, Fromm is optimistic in his conviction that the human

forces of reason and love will prevail. It is when Fromm views what the cultural influences have been and continue to be on man's human potentialities that a pessimistic tone appears.

He sees man as caught on the horns of a specifically human dilemma. On the one hand, man is an animal like all other animals in nature. On the other, he is a reasoning, self-aware, and imaginative creature. These latter characteristics preclude an automatic instinctive accommodation to nature that is available to other animals. The result is a feeling of disunity with nature, of loneliness and separateness. As Fromm sees it, man strives to escape these feelings by finding some other kind of unity with the world. He can do so in productive ways by developing his human capacities for reason and love to the fullest, or in regressive and nonproductive ways that lead to a constricted and neurotic relatedness both to the world and to himself.

In addition, Fromm sees in man the development of characteristic ways in which he acquires or assimilates what he needs from the world. Fromm has stressed in particular the influence of the economic and political structure of society on the development of these orientations, but he does not emphasize this aspect to the exclusion of constitutional and temperamental determinants.

He describes a number of nonproductive orientations (or character types), all of which he attempts to relate historically to the economic social structure prevalent at the time these character types first appeared.

The influence of our contemporary Western economic system is seen in what Fromm describes as the *marketing character*. This person experiences himself as a product to be marketed and shaped to bring about the greatest rewards. He views himself as an object to be manipulated, a commodity to be transformed to the demands of the marketplace. In the construction of this kind of nonrelatedness to the world, he loses any sense of his true self and is left with feelings of futility and emptiness.

Then there is the *receptive character*, who is basically passive and dependent upon being given things from the world outside. There is the *exploitative character*, who also sees everything that is good and nurturant as existing outside himself, but who uses force, manipulation, and guile instead of dependence to gain his ends. The *hoarding character* has little trust in the outside world and thus entrenches himself in what he considers a safe position by hoarding and saving—not only material items but such intangibles as love.

In his more recent writings, Fromm has introduced another nonproductive orientation, which he calls "necrophilous" (which he contrasts to "biophilous": life-loving). The *necrophilous* orientation is the most pathological of those he has described, for here there is a love of death, decay, and destruction. It is in the description of this orientation that Fromm seems to emphasize the presence of a significant constitutional component. Fromm points to the relationship between this conception and Freud's view of a death instinct.

Except for the marketing orientation, Fromm's descriptions of character are very similar to portions of those presented by Freud many years earlier. The receptive character is very much like Freud's description of the oral-passive type; the exploitative character is similar to Freud's oral-aggressive type; the hoarding character is like Freud's anal-retentive type; and the neocrophilous character is very similar to Freud's anal-sadistic type.

The difference between Freud and Fromm in their view of character types is, therefore, not so much on the basis of the clinical descriptions, but in how each views the causes for the development of a specific type. Freud sees character as coming primarily from fixations that result from traumatic experiences—deprivation or even overgratification—at various stages in the development of the sexual instinct. Thus, if such occurrences are experienced at the first oral stage of psychosexual development, then a fixation could result in an oral-passive character. At the later anal stage, then, an anal character would be the outcome. Fromm, on the other hand, emphasizes sociocultural factors in the determination of character.

Neither Freud nor Fromm neglects a description of the ideal adult character. Fromm labels this the productive character, and Freud's term is the genital character. Although referring primarily to the same traits, Fromm describes more richly a productively active, reasoning individual who relates truly to himself and to others and who is capable of realizing his human potentialities. Freud's emphasis is on heterosexual adjustment in the adult.

Both Freud and Fromm have pointed to the long dependency of the child on his mother and the role such dependency plays in his development, but they differ as to the important aspects of such dependency. Freud singled out the Oedipus complex as a momentous event in the life of the child, especially the male. The child desires to possess his mother sexually, but he fears his father's revenge (castration) for harboring such wishes. As a result of this complex, the child's sexual development is interrupted and remains latent from about the sixth to the twelfth year. Then, assuming the normal psychosexual development, hormonal changes accompanying puberty reawaken his sexuality and lead to an adult heterosexual orientation. The importance of the mother as the original love object of the child is stressed.

Fromm's emphasis goes beyond the sexual one. He stresses the importance of the burgeoning opportunities for growth and independence that the child encounters. If the threat of leaving behind the all-protective love of the mother is great and the child's experiences are constricting, then his development is stunted in that he regresses to a symbiotic-like dependency on the mother. Unless there is a push to greater independence, such a regressive orientation can result in an emotionally crippled adult who is not free and who remains dependent on any motherlike figure for nurturance. This dependence can be on authorities or on symbols of authority, such as "God" or "country." Fromm sees the child's sexual desire to possess the mother as a positive rather than a regressive sign, for in the wish is a sign of separateness from the mother and an attempt to assert one's independence and self-sufficiency.

Freud and Fromm differ in their conceptions of love. For Freud, all love stems from the sexual drive. He sees the love for friend, for parents, and for ideals as an inhibited expression of the basically sexual aim of love. Furthermore, he sees a basic incompatibility between love of others and love of one's self. He described a situation in which the individual possesses a limited fund of energy for love. The more narcissistic and self-loving the person, the less love remains for objects outside himself.

Fromm does not make this distinction between self and object in considering the capacity to love. He sees love as an expression of care and respect that cannot be divided between outside objects and one's self. In other words, we are incapable of loving others without also loving ourselves. Fromm's view of love is tied less narrowly to a sexual aim. He proposes a number of different kinds of love, only one of which has an erotic base. The capacity to love, he says, is as important in man as the capacity to reason, and only in the realization of these capacities does man become truly human.

It is now commonplace to refer to the current era as the "age of anxiety," and it is only a short step from a discussion of love to one on anxiety. Freud's theory of anxiety went through two stages. Initially, he saw anxiety as a transformation of sexual energy that is blocked in its aim of direct discharge. He later changed this view and explained anxiety as a warning signal of a potentially threatening situation. Such threat could come from the external environment—in which case it corresponds to what we call fear—or it could emanate from unconscious internal sources, such as the potential breakthrough of repressed material into consciousness.

Fromm's approach to anxiety is related to his view of man's separateness and aloneness. Each step away from the security of a regressive and dependent relationship is accompanied by anxiety.

How does a person learn to think and what is the nature of consciousness? The concept of the unconscious was known by philosophers and writers long before Freud, but it was he who gave us a systematic rendering of its contents and workings. In his distinction between conscious and unconscious, he described two types of thought processes: primary process thought, found in the unconscious; and secondary process thought, a function of consciousness. He has described primary process thought as unconscious, illogical, symbolic, and as present from infancy. The only reality for this primary thought process is the inner, unconscious one. Psychotic thought, dream thought, and the symbolic thought of the artist are all examples of primary process thought. On the other hand, secondary process thought is logical and coherent and attuned to outer reality. It develops from the necessity of dealing with the outside world in order to attain need satisfaction.

Fromm has not yet detailed his conceptions of various thought processes, but he has emphasized cultural influences in his view of a social filter that both acts upon the development of the capacity to think and distorts the content of thought to fit the values of the culture. In his view, the productive person is a critical thinker who can transcend the limiting effects of socially determined thought. Fromm also is reluctant to equate an artistic thought process with a psychotic one.

Some of the more orthodox Freudian theorists also have been reluctant here, and one, Ernst Kris, proposed the view that although artistic thought is of a regressive, primary process type, it nevertheless can be viewed as serving the individual in a creative and reality-oriented manner.

Freud's emphasis on understanding the dream relates to its latent content (the true meaning of the dream), not to its manifest content (the dream as related by the dreamer). The latent dream content is distorted by various primary process mechanisms in its transmission from the unconscious to the dreamer's awareness. Freud saw the interpretation of dreams as the most direct access to the contents of the unconscious. When the latent dream content finally emerges via the analytic process, it is seen to be an attempted fulfillment of some repressed wish relating to the formative stages of personality development.

Fromm also emphasizes the importance of understanding the unconscious through the dream, but his attention is directed more narrowly to the manifest dream content. For him, this content communicates an unconscious message in symbolic language, and the understanding of this language makes the message clear. In addition, he does not view all dreams as based on repressed childhood wishes.

Both men agree on the presence of universal symbols of dreams, but while Fromm might interpret such a symbol directly to the patient, Freud would have been hesitant to do so. Freud pointed to the necessity for the dreamer to associate to each portion of his manifest dream—no matter how inconsequential—in order to arrive at its latent content. Fromm does not neglect the importance of such associations, especially for those parts of the dream containing accidental symbols—in which meaning is found only in relationship to the dreamer's personal life experiences.

Psychotherapy

Psychoanalysis refers to a psychology of personality, to a research tool for the investigation of human behavior, and, finally, to a psychotherapeutic method. The term is most usually used in the last sense. (One oftentimes finds surprise among people who are being analyzed when they are faced with the fact that there exist other approaches to psychotherapy besides the analytic one.) The preceding sections have been concerned with some of the psychological, rather than psychotherapeutic, views of Freud and Fromm. In going on to describe their respective approaches in therapy, we are limited by the fact that as yet Fromm has said little publicly on this topic.

Freud indicated several goals for the person under psychoanalysis, and each of these is based on different ways of viewing the personality system, but he was not optimistic about their attainment. Most broadly stated, the primary goal in psychoanalysis is to help the patient resolve the unconscious conflicts relating to his early childhood experiences, which, as Freud viewed it, are the most significant causes for the adult neurosis. To accomplish this, it is necessary to bring into consciousness as much unconscious material as possible. Freud also saw psychoanalysis as a method whereby the energy in the various structural systems of the personality is balanced so that the reasoning, reality-oriented faculties are enhanced. He was quite aware of the dangers of an interminable analysis and warned about this.

Fromm's primary goal for his patient can be put into his more general humanistic perspective: to help the person realize to the fullest degree possible his human and individual potentialities for productive relatedness to the world, for self-awareness, for reason, and for love. For Fromm, as it was for Freud, the curative effect is based on bringing into awareness the unconscious forces that have molded and continue to direct the patient's behavior. (It is for this reason that Fromm considers himself a follower of Freud, and not the founder of a different "school" of psychoanalysis.)

The major difference between Freud and Fromm here lies only in what is considered to be the main area of repression. In the earlier phase of Freud's theory, repression was found to operate primarily in the area of sexual instincts; in the later phase, he emphasized the importance of repressed aggression. Fromm does not give a central role to the repression of sexual desires and believes the repression of various types of aggressiveness to be more important. But, going far beyond that, he believes that anxiety, aloneness, alienation, and narcissism are among the most significant areas of repression.

It should be added that for Fromm the main problem is the person's total response to the question of human existence, which each one has to answer by the very fact of having been born. The answer is not essentially one of ideas but one of character: everyone wants to make some sense out of his life, in fact, to "make the best of it." But there are better and worse forms of responding to the problems of existence. The better ones increase energy and vitality and make for a person's sense of unity. The worse ones create anxiety, insecurity, submission, and sadism, and cause suffering. Symptoms are signs of the contradiction between optimal or ideal character structures and the particular form of character that a person has adopted, under the influence of constitution, early upbringing, social structure, and accidental experiences. Fromm holds that awareness of one's inner reality is a crucial factor in change, together with the effort to practice a different kind of life.

What are the characteristics of the patient most likely to benefit from psychoanalysis? Freud believes that there must be good capacity for reality-contact in the prospective patient, especially in those areas in which his neurosis should not limit his perceptions. Thus he does not see psychoanalysis as the treatment of choice for a psychotic disorder. Both Freud and Fromm see traumatic experiences in the patient's past life as a good sign. Without such indications there is greater likelihood that constitutional factors are operating in the development of the neurosis, and such factors are not greatly amenable to change through psychoanalytic treatment.

Fromm also has pointed to the need for what he terms a "vitality" in the prospective patient. He sees this as indicating an energy oriented toward growth and life, love of life as opposed to a hate of or indifference to life. He means more than simply a high energy level, for he points out that destructive people also can be viewed as possessing a great amount of energy. Finally, Fromm and Freud—as well as analysts of all persuasions—are interested in gauging the underlying seriousness and intensity of the patient's motivation for analysis. Without strong motivation, there is little hope that the patient will stay on to work through anxieties as they emerge in his analysis.

Both Freud and Fromm have emphasized the importance of understanding the patient's childhood history, but Fromm does not appear to dwell as long on this stage of the patient's life in the analysis as do those who follow the more orthodox Freudian approach. The past is used to help in the understanding of the patient's present behavior and as an aid in uncovering the unconscious resistances to the analysis. Freudians might object that this is their emphasis as well. But in practice, too often their approach leads to a minute and overly intellectualized investigation of childhood experiences, particularly those relating to psychosexual development.

Freud emphasizes a continual focus on the patient's conscious and unconscious resistances to the aims of the analysis. The analysis must become an integral, ongoing part of the patient's life, and the orthodox Freudian analyst generally sees his patient for no less than one hourly session each day, five days a week. To attempt an analysis on a less frequent basis is seen as only complicating the problems of dealing with the patient's resistance. Depending upon the defenses and repressions of a particular patient, an orthodox analysis can continue for five or six years or even longer.

Fromm's view on the frequency of visits corresponds with those who generally are considered to be neo-Freudian: a successful analysis is possible in as few as three sessions—for some patients, even two sessions—each week. What matters for Fromm is not the number of hours but the aliveness or intensity of each session and the kind and degree of the patient's resistance. However, like Freud, Fromm has expressed doubts as to how many people really can be analyzed "successfully." Since the patient is seen less frequently, Fromm's approach emphasizes—as does that of Harry Stack Sullivan—the active participation of the analyst in the therapeutic process.

Free association is the tool on which Freud bases his approach to treatment. The patient is instructed to say everything that comes into his mind without withholding, judging, or distorting the content. A second tool in the orthodox Freudian approach is the use of the transference relationship to gain an understanding of the patient's unconscious processes. Freud describes transference as a process in which the patient projects onto the analyst a complex of conscious and unconscious feelings that existed for significant figures—usually his parents—in his past life. Freud found that the best condition for the development of transference and for free association was to have the patient lie on a couch while the analyst sat in a chair behind him. In this arrangement, the analyst's presence interferes less with the free associations of the patient and enhances the development of the transference.

The approach suggested by Fromm—and by most neo-Freudians—is to have the patient sit in a chair while the analyst sits across from him. This face-to-face confrontation is maintained throughout the analysis and enables the analyst to attend directly to nonverbal cues such as body movements, which are seen as important aids in understanding the patient's unconscious. Fromm does not believe that this arrangement interferes with the development of a transference relationship. He points out that important elements of transference emerge even before the patient sees the analyst, for, in his fantasies about what kind of person the analyst will be, the patient already has begun to project transference elements.

Besides transference, Fromm also emphasizes another aspect of the relationship between therapist and patient: the reality factor of two separate individuals reacting to each other. He stresses that the analyst should not disregard this aspect of the relationship. In other words, he does not agree that every feeling of the patient for his analyst necessarily is based on transference. Fromm, too, wants the patient to express his uncensored thoughts and feelings. But he is concerned that free association should not deteriorate into "free chatter," and he interrupts the patient when this happens. He also actively suggests the patient associate to problems Fromm considers relevant, based on the analysis. Fromm believes it is important to tell the patient what unconscious trends he detects; then the focus is turned to an analysis of the patient's response. Fromm

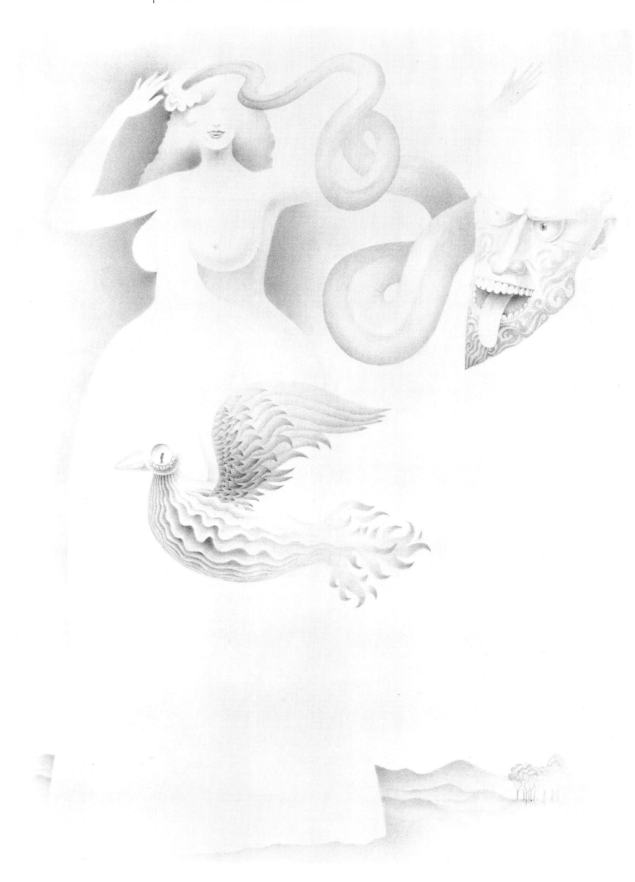

is much more active than the Freudian analyst, not in the sense of offering the patient advice about the "right" way of acting, but in his insistence on the production of unconscious material and on the analysis of resistance.

The Freudian approach, especially early in the analysis, is to remain silent, allowing the patient uninterrupted reign with free association. The analyst neither comments nor interprets. He does not respond to complaints that he is doing nothing, saying nothing, being of little help. It is only at a later stage that the analyst becomes more active in making interpretations based on his observations of the patient's transference, associations, and dreams.

In Fromm's view, the patient-therapist interaction is the primary tool that furthers the work of analysis. He emphasizes the urgency that the patient must feel about his manner of relatedness to the world if there is any possibility for productive change. He sees the analyst as a sensitive and trained instrument who uses his full self—both reasoning and affective—in the analytic interaction. As Fromm sees it, for the analyst to sit back making unverbalized theoretical constructions to himself about the nature of the patient's problems without a continual active participation in the analysis leads only to an intellectualized and nonproductive experience that can drag on for years. Freudians criticize this active involvement from the very beginning of the analysis as an almost naive approach to an understanding of the nature and forms of unconscious resistance. Indeed, some liken this approach to an exhortation that can have no real effect on unconscious material.

Finally, we can say that Freud's theories were presented in a highly systematized and rigorous manner, whereas Fromm's writings exhibit a less exacting and less exhaustive presentation. Some account for this by saying that Freud was primarily the psychologist, while Fromm is more the social philosopher. But because of his broad social views, Fromm's concepts are of interest not only to psychoanalysts but to people of many persuasions in the social sciences and in the humanities. Whether Fromm's views can equal the rigorous nature of those found in Freud awaits his more formal, systematized presentation of humanistic psychoanalysis.

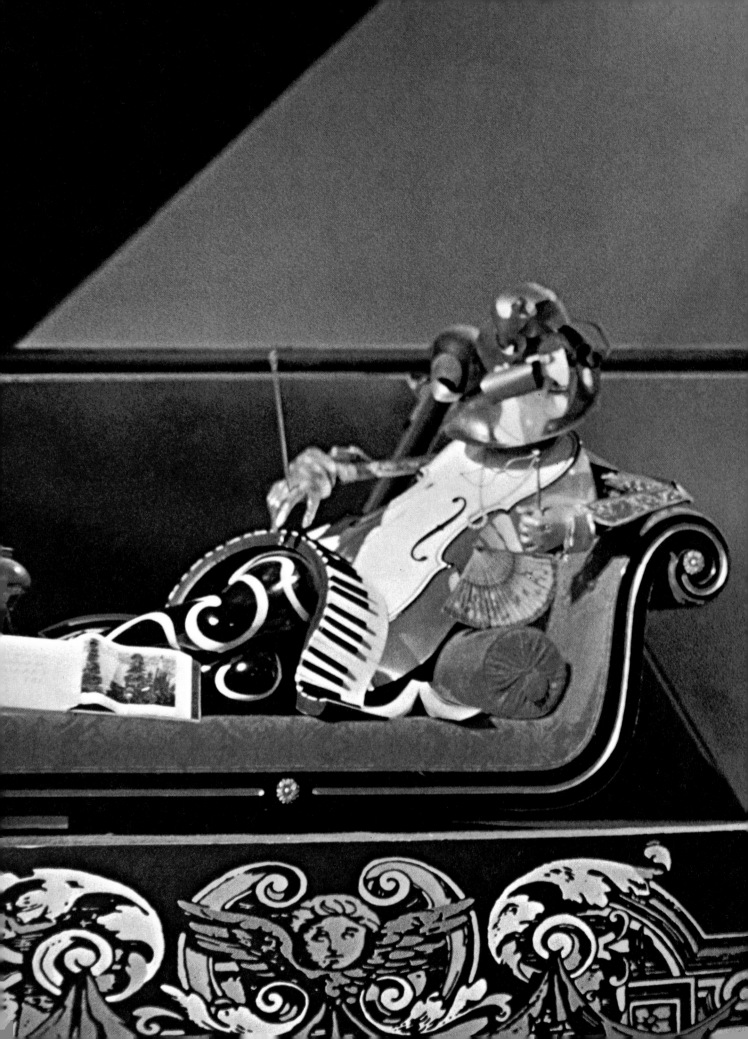

New Ways in Psychotherapy

Hans J. Eysenck

Behavior therapy has sprung from a disenchantment with the predicates and results of traditional psychotherapy, especially psychoanalysis. Its principles and concepts are derived from laboratory observations of animals rather than from assumptions about internal processes. The importance of reward and punishment is stressed. Symptoms are seen as significant in themselves rather than as expressions of internal conflict. Symptom removal is to be achieved, not avoided.

Hans Eysenck outlines the history and current status of one major kind of behavior modification: Wolpe's systematic desensitization. He also covers, though less thoroughly, aversion therapy and operant conditioning. His discussion mirrors the dispute between clinicians and experimentalists. In his opinion, the clinician who works with a behavior therapy approach can attain scientific rigor and, thereby, respectability.

To be sure, Eysenck's viewpoints are hotly debatable, having been questioned by both experimental and clinical psychologists. Nevertheless, behavior therapy, with increasing diversity and sophistication, speedily continues its gain in popularity.

For the past fifty years neurotic disorders have been viewed almost exclusively in the light of Freudian theory. Very briefly, this theory states that neurosis originates in early childhood when an experience arouses fear or anxiety too great to be borne. The experience is repressed into the unconscious—that is, conscious memory of it disappears. Later, however, something associated with the forgotten experience arouses the original intense emotions in an obviously inappropriate or inexplicable way. For example, a woman reacts so intensely to cats that the mere picture of a cat causes her to tremble, perspire profusely, become nauseated. A man finds that what he has regarded as a natural though unusual fastidiousness has gradually been transformed into an obsession that makes it impossible for him to touch anything handled by others—money, doorknobs, tableware, books.

According to prevailing Freudian theory, neurosis can be cured only through a therapy that, by painstaking probing in the course of many sessions, uncovers the repressed experience as well as the unconscious motives and conflicts associated with it. Now able to understand why the experience aroused such overwhelmingly painful emotions, the patient is cured. Without treatment, it is claimed, neurotic disorders will persist or get worse. Ridding the patient of the symptoms while ignoring the underlying causes will only complicate matters: There will be a relapse, or the underlying fears and anxieties will attach themselves to a different object, or a different set of symptoms will appear. The patient may, for example, be relieved of a neurotic fear of rats only to find himself even more seriously incapacitated by a fear of automobiles; the patient cured of his claustrophobia may be plunged into a deep depression.

It is generally believed that even though psychotherapeutic treatment may take years, it is thorough and will eventually lead to a permanent cure. These beliefs have seldom been contested, and there is virtually unanimous agreement—even among adherents of nonanalytic psychotherapy—that neurotic disorders can best be understood and treated on the basis of Freudian or neo-Freudian theory.

The casual reader of modern textbooks of psychiatry or clinical psychology is scarcely aware that there is, in fact, no evidence to support Freudian theory, while there is considerable evidence that all the foregoing beliefs are actually false.

I wish to discuss only briefly some of the studies that disprove psychoanalytic dogma, and to focus on "behavior therapy," a new approach that offers an effective alternative, both in theory and in practice, to conventional "insight" or "dynamic" psychotherapy and that promises at long last to bring scientific method to bear on a field until now ruled by faith and dogma.

Does Psychoanalysis Cure?

One of the most striking features of neurotic disorders is the fact that in the majority of cases they are subject to spontaneous remission—that is, in time the symptoms disappear without therapy. I have combined the results of four independent studies to show the percentage of severely neurotic patients whose symptoms disappeared without any psychiatric treatment whatsoever (see Figure 1).

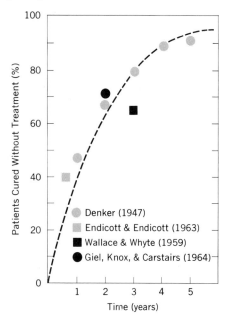

Figure 1. A curve fitted to the combined data of four independent studies of patients who recovered from neuroses without treatment.

In three of the studies, spontaneous remissions occurred in from 65 to 75 percent of the cases over two to three years; in the fourth, a long-term study, 90 percent of the patients were free of symptoms at the end of five years. There is much other evidence in the literature to substantiate the claim that neurotic symptoms sooner or later disappear spontaneously in many cases.

This raises a serious question about the effectiveness

of psychotherapy. To prove its worth, proponents of psychotherapy must show that the percentage of cures following treatment is significantly greater than the percentage of spontaneous remissions. In 1952 I analyzed a number of reports on the effects of psychotherapy and found that the figures for cures did not differ from those for spontaneous remissions. Statistically speaking, therefore, treatment had contributed nothing. Analyses of later studies on adults and children, including much more data, tended to support this conclusion.

It might nevertheless be argued that even though psychotherapy does not produce more cures than does the passage of time alone, the cures it does achieve are more permanent—that is, there are fewer relapses. However, a ten-year follow-up study by Johannes Cremarius showed that this is not the case. Of more than 600 neurotic patients treated by various methods, including psychoanalysis, 73 percent were considered to be improved or cured when treatment ended. Eight to ten years later, only 25 percent of this group were still considered improved or cured. In other words, of those patients declared to have benefited from treatment, two out of three suffered a relapse.

To date, then, there is no real evidence for the effectiveness of psychotherapy—as is now admitted even by leading psychoanalysts and psychotherapists—though with further search such evidence might be uncovered.

Pavlov's Dogs

The theory and practice of behavior therapy are grounded on modern knowledge of learning and conditioning. Classical behaviorist theory holds (1) that behavior can be understood as a response to a stimulus, and (2) that most behavior is learned through a process called *conditioning*, by which links are established between certain stimuli and responses.

To illuminate the meaning of these terms, let us recall Pavlov's salivating dogs. A hungry dog responds to food in its mouth (an unconditioned stimulus) by salivating (an unconditioned response). This is but one example of the many "built-in" responses or reflexes over which the organism has little or no control. Pavlov found that if an experimenter consistently rings a bell (a neutral stimulus) just before he puts the food into the dog's mouth, the dog will gradually associate the sound of the bell with the presence of the food. Eventually the sound of the bell (the conditioned stimulus) will alone be sufficient to cause the dog to salivate (now a conditioned response).

Much behavior is learned through conditioning of this sort; it is involuntary and may take place without the organism's being aware of it. But it must be *reinforced*; if it is not, the conditioned response will *extinguish*. In other words if, after the dog is conditioned to salivate at the sound of the bell, the bell is repeatedly rung but no food appears, the association between the conditioned and the unconditioned stimuli will extinguish and the dog will no longer salivate at the sound of the bell. These principles of conditioning and extinction are fundamental to classical conditioning, the basis for much of behavior therapy.

"Unscaring" Scared Cats

Behavior therapy has its roots in the early studies of John B. Watson, Mary Jones, and other behaviorists, but it may be said to date from the end of the 1950s with the publication of Joseph Wolpe's book, *Psychotherapy by Reciprocal Inhibition*, and my paper, "Behavior Therapy." Since Wolpe's method is an important part—though only a part—of the general theory and practice of behavior therapy, it serves as an excellent starting point for discussion.

Increasingly dissatisfied by his lack of results with conventional psychotherapy, Wolpe set out to see if the behaviorist approach, so successful in changing the behavior of laboratory animals, could erase neurotic behavior in humans. In a series of exploratory experiments with cats, Wolpe gave them a mild electric shock at the same time he presented them with a variety of neutral stimuli such as a toy mouse, a rubber ball, flashing lights. Thus he was able to induce a "neurotic" fear of the previously neutral stimuli. He then conducted another series of experiments to see if he could erase their neurotic fear by reversing the conditioning process. He concluded that the most satisfactory treatment was to expose them to the fear-provoking stimuli under conditions that were incompatible with fear.

He began by feeding his cats in a "safe" environment in which there were no fear-provoking stimuli. Gradually, through a series of carefully worked-out stages, the safe environment in which they were fed was made more and more similar to the original traumatic situation, by adding, one at a time, the stimuli associated with fear. Now, however, each stimulus became associated with gratification, and since gratification is incompatible with fear, Wolpe was able to extinguish the fear response and restore the cats to apparent normality.

Just Relax

Wolpe next applied this approach, which he called *desensitization*, to problems of human neurosis. To start with, he looked for a practicable method of desensitizing his patients. He needed to find a response that would be incompatible with fear or anxiety. His search led him to the work of E. Jacobson, who had developed a method for relaxing patients and recommended it as a treatment for neurotic disorders. Because it is impossible to be relaxed and anxious at the same time, Wolpe decided to use relaxation as the essential response that might damp down anxiety reactions in his patients.

At first he attempted to relax his patients in the presence of the objects that were producing their fear. But it was soon evident that this procedure would be both tedious and impractical. Not only would it involve gathering a large collection of objects to meet his patients' varied needs, but what of the patient who was terrified of horses, or was compelled to dive under a table at the sound of an airplane? Furthermore, in some patients the anxiety was not associated with an object but with an experience—for example, riding in an elevator or a subway.

Wolpe therefore began to experiment with the imaginary evocation of the anxiety-provoking stimuli, a method that was easy to manipulate in the consulting room and allowed a great deal of flexibility in planning treatment. In practice, Wolpe's desensitization technique works as follows. Before the desensitization treatment is begun, the therapist takes a general history of the patient and a complete history of the disorder. Next, he attempts to reduce or eliminate any conflicts or anxiety-producing situations in the patient's life that do not directly bear on his neurotic symptoms. Then he trains the patient in Jacobson's method of progressive relaxation, where the subject is taught to relax first one muscle, then another, progressing from one part of the body to other parts. Finally, patient and therapist discuss all the stimuli and situations that might possibly produce anxiety, grading them in a hierarchy ranging from the most to the least disturbing.

The Lady and the Cat

Now the patient is ready for desensitization. Let us illustrate this process through the story of a woman who suffers unbearable anxiety at the sight of a cat. In the course of discussions with her, the therapist has found that she is least disturbed at seeing a small kitten in the arms of a child. When treatment begins, she is asked therefore to imagine this sight as clearly and vividly as she can. Though she feels some anxiety, it is bearable. Still keeping the picture firmly in mind, she is instructed to relax as she has been taught. She finds that when she is thoroughly relaxed, her anxiety disappears. She repeats this exercise in subsequent sessions until she never experiences any anxiety while imagining a kitten in the arms of a child. Now the therapist asks her to imagine a slightly more disturbing situation—a kitten playing with a ball of wool, pouncing on it, biting it, and so on—while she relaxes. When this imaginary situation ceases to provoke anxiety, the therapist asks her to evoke a still more disturbing image, moving up the hierarchy that had been established prior to treatment. Eventually she is able to imagine with tranquility a big black tomcat stalking through the grass or curled up on her bed. And finally at the end of treatment, she is able to confront cats in real life as tranquilly as she can evoke their images in the consulting room.

Indeed, at each stage of treatment she finds she can transfer to real life her new ability to tolerate the stimulus. Thus when our hypothetical patient reaches the stage at which she can evoke the image of a playful kitten without anxiety in the therapist's office, she no longer experiences anxiety at the actual sight of a kitten frolicking in the neighbor's yard.

In behaviorist terms, desensitization, as well as the other therapeutic procedures used by Wolpe, is based on a general principle that he states as follows: "If a response antagonistic to anxiety can be made to occur in the presence of anxiety-provoking stimuli so that it is accompanied by a complete or partial suppression of the anxiety responses, the bond between the stimuli and the anxiety responses will be weakened." In somewhat simpler terms, we can say that because relaxation suppresses, or inhibits, anxiety, the lady was desensitized to cats by gradually conditioning herself to respond with relaxation. The "cat-anxiety" association has been replaced by a "cat-relaxation" association.

Does Behavior Therapy Work?

Wolpe claimed that desensitization was not only much more effective than psychotherapy, but was also quicker. In an unselected series of more than 300 cases he found that 90 percent were improved or cured after an average of thirty sessions. Reports by his students and followers on the whole corroborate his findings. None of these clinical studies, however, included the proper control groups—patients with similar disorders who were not treated, or patients treated by other methods. Thus questions about the superiority of desensitization to psychotherapy could not be effectively answered in terms of percentages, treatment times, and so on.

Recently, however, James Humphery carried out a study specifically designed to compare the results of behavior therapy with those of traditional psychotherapy. Formerly director of a child guidance clinic and a psychotherapist of many years' experience, Humphery was trained in behavior therapy specifically in order to conduct the investigation. His subjects were seventy-one children who had been referred to London child-guidance clinics for all types of disorders except brain damage and psychosis. The children were divided into matched groups: The thirty-four in the control group received no treatment of any kind; the thirty-seven children in the treated group were then divided into two groups, one of which received behavior therapy and the other traditional psychotherapy. A five-point rating scale was used to establish the severity of each child's disorder (his clinical status) and to evaluate the success of the treatment. Each child was rated on this scale at the beginning of the study; the children in the treatment group were rated immediately after treatment, while those in the control group were rated ten months after the start of the experiment. Experienced psychiatrists, who did not know to which group a child had been assigned, did the rating. The decision to end treatment was made in consultation between Humphery and the psychiatrist assigned to the case. A rise of two or more

points on the clinical rating scale was taken as an arbitrary criterion of "cure."

All children were again rated ten months later. Of the children who received behavior therapy, 75 percent were rated cured at the close of treatment, as compared with only 35 percent of those who received psychotherapy. At the ten-month follow-up, 85 percent of those who had received behavior therapy were rated as cured—an increase of ten percentage points—but only 29 percent of those in the psychotherapy group were still considered cured. Of those who had received no treatment at all, 18 percent were found to be cured (see Figure 2).

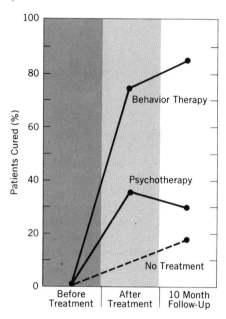

Figure 2. In the follow-up study of 71 children, some of whom were treated by behavior therapy, some by psychotherapy, some not at all, behavior therapy proved to have effected more and longer-lasting cures.

These results are even more impressive when differences in the length of treatment are taken into account. The children receiving psychotherapy required twenty-one sessions spread over thirty-one weeks before it was thought that treatment could be terminated, but those receiving behavior therapy required only nine sessions during eighteen weeks. Thus behavior therapy cured twice as many cases as did psychotherapy, and in less than half the number of sessions. By happenstance, moreover, the children assigned to the behavior therapy group were the more seriously ill, which would seem to militate against the success of behavior therapy. On the other hand, because the children given psychotherapy began treatment with a higher clinical-status rating, they were less likely to achieve the two-point rise necessary to denote cure. These factors were undoubtedly important in accounting for the startling difference between the two groups. It should be noted, however, that the percentage of cures resulting from psychotherapy in this experiment did not differ from that usually obtained in the clinics involved in the study.

Interesting as the study may be, it can be criticized on various grounds. From the standpoint of this article, however, the most interesting focus for examination is the assumption that the crucial therapeutic element for the children treated with behavior therapy was the *combination* of desensitization and relaxation. This may not have been the case. At least three alternative hypotheses could be put forward. One, simple extinction might be involved. According to the laws of conditioning, if the anxiety-provoking stimulus is repeatedly evoked without any distressing consequences, the response should eventually be extinguished; thus we might conclude that desensitization—without relaxation —is sufficient to produce a cure. Two, since relaxation lowers the intensity of all responses (drive level), this in itself would reduce the intensity of the conditioned fear response and might suffice to bring about a cure. Hence relaxation—without desensitization—might be the crucial therapeutic element. Three, it might be that the sympathetic attention of a person in authority is, by itself, all that is needed. Indeed, this view has often been expressed by those who claim that behavior therapy embodies important but standard psychotherapeutic procedures. For example, during the preliminary interviews the behavior therapist, despite his radically different approach to treatment, in fact employs such elements of psychotherapy as sympathy, acceptance of deviant behavior, and movement toward insight.

Clearly, questions such as these cannot be answered in the "clinical trial" type of investigation but must be dealt with in formal experimental studies. Fortunately, a number of such studies have been made in the last ten years.

Neurosis in the Laboratory

Behavior therapists, taking these problems into the laboratory, have designed experimental studies previously thought impossible in so complex a field as human emotion and interaction. To compare the effects of differing treatments, it is essential that the pre- and post-treatment states of the patient be measured as accurately as possible. Studies have usually focused therefore on such relatively simple disorders as phobias for snakes and spiders.

Is it possible to measure fear with any degree of precision? To be sure, the patient confronted by a snake can be asked to rate his own fear on a numbered scale ranging from "intense" to "slight." But while his subjective feelings are certainly relevant, they are not objectively "observable" enough to meet scientific criteria. Objective measures of fear, based on involuntary physiological reactions, have therefore been devised. We are all aware that fear is accompanied by a temporary increase in heartbeat (our hearts "pound"), by a temporary restriction or collapse of capillary blood vessels (we "turn white"), by profuse sweating, a dry mouth, and other changes—all of which can be measured with suitable instruments. Indeed the polygraph, or so-called lie detector, does nothing more than measure several physiological concomitants of changes in emotional reaction.

In addition, it is possible to measure a patient's actual behavior vis-à-vis the fear object—his *approach-avoidance* behavior. Fright is accompanied by an involuntary retreat from stimulus. How near will the patient approach the feared object? Will he touch it for a moment only? Will he handle it?

We can thus measure with some degree of accuracy the behavior we wish to modify and the degree of our success. This approach has enabled researchers to isolate specific components of behavior therapy and see which is the active ingredient. A study conducted by Stanley Rachman at Maudsley Hospital illustrates how this can be accomplished.

Rachman attempted to answer some of the questions posed by Wolpe's "reciprocal inhibition" theory, using as subjects a number of persons who feared spiders. He divided his subjects into four groups. One received behavior therapy (desensitization plus relaxation), a second desensitization only, a third relaxation only, and a fourth no treatment at all. Rachman used two independent measures of anxiety: the subjects' own estimates of their fear and a scale based on the subjects' physical avoidance of spiders (see Figure 3).

The results show very clearly that only the *combination* of desensitization and relaxation significantly decreased the fear of spiders.

Behavior Therapy versus Psychotherapy

In addition to testing out the effectiveness of different components of behavior therapy, recent laboratory experiments have enabled us to compare different treatments. The work of Gordon Paul at the University of Illinois is an example. Persons suffering from severe stage fright were divided into four groups: some received the desensitization-relaxation therapy, some received conventional psychotherapy, some received a placebo (in this case, non-therapy-oriented meetings between patient and therapist), and an untreated control group. Paul used four general measures of anxiety: (1) observable manifestations of anxiety during public speaking, as rated by trained observers; (2) the subjects' own ratings of their experienced anxiety; (3) pulse rate; and (4) palmar sweating.

Ratings made before and after treatment demonstrated that on all four criteria the group receiving behavior therapy showed the greatest average reduction of anxiety (see Figure 4). Indeed, only in this group was there a noticeable reduction in pulse rate after treatment,

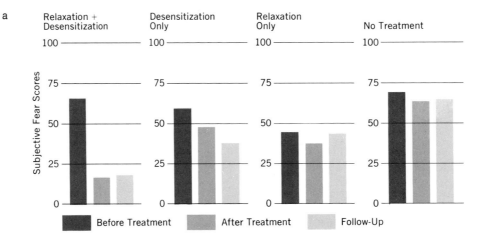

Figure 3. The importance of both desensitization and relaxation in behavior therapy is shown with patients suffering from an extreme fear of spiders. The effectiveness of desensitization plus relaxation is compared with desensitization only, relaxation only, and no treatment at all (controls). Estimates of fear were obtained before treatment, after treatment, and in a follow-up evaluation. Two measures of fear were employed: the patients' own estimates of their fear (a) and a scale of the physical avoidance of spiders (b).

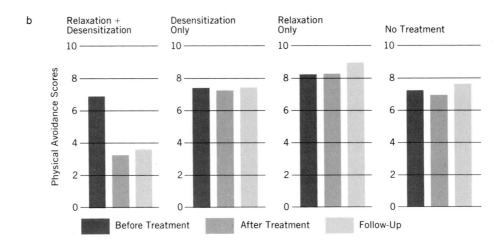

while pulse rate actually increased in the control group. Results with psychotherapy and the placebo were about the same, while the control group showed little change. It should be added that the behavior therapy was carried out by psychotherapists (specially trained in Wolpe's method for this experiment), who continued to prefer psychotherapy and its associated doctrines.

Gordon Paul and Donald Shannon later carried out a similar study in which they added a fifth experimental condition: Five patients were given behavior therapy as a group. This treatment was as effective as individual treatment. In addition, it was found that the academic performance of those given behavior therapy greatly improved, indicating that the specific reduction in anxiety achieved in the experiment may have generalized to other life situations.

Many more questions raised by behavior therapy are being studied in similar experiments, questions such as: Which is more effective, the presentation of the actual anxiety-producing stimulus or its imaginary evocation? Is it better to space the treatments or to compress them into short periods of time? How quickly does desensitization transfer to real-life situations?

These questions have not yet been definitively answered. Nor can it yet be claimed that the experiments I have described clearly show the superiority of behavior therapy. What may, I think, be claimed is that for the first time therapeutic methods are being tested in properly designed and controlled experiments, using objective criteria of known reliability. Vital questions that were until now discussed only in a subjective fashion are being brought under experimental control.

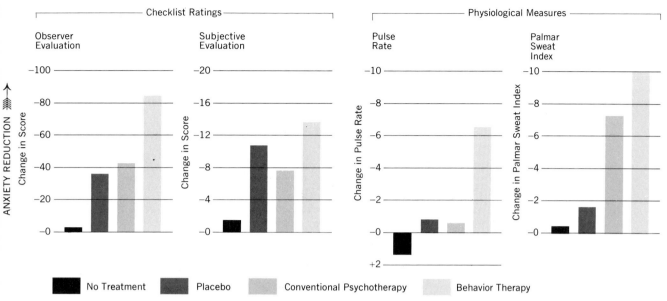

Figure 4. Groups of patients suffering from anxiety caused by severe stage fright were given conventional psychotherapy, behavior therapy (desensitization plus relaxation), placebo treatment (non-therapy-oriented meetings with a therapist), or no treatment (controls). Anxiety was measured before and after treatment by observer and subjective ratings and by physiological measures of pulse rate and palmar sweating. (Scale values are not identical.) In all cases, behavior therapy produced the greatest amount of anxiety reduction.

"Treatment Machines"

Psychoanalysts hold that an essential element in therapy is the transference—the interaction in which the patient transfers to the analyst his feelings toward significant persons in his life. Experimental studies of Wolpe's method suggest, however, that since the important ingredient in behavior therapy is the combination of conditioned stimulus and relaxation, the presence of the therapist may not be necessary. Could learning machines be substituted for the therapist? Properly programmed, they might be used both to teach the patient how to relax and to carry him through the desensitization process, based as it is on the patient's visualization of the fear-provoking stimulus.

Machines may indeed replace the therapist. Peter Lang, at the University of Wisconsin, has shown not only that behavior therapy can be programmed, but that it can be as effective as personally administered treatment. So far this has been demonstrated only with patients suffering from neuroses involving a single symptom, but an extension of this approach is inevitable. In the first place, there are very few trained behavior therapists and very many neurotics. Any method that shortens treatment and makes it possible to treat more patients is sure to be employed. In the second place, once patient and therapist have constructed the stimulus "hierarchies," the rest of the treatment is repetitive and mechanical. Most therapists would, it seems safe to say, gladly turn this part of their work over to a machine.

To be sure, much more study is needed before we can know whether, and to what extent, treatment by machine is feasible with the more complex neuroses, or with psychoses. It is possible, too, that the use of machines will be governed by the patient's personality type or emotional needs. It might be that introverts would do well with programmed treatments while extroverts, or those particularly in need of personal support and human contact, would prefer to work only with the therapist.

Neurotic Symptoms or Bad Habits?

So far in this discussion we have dealt only with one type of neurotic disorder and with one type of behavior therapy. This is justifiable because most neurotic patients who seek psychiatric help are suffering from disorders that produce distressing symptoms—negative emotional states such as anxiety, phobic fear, depression, obsessional or compulsive reactions, and so on. In all these disorders—which I have called "disorders of the *first* kind"—behavior therapists hold that classical conditioning is implicated, either through a single traumatic experience or through a long series of subtraumatic events in which emotions of terror or anxiety are associated with some previously neutral stimulus.

Behavior therapists agree that neurotic symptoms are learned. That is, they are neither innate nor due to lesions in the nervous system. Consequently, any explanation of neurotic behavior ought to proceed from the firm basis of our knowledge, gained in the laboratory, of learning and conditioning. According to these theories, there is no "neurosis" or "complex," as such, that causes the symptoms. There are only symptoms. A patient's response of overwhelming anxiety to so neutral a stimulus as the picture of a cat is, for example, in a real and literal sense *learned*. It is a "bad" (or maladaptive) habit, acquired through the processes of classical conditioning. The so-called symptom *is* the neurosis—I say "so-called" because the anxiety response is not in fact symptomatic of anything. Behavior therapists are not pained, therefore, when psychoanalysts accuse them of curing only the symptoms. They answer that there is no disease other than the symptoms. And in any case, as someone has said, "It ill becomes those who cannot *even* cure the symptom to complain that others *only* cure the symptom."

Learning and conditioning theory can explain the otherwise puzzling fact of spontaneous remission. It has often been said that "time the great healer" is responsible for such cures. Clearly, however, it is not the mere passage of time that alone works the cure. It is the events that transpire during time. What are those events? If the symptom is in fact a conditioned response, then the response should gradually be extinguished if the sufferer, over a period of time, encounters the original fear-provoking stimulus without its being reinforced by a traumatic event. The woman who is terrified of cats will, from time to time, encounter cats, and if nothing happens to reinforce her fear, it should gradually die away.

In many cases, however, this cannot come about because the patient refuses to encounter the conditioned stimulus. By taking great pains to avoid it, he evades the possibility of testing reality. Furthermore, each time he avoids the stimulus he is consolidating the very behavior pattern that is the neurosis.

A striking example of this is the case of a woman we recently treated for a cat phobia so severe she was unable to leave her room. The phobia had developed when, as a very young girl, her father drowned her favorite kitten before her eyes. So traumatic was the experience that every time she saw a cat, she ran away. Doing so reduced her anxiety—and reinforced her avoidance behavior. The conditioned habit, feeding on itself, became so dominating that eventually she immured herself in her room. Behavior therapy, by gradually exposing her to the sight of cats while she was thoroughly relaxed, completely restored her to a normal life within a few weeks; there was no relapse, nor was there any indication that her anxiety had been transferred to some other object or had expressed itself in some other form. This freedom from relapse and symptom substitution after behavior therapy has also been observed many times by other therapists, even by some who were unsympathetic to this approach. Nevertheless, long-term, follow-up studies are needed to put this point beyond argument.

Aversion Therapy

In addition to disorders of the first kind involving distressing symptoms such as anxiety, phobic fear, or depression, there are neurotic disorders of the second kind. They may arise when some socially desirable conditioning has failed to occur, as with psychopaths or sociopaths. Such people are characterized by an almost complete lack of social responsibility; they are the pathological liars, or those who steal or murder regardless of the fact that they will almost certainly be found out and punished.

Disorders of the second kind also arise when some socially undesirable or unacceptable behavior has become associated with positive emotions such as pleasure, comfort, happiness, sexual arousal. The most obvious examples are associated with the sexual impulse—homosexuality, fetishism, transvestism, among others. For instance, an ordinarily neutral stimulus such as a shoe may accidentally become associated with sexual pleasure and through subsequent reinforcement come to serve as a conditioned stimulus that calls forth a sexual response (shoe fetishism).

In cases of this kind the aim of the therapist is to break the association between the conditioned stimulus —a woman's shoe, for example—and the conditioned response—aberrant sexual satisfaction. The dissociation process is often called "aversion therapy," and is the opposite of desensitization. In desensitization therapy, the link between the conditioned stimulus (a cat) and the conditioned response (fear) is replaced by a new link between the conditioned stimulus and a pleasant response (relaxation). In aversion therapy, the link between the conditioned stimulus (a woman's shoe) and the pleasant sexual response is broken by linking the shoe stimulus to an unpleasant experience.

The classic example of aversion therapy is the use of apomorphine to cure alcoholism. The patient takes the drug, which causes nausea and vomiting. Just before the onset of nausea, he is given a drink of liquor. The drink (conditioned stimulus) is now followed by a very distressing conditioned response—nausea. Behaviorist theory predicts that after many such repetitions, the mere sight of a drink will evoke the newly conditioned response.

In spite of its apparent crudity, aversion therapy works surprisingly well if properly carried out. However, research reports show that much useless effort has been expended by medical people with little knowledge of conditioning procedures. To take but one example: In treating alcoholism many would-be therapists have administered the drink *after* nausea has set in. Behaviorists know that conditioning will be effective only if the conditioned stimulus *precedes* the response to be conditioned; backward conditioning just does not occur.

Modern behavior therapists prefer to use electric shock rather than drugs in aversion therapy. The intensity of the unconditioned stimulus (the shock) can be much better controlled; it is less messy; and it can be administered at a precisely chosen moment. Where the patient urgently requests such treatment, electric shock has been used to cure certain sexual deviations, including homosexuality and transvestism.

Typically in such treatment, while the male homosexual is looking at pictures of nude males, he is given a moderately intense shock. The combination of the male picture (conditioned stimulus) with shock (unconditioned stimulus) should lead to an aversion to men as sex objects (conditioned response).

The treatment is not yet complete, however. The next step is to condition a positive response to women: the picture of the nude male is suddenly replaced by the picture of a nude female—and the shock is terminated. Since the cessation of shock is pleasurable, a favorable response to women is now established.

Techniques such as these offer a potentially powerful therapeutic approach. However, the effectiveness of these conditioning methods cannot as yet be judged because too few cases have been studied, and there have not been enough long-term, follow-up studies.

"Operant" Conditioning

No article on behavior therapy would be complete without some discussion of *operant conditioning* as a technique for changing behavior. Because the theories of operant conditioning underlie such revolutionary new pedagogical methods as the use of teaching machines, as well as new approaches to therapy, I should like to describe this method briefly.

Operant conditioning was originally worked out by B. F. Skinner, who succeeded in shaping the behavior of pigeons by reinforcing bits of behavior that were originally quite random. In one of Skinner's early experiments, he fed a hungry pigeon whenever it happened to stretch its neck above a predetermined point. Gradually it "caught on" and spent most of its time raising its head just as high as it could. This method of changing behavior is also called "instrumental conditioning," since the organism's behavior is instrumental in obtaining the "reward."

The notion that psychotics can learn to control their delusions or their unacceptable behavior is rejected by almost all knowledgeable people. Nevertheless, the technique of shaping behavior, originally worked out with pigeons, has been used with startling success to change the behavior of psychotic adults and disturbed children. Hardcore schizophrenics, considered hopeless, who had been vegetating for years in the back wards of mental hospitals, have been taught to relinquish the behavior that identified them as insane. An example is reported by Colin Blakemore of the Maudsley Hospital.

A middle-aged woman, suffering from severe paranoid delusions that communists were following her everywhere trying to kill her, was asked to wear earphones during her meetings with the therapist. Every time the woman mentioned her paranoid ideas, the therapist pressed a button that enabled him to deliver an unpleasant noise into the earphones. Whenever she talked normally, the therapist turned off the noise. Gradually the paranoid topic dropped out of her conversation completely—not only in the presence of the therapist but in the ward as well.

As further proof of the efficacy of this technique, Blakemore reversed the process. He brought back her paranoid talk by punishing her whenever she spoke of normal topics; then he again taught her to leave communists and persecution out of her conversation. Thus he showed that by employing this technique, he could bring her talk under complete experimental control.

This experiment, like many similar operant conditioning experiments with mental patients, raises more questions than it answers. Hopefully, these questions will be answered in the future with more experiments using many subjects and rigorous controls. In the meantime, however, operant conditioning has opened many new and undreamed-of avenues to the therapist.

Action Before Thought?

Some of the most important consequences of behavior therapy are its effects on theory. For example, it has long been held that thought precedes and controls action. Behavior therapy suggests that the contrary may often be true, so that changing a person's behavior through some form of conditioning process may actually change his thought or mental set.

For example, Teodoro Ayllon, at Anna State Hospital in Illinois, reports the case of a woman who was committed to a mental hospital because she would not eat for fear her husband would poison her. She refused to feed herself in the hospital and had to be fed by a nurse. Finding that she was very fastidious about her personal appearance and her clothing, Ayllon told the nurse to spill food on the woman's dress whenever she fed her, and to explain that it was very difficult to feed another person. Gradually the patient began to feed herself—and at the same time her delusions about being poisoned began to disappear. Her *actions* in feeding herself had changed her *thought* that she would be poisoned.

Of course, not too much should be read into isolated experiments of this sort. On the other hand, when we keep in mind that psychotherapists have had almost no success with cases such as these, it seems reasonable to suggest that behavior therapists are opening doors and windows, bringing fresh air into a room in which the atmosphere had grown very heavy, stale, and musty.

Science and Psychotherapy

The work of the behavior therapists has important implications for the treatment of neurotic and psychotic disorders, and has opened new paths toward understanding them. I would like to suggest, though, that their chief contribution has been to bring this hitherto mysterious realm under the discipline of scientific

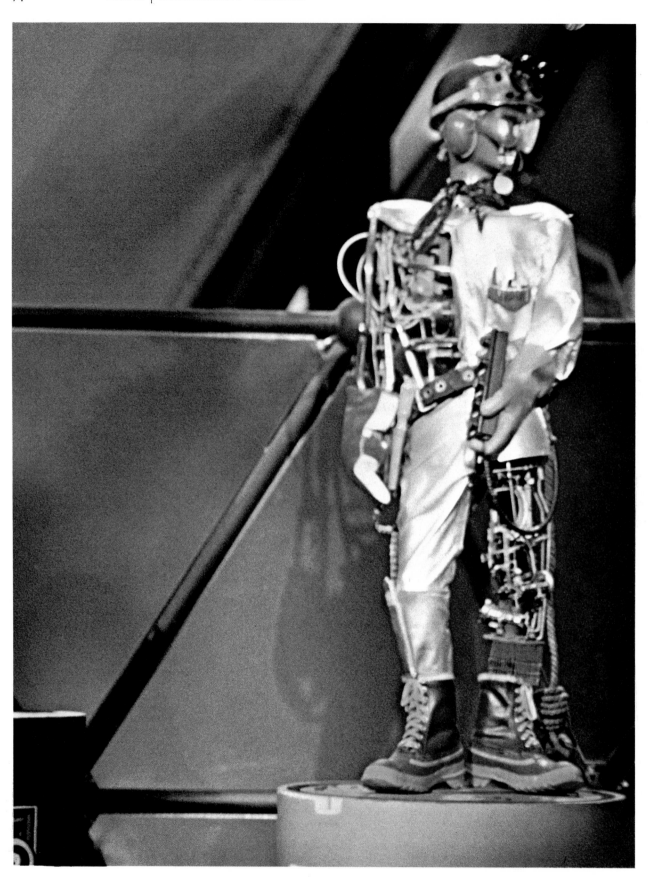

method. It is possible, though unlikely, that all the theories of conditioning discussed in this paper are wrong. But by insisting that both theory and practice be experimentally tested, behavior therapists are trying to ensure that errors will be exposed, and that new evidence will be obtained on which new and better theories can be based.

Behaviorist objections to psychoanalysis and its allied psychotherapeutic theory and practices are not based solely on opposition to Freudian *theory*. They are based on an opposition to the Freudian *approach* as well; it must be ruled out of court, as far as science is concerned, on two grounds. In the first place, Freudian theories are not stated in terms that permit them to be tested and verified; indeed it is almost impossible to think of experiments by which they could be either confirmed or disproved. In the second place, practitioners have made no effort to gather the kind of data, based on experience and observation with patients, that alone could give us a factual basis for evaluating their work. They demand belief, but they do not offer proof.

Behavior therapy is based on applying fundamental discoveries gained in the laboratory to practical problems—curing neurotic patients. The Freudian approach reversed this process. Freud's dynamic psychology was based on "discoveries" made in the course of treating patients. He and his followers universalized these ideas by applying them to all human beings. They manufactured new theories to bolster the original assumptions and attempted to fit all aspects of human behavior into their untested theoretical framework.

Behavior therapists hold that theories that attempt to explain behavior, neurotic or otherwise, should be based on fundamental scientific knowledge that is susceptible to experimental proof. They are attempting to test how well learning and conditioning theory can be applied to human problems, and they ask that judgment be suspended until the proof is conclusive. If their experiments are subject to criticism, better experiments will be designed in accordance with the criticism. If the theories do not stand up to experimental test, then better theories will be put forward to fit the established facts. As I see it, this is nothing more—nor less—than the long-delayed introduction of scientific method into the murky and emotion-ridden field of psychotherapy. In essence, psychotherapy involves changing those maladaptive emotional states and behavior patterns that interfere with adequate functioning. The new approaches and results I have described hold promise that, after fifty years in the twilight zone of unverified claims, unjustified beliefs, and passionately held dogma, psychotherapy will at last become truly scientific.

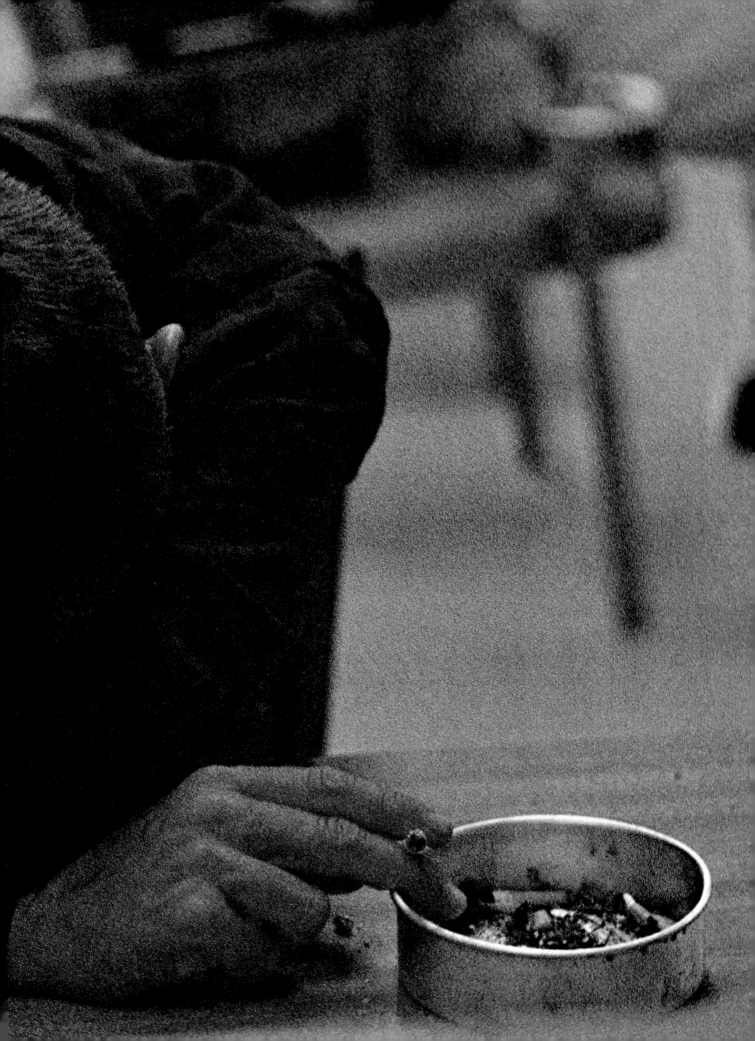

For Helplessness: Can We Immunize the Weak?

Martin E. P. Seligman

Laboratory analogs of psychopathology have been created and studied for decades. Animals can be subjected to more extreme environmental manipulations than can humans. They can be deprived of food, toys, or mommy. They can be exposed to cold, insoluble problems, or electric shock. When the effects of these manipulations have been measured, methods of reversing or undoing the damage can be developed. As Eysenck pointed out in the preceding article, the techniques of desensitization, aversion therapy, and operant conditioning were tested in the laboratory before they were added to the therapist's armamentarium.

The usual focus of laboratory methods is on active emotional and avoidance responses. Martin Seligman expands it to passivity and helplessness as well. In a study in which a dog's effect on its environment is controlled, Seligman shows one possible cause of passivity and points to ways of modifying, perhaps even preventing, the development of such behavior. How analogous the learning processes of dogs and humans are has not been established; nevertheless, the studies Seligman describes yield valuable clues to the etiology and treatment of maladaptive passivity. After all, the primary contribution of such studies lies in the testable hypotheses they suggest, not the quantitative data output.

Archie has turned fifteen and is moving toward total dropout. Soon he will quit school, where he feels increasingly ignorant, useless, and helpless, and enter the larger world where he is guaranteed to feel similarly ignorant, useless, and helpless, and where the consequences will be more serious.

Archie has been shaped for this from infancy. He never knew his father, his mother was seldom at home, and Archie grew into childhood almost alone in an ugly, monotonous, bullying, nonverbal world. At five-and-a-half he was far behind his schoolmates in handling standard English; he wanted to follow the teacher's instructions, but she used too many words he didn't

know and he was afraid to ask what she meant. As he dropped farther and farther behind in verbal skills, school became more and more incomprehensible. But every year or so he was pushed on to the next grade.

Archie's vicious circle of failures has begun, and it seems almost inevitable that a series of horrors awaits him in the outside world. The outcome is almost predestined.

A few years ago, Mr. Thompson was a grocer in a small Midwestern town. His business was never very good; despite his frantic efforts, his credit dried up, his debts grew, and his customers went away. His wife of seventeen years left him. Soon after this his only son was run over by a truck, and his crumbling world at last collapsed. Mr. Thompson lies curled up in his bed in a back ward of a state hospital, staring at a wall. He hasn't spoken for a year and a half. He is not much trouble—it is fairly easy to feed and clean him. He probably will be kept alive for many years.

Archies and Mr. Thompsons are little more than statistics. They are creatures of the welfare roll, the state or federal mental-health budget, the police blotter, the editorial, the casebook in psychopathology. In almost every Archie or Mr. Thompson we can find failure, depression, the feeling of powerlessness, some final giving up that requires institutional notice by society.

What can be done for the Archies and Mr. Thompsons of this life?

That such patterns of helplessness are today so widespread and recurrent suggests that we know very little about preventing or curing them. One thing that experimental psychologists can do is call attention to the events taking place in their laboratories and suggest functional analogies—or at least intriguing ones—that may be useful when society is ready to be truly serious about cures and prevention of helplessness. A few years ago Bruce Overmier, Steve Maier, and I stumbled onto a behavioral phenomenon that suggests such an analogy.

Shock

In the laboratory of R. L. Solomon, we had been using dogs and traumatic electric shock to test a particular learning theory. We strapped dogs into a Pavlovian harness and gave them electric shock—traumatic, but not physically damaging. Later the dogs were put into a two-compartment box where they were supposed to learn to escape shock simply by jumping across a barrier from an electrified section into a nonelectrified section. We found that if a harnessed dog first experienced shock over which it had no control (that is, nothing it did affected or related to the shock), something bizarre happened when we put it in the shuttlebox. But first let me tell you what a nonshocked, or naive, dog does in the shuttlebox.

When a conditioned stimulus (CS) comes on—for example, the lights go dim—the experimentally naive dog looks around. Ten seconds later strong electric shock comes through the floor. The dog howls, runs around frantically, defecates and urinates, and finally throws itself over the barrier. This response gets it out of shock and turns off the conditioned stimulus (the lights come back on). A few minutes later the second trial occurs. When the CS goes on this time, the dog looks afraid. Ten seconds later when the shock comes on again, the dog goes through a shortened and more purposeful or adaptive version of the first howling-running behavior, and jumps over the barrier faster than before. After a few more trials, the dog stands poised at the barrier and leaps over at the instant of shock.

Eventually it avoids shock altogether by jumping as soon as the lights dim.

However, if a dog receives inescapable shock in the harness twenty-four hours before escape training, its behavior is dramatically different. At the onset of the first shock in the box, the dog howls, runs around, defecates and urinates—but only for a few seconds. It then settles down and takes the shock, whining and howling but making few escape movements. Typically, it does not get across the barrier. (We terminate shock after sixty seconds if the dog doesn't jump.) On the second trial, the dog runs around a little, but soon stops; it again stands or sits, howling and whining. After a few more trials, the dog makes virtually no escape movements, and appears to have given up.

Occasionally, one of these passive or helpless dogs, after enduring three or four shocks, will jump over the barrier and escape shock. A naive dog's first escape response reliably predicts that it will continue to escape shock in increasingly adaptive ways. Most helpless dogs, however, do not catch on after one escape; they soon revert to taking shocks.

We have concerned ourselves with three questions about this striking phenomenon: (1) Why does it occur? (2) How can such passivity be cured once it has set in? (3) How can victims of inescapable shock be prevented from passively accepting subsequent trauma?

To find what causes helplessness, we must look closely at what a dog can do during inescapable shocks. It can turn its head, pull on the restraining straps, bark, wag its tail, and the like. What these voluntary responses have in common is that they haven't the slightest effect on the shock.

Traditional learning theorists have supposed that animals could learn only two relations between their responses and rewards: either that a certain behavior produced a reward, or that the behavior no longer produced a reward, and was thus extinguished. We now think that animals can also *learn* a third relation—that in certain situations no response makes any difference. It is, we think, this third learning that is behind the seemingly unnatural passivity to trauma that the helpless dogs display.

What might be expected of a dog that learns that its entire response repertoire is irrelevant? Such a dog might simply stop trying to do anything about shock. We think our passive dogs just do not try because they have *learned* that it does not pay. Learning that reward and response are unconnected is an *active* form of learning, and as such can interfere with the learning of new relationships. This may account for the fact that when passive dogs do jump the barrier, they do not learn that their response has in fact produced shock termination.

We are suggesting therefore that it is not that trauma per se produces helplessness, but rather that helplessness results from a learned relationship to trauma; the animal has learned that trauma is always inescapable and uncontrollable. To test this idea, we worked with two groups of dogs in the harness. For one group, shock was independent of all responses. The other group could turn off shock merely by pressing panels beside their heads. We theorized that if dogs learned to stop shock by turning their heads, they later would escape and avoid shocks in the box. The group undergoing uncontrollable shocks would have learned, conversely, that they were helpless and would be passive or helpless in the box. This is exactly what happened.

Cure

Learning that the environment cannot be controlled is central to developing the helplessness syndrome. This idea suggested to us that canine helplessness could be prevented and, once it happened, broken up.

Suppose a dog sits on one side of a box, session after session, and takes shock without trying to escape. How can you make it begin to respond successfully? Obviously, you must get it to learn that the relationship between its responses and shock termination could be one of control. We dropped meat on the other side of the barrier to encourage helpless dogs to escape shock; we took the barrier out altogether; we called to the dogs from the nonelectric side. Nothing worked. As a last resort, we pulled them back and forth across the box on leashes, forcibly demonstrating to them that movement in a certain direction ended shocks. This did the trick, but only after much dragging. Dogs so treated finally learned to escape shock on their own.

Prevention

Modern psychotherapy uses retroactive measures almost exclusively; it attempts to cure ills that are well established. This has given the entire therapeutic discipline a pronounced backward-looking character. It's worth pointing out once again that some of the most spectacular successes in medicine have been scored with future-looking or preventive therapy, that is, with immunization. Could we immunize dogs against the effects of inescapable shock? If a dog's first experience with shock is with *controllable* shock, will this exposure in and of itself prevent later inescapable shock from producing

helplessness? The answer is yes. If a dog first gets escapable shock in the box, and then gets uncontrollable shock in the harness, it will escape normally when it is returned to the box. Such a dog will also struggle much more in the harness than naive dogs, trying to gain control over shock that actually is uncontrollable.

The Analogy

In actual or scientific and ethical terms, the distance is vast between the Archies and Mr. Thompsons on one hand and dogs in a box on the other. All such distances must be crossed by speculation or imagination; the most we can ask is that the imagination be educated, and that the speculation touch a few testable signposts.

Take Mr. Thompson. To what extent did his history of failure, of independence between what he did and what happened to him, cause his present state? To what extent would a lifetime of experience controlling his environment have prevented failure from reducing his response repertoire to nil? Could he even yet be cured by a leash-dragging technique similar to ours? Our analogy suggests that he might be. (It says nothing about whether he *ought* to be—whether we should undertake to deny the human mind its last refuge of dissolution or madness.) But the present way of treating patients like Mr. Thompson, with its emphasis on keeping them quiet and docile, only encourages passivity.

And Archie? From the cradle on, if mother (a combination of affection and intelligence) isn't around to feed you and change you when you cry, crying becomes an irrelevant response. (We might consider crying to be a kind of speech.) If affection and intelligence don't respond, whatever you try, then trying becomes irrelevant. Would it be possible to bypass parental neglect, and an entire generation of shamelessly incompetent teaching professionals, and teach the Archies of this world that there are many situations in which response does control the environment? Could we inoculate Archies against helplessness?

Our canine analog suggests very strongly, I think, that such immunization is possible.

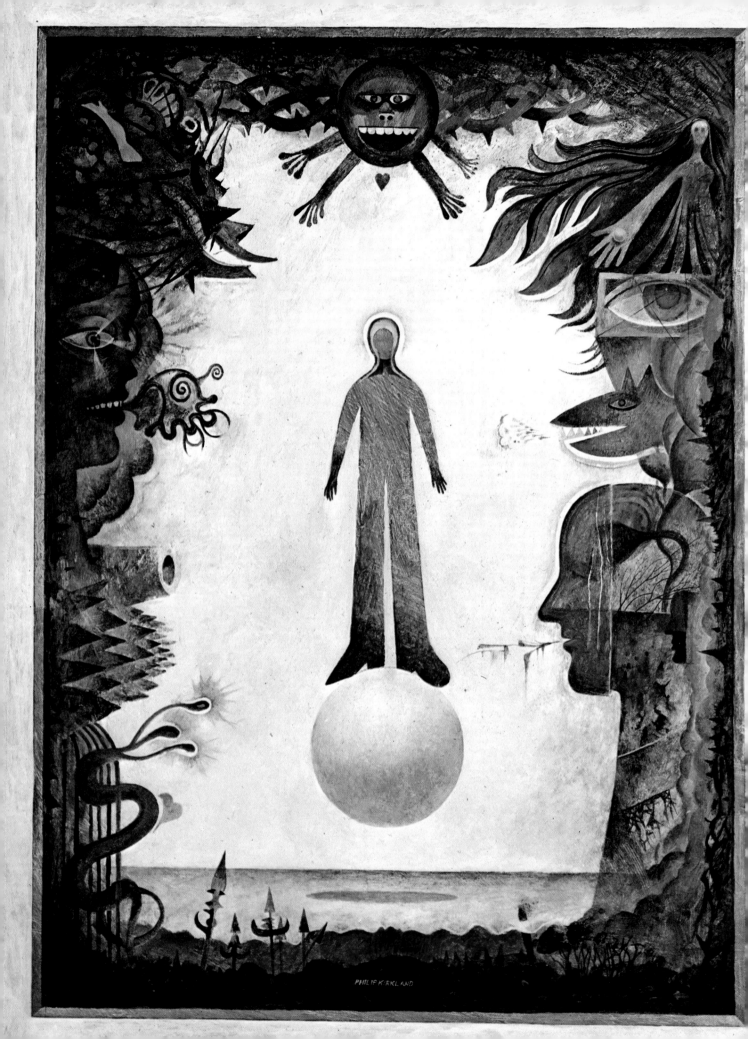

PHILIP KIRKLAND

Morality in Psychotherapy

Marvin Frankel

What is psychotherapy good for? According to Marvin Frankel, traditional psychotherapy is perfect for dealing with the neurotic who wishes to be absolved of any responsibility for his behavior and its consequences. The psychoanalytic model is designed to convince the neurotic (who needs but a little persuasion) that he is indeed at the mercy of his own unconscious forces. Thus absolved, he is able to rest in peace or to act without guilt.

Is peace of mind the essential goal in therapy? There are alternatives to the passive acceptance of one's own blamelessness. Frankel's approach, integrity therapy, stresses man's freedom of action and responsibility for the consequences of his acts. It would apprise the neurotic of motives in his maladaptive or self-destructive behavior, and it would regard guilt as a healthy indicator of a lapse in personal ethics.

Frankel's views suggest that today's psychotherapist should reexamine his own aims and needs in the therapeutic relationship. As for the patient, given the solid entrenchment of the traditional approach, is he free to choose to be free?

The year is 1930. The place, Berlin. You are a practicing psychoanalyst confronting an interesting new patient in your office. His name, Adolf Hitler. He is a professional politician regarded as one of the country's rising young men. Now he has come to you because he is troubled by persistent anxieties. He speaks confidently about his plans for Germany, yet he admits to fear of failure and therefore punishment by "lesser" beings. Lately, however, when he considers some of the harsh deeds demanded by his grandiose plans, he has been bothered by feelings of guilt. Nevertheless, he is convinced that the ends he has in mind fully justify the means. He is bothered only because his increasing anxieties and guilt feelings may impede him in the execution of his designs. Hitler asks you to put an end to these disturbing feelings. Can you help him?

For many, the answer would appear to be obvious—for certain actions, guilt necessarily is the result. Hitler must be convinced that his anxiety and guilt are altogether realistic in light of his harsh intentions; that such disturbing feelings occur not without reason, but come about directly from his grand designs because these designs are wrong. Hitler, one might say, feels guilty because his schemes violate his basic principles. As

Hitler struggles with guilt, he is admitting, if only to himself, that he does indeed contemplate violating his every moral principle.

But he had come to the analyst to buy himself moral carte blanche, not to have his plans imposed upon. Given such a case today, we have reason to believe that many of our contemporary psychotherapists would be able to oblige an Adolf Hitler. This is because of the *kind* of values they bring to bear upon the psychotherapeutic relationship. What are these values?

An inkling is provided by the recent book by Joseph Wolpe and Arnold Lazarus, *Behavior Therapy Techniques*, which devotes seven pages to "tactical principles." Using these "principles," we may theorize how they might have been applied to the neurotic German politician. Regarding the patient's fears, Wolpe and Lazarus undoubtedly would have invoked their third tactical principle, which says in effect that the patient should be made to realize that there is no "virtue" in confronting one's fear. Then, Hitler would have undergone the treatment the behaviorists call "desensitization," in which, with muscles relaxed, he would have learned to overcome his fear of certain authority figures. Thereafter, in any confrontation with authorities, although they well might fear this wild-eyed upstart, he no longer would need fear them; he could dismiss them from his life and from his dreams.

As for the patient's growing sense of guilt, Wolpe and Lazarus state explicitly on page 16 of their book that a patient has no choice in becoming what he is. Hence, blame and culpability are incongruous. Hitler, now fully confident and secure in the knowledge that he really shouldn't be blamed for the political tack he yearns to take, presumably would have given his mustache a touch, paid his bill, and trooped out of the office.

Mental treatment from Freudian analysis to behavior therapy has declared that it is wrong to censure the blameless patient—a patient without free will, without responsibility, a patient whose acts are determined by his history.

Free Will and Decision Making

The epistemological question of whether free will really exists had best be left to philosophers. What is important for psychologists to realize is that people do, in fact, feel free. Every man makes choices every day. A hostess asks: "What will you have to drink?" The individual makes a decision not only on what to drink but whether he will take an alcoholic drink. Aside from the oft-reported social pressure to imbibe, he is under no compulsion to drink, or at least he would not recognize such a compulsion. He *feels* that he has made a free decision to have a drink.

This feeling becomes important to him when he recognizes that by his decision making he can alter consequences. During the course of the evening, our guest may accept more drinks. Then comes the time when he thinks about his automobile and about the drive home. Here he faces alternatives: He can switch to coffee and drive home himself; he can have another drink and hand the car keys to a sober wife; or he can take another drink and drive home anyway. Whether he drives home or not, in this instance he will know that he has affected consequences. If he ends up drunk and driving and then has an auto accident, his reaction—superficially at least—may be to blame the "other guy"; but if subsequently he is burdened with remorse, can it be said that he has no reason for his guilt?

I am not denying any of the usual symbolism—that the car represents his masculinity and that to surrender the keys would be castration, or that by drinking and driving he is overcoming a feeling of inadequacy. But if this man should seek psychotherapy because of guilt over the accident, it seems primary to me that he jolly well knew the risks he was taking, that he took them, and lost. And *he*, not his masculinity, is responsible.

For contrast, let us consider another example. The same man dreams of being at a party, then drinking too much, and then crashing his car. He need feel no guilt, no responsibility for this nightmare. Before he goes to sleep, he cannot make a decision about what he will

dream. Such a feat is beyond human control. Neither can he alter the events in his dream; obviously they too are beyond control. The preconditions for decision making are not present in dreaming, either in fact or in the individual's feeling about them. Without the possibility of decision making, there can be no responsibility and no freedom.

A person acts as though he possesses free will to the extent that he engages in decision making, and he experiences freedom to the degree that he feels responsible for the consequences. Decision making takes place only when the individual, whether *rightfully* or not, decides that he can critically alter the outcome of an event. It is a clinical cliché, but nonetheless true, that some people assume responsibility for behavior that others would consider to be outside the margin of personal control. Clearly the boundaries of culpability are subjectively established, and this analysis also directly implies that free will is not intrinsic to the nature of man. When an individual cannot make decisions with a sense of responsibility, he simply is not free. There are many people who cannot bear the feeling of responsibility and of possible guilt for their active decisions. And a person who will not pay the price of guilt cannot accept the cost of free will. One can say that free will is not an essential characteristic of the individual but resides instead in man's active capacity for registering his choices and preferences. A person can jail himself psychologically as easily as he can lock himself in a cell. A man may be quite capable of acting freely and yet at the same time suffer because the act of decision making *necessarily* carries in its wake the responsibility for error and failure. Indeed, it may be argued that happiness often can be purchased at the expense of freedom.

| TRADITIONAL PSYCHOANALYTIC VIEW | Actually, patients in psychotherapy, and particularly in traditional psychoanalysis, may be said to be trading precisely in this kind of currency—often purchasing a form of security at the expense of freedom. Let us examine traditional psychoanalysis and the nature of the help it offers to the neurotic.

The patient who walks into the psychiatrist's office is a desperate man. As a neurotic, he exists in a rapidly diminishing life space in which he becomes more and more uncertain of his powers and of his responsibilities. He feels pushed or pulled by maternal sighs, wifely cries, employer ties. He sees himself as a creature enfeebled by circumstances—a victim. And he has come to the analyst when everything else has failed him.

Yet the very act of seeking help indicates that the neurotic still can make a decision and follow a course of action, that he still feels some sense of responsibility for his condition. He is uncertain about what is properly within and beyond his control. But does the analyst utilize and build on the remaining nodule of responsibility? No.

First, the patient is invited to free-associate. In doing

so, he is asked to suspend his critical judgment, his powers such as they still may be to discriminate reality from fantasy. Then, of course, the patient's dreams are gone over in great detail, with emphasis on the meaningfulness of their content, despite the fact that they come without the patient's consent or control. His volitional, responsible communications thus are made subordinate to his involuntary productions. The patient initially was concerned with the extent of his responsibility for—and his increasing failure to exercise control over—his circumstances. In psychoanalysis, he is instructed that he best can understand his predicament through exhaustive examination of behavior generally regarded as outside his control.

Not only that, but the patient is invited to detail his woes while lying on a couch. Thus supine, with the analyst out of sight so that the patient will not be able to intuit approval or disapproval as indicated by facial expressions, he may "freely" associate. He will be free, that is, from noting the consequences of his behavior. Psychoanalysis is, of course, a private affair. And if an individual is having trouble coping with his life, what better place than the quiet, reflective atmosphere of the analyst's office? The patient immediately is instructed to postpone all major decisions. He gains the respectability of a prescription for what may be his trouble in the first place—inability to make a decision and to accept the consequences. And he is cut off from the significant people in his life—for him, probably a big relief.

The contemporary analyst may object that the above techniques have been much modified today, and that in any case treatment hardly stops with free association and with dream analysis, used for insights into the patient's general life style. In answer, we might say that, while methodology today may be different, there still remains the basic assumption that the behavior of the neurotic is not motivated responsibly but instead is the result of unconscious processes. When the patient leaves psychoanalysis, he is firmly assured that in all or almost all he personally is blameless.

At fault here, of course, is the general psychoanalytic conception of the origin of neurosis. Briefly, the neurotic is characterized as an individual unable to translate his instinctual impulses into proper social channels as a result of the overly restrictive and punitive child-rearing practices of his parents. According to such thinking, the patient's freedom to determine his own circumstances and life style was stunted before he could be held accountable for any action. The repressed sexual wishes of childhood haunt the man throughout his days, rendering him unable to cope adequately with his life.

If there is a strong element of predestination about my description of such thinking, let us consider from Freud's own writings just how much predetermination there is in his theories. In his analysis of a phobia in a five-year-old boy, Freud writes of Little Hans, who suffered a phobic fear of horses. Specifically, Hans was afraid that he would be bitten by a horse. Freud, taking his symbolic lens, viewed the phobia as the boy's terror of being punished (castrated) by his outraged father for sexually desiring his mother. Freud, of course, pointed out that Hans was quite unaware (unconscious) of his lust for his mother and of his fear of his father. Thus, neither in choice of symptom (the fear of horses) nor in its underlying cause (the classic Oedipus situation) did Freud make any effort to show how Hans could have avoided his neurosis. Quite the contrary. Freud describes how he allayed Little Hans' anxiety by relating that, long before Hans came into the world, he, Freud, knew that a Little Hans would be born who would love his mother and fear his father's anger. Little Hans, having no responsibility for all that happened, was introduced to predestination and was absolved. Then Freud says that upon leaving the office, the little boy looked up at his father and asked, "Does the professor talk to God?" If nothing else, one must admire the boy's powers of connecting concepts according to the evidence he was given.

Integrity Therapy

Until 1945 psychotherapy and psychoanalysis were virtually synonymous terms. In the past few years, however, there has been a very healthy development of both theory and practice in the field of psychotherapy in particular: the approach of *integrity therapy* as expounded by O. H. Mowrer, of the University of Illinois, in a series of provocative articles. As its name implies, integrity therapy epitomizes a curative process that articulates how neurosis results from the patient's active decisions, decisions for which he alone can be held accountable. During therapy, the important distinction is drawn between behavior that simply is caused and behavior that indeed is motivated. The analytical and practical importance of distinguishing between a motive and a cause perhaps can be made clear with a brief example taken from clinical practice:

Mr. A, a psychotherapy patient, disclosed in the first interview that he unconsciously did many things that indicated that he wanted to fail. To illustrate, Mr. A told of having completed a write-up for a research design for which he needed the support of his two immediate supervisors. Mr. W, the first supervisor, rejected the proposal; Mr. A was somewhat dismayed, but he took his proposal to Mr. X, the second supervisor. And then, without even being asked, he volunteered to Mr. X the information that Mr. W had rejected his write-up. The following day, the second supervisor also turned down the proposal. Mr. A felt that he literally had doomed himself. Asked why he felt that way, he replied he once had been a successful salesman. "If there's one thing a salesman knows, it's that you don't tell the customer how unsuccessful you have been trying to sell the product," he said.

Of course, Mr. A did not chide himself with a motive

for failure. Instead, he inferred an invidious operation, beyond his control, of unconscious motives (causes, really) that affected his behavior in self-defeating ways. He assumed that he was victimized by unconscious forces and thus avoided responsibility for his defeat.

I am not inclined to view the unconscious as a necessary adjunct to psychotherapy and so I simply commented to Mr. A that, since he was of the opinion that he wanted to fail, we had what amounted to a success story. He was nonplussed. "You have succeeded in failing," I said. "What is the problem?"

It soon became clear that Mr. A did everything he could to sustain his hope that he could succeed if only he didn't stand in his own way. Mr. A began to cry. It was evident that he was experiencing the full shame of his decision to avoid facing the truth about his abilities. Moreover, he knew that he still was *freely unwilling to change*, and hence the tears. Suddenly Mr. A, the same patient who moments before had aloofly related the unconscious causes for his failure, was crying bitterly. How much happier he would have been, I thought, had I been of traditional psychoanalytical persuasion and had joined with him to affirm his defense of unconscious victimhood. Instead, my therapeutic response was designed to make him face the possibility that he was being *motivated* to fail rather than merely being the innocent victim of hidden causes.

Integrity therapy tries to focus on the patient's "free" choices—his motives and decisions. Thus, although Mr. A assuredly had a history of former conflicts, we did not plunge into a distracting examination of them for their own sake. Within the framework of integrity therapy, the historical problem is viewed as contemporary in the most vital sense—the patient currently is behaving in a way that ensures the perpetuation of his neurosis. Mr. A, for instance, was motivated in his conduct neither by instinctual gratification nor by sex phantasy, but simply by the need to sustain hope for a success that he secretly feared was beyond him. Unable to accept this, he intruded his "inadvertent" mistakes that ruined things for him. Then he further intruded an imagined mental problem that he had no way of knowing or controlling.

| MOTIVES AND CAUSES | The basic point is that a distinction between motives and causes has been ignored in the deterministic approach to therapy. In his stimulating monograph, "The Concept of Motivation," R. S. Peters, of the University of London, argues that, while we can say that all motives are causes, the converse, that all causes are motives, is not necessarily so. An ankle broken while a boy plays basketball is a *cause* of his being allowed to stay home from school to rest up and soak up both the service and sympathy of his family. But a reluctance to take up again the rigors of school work, coupled with a desire to continue as the recipient of the family's service and sympathy, well may be the *motive* for a suspiciously lingering convalescence.

Freud, acute observer of the human scene that he

was, failed to make this distinction: motive involves responsibility on the part of the patient; cause, despite its psychic origins, does not necessarily relate to personal responsibility.

To Freud, the etiology of neurosis could be compared to a flu victim's being infected with virus. The flu victim fails to know what his symptoms mean simply because he is not a doctor and hence lacks necessary understanding. In the same way, the neurotic, according to Freud, has a faulty understanding of his conflict; "unconsciously" he does not want to know what it is. In Freudian theory it follows that because the neurotic's ignorance is unconsciously caused, he no more can be blamed than can the flu victim. Further, says Freud, the neurotic even carries on in his unconscious way and himself distorts the symptoms. Thus he will complain of feeling guilty because he has broken personal rules.

The Freudian psychiatrist "knows" that guilt is the result of unconscious wishes for which the patient is blameless. After all, did Little Hans really attempt to seduce his mother? If we ask why the neurotic stops short of acting upon his supposed wishes, we are brought back to the "unconscious." We are told that too-exacting practices in rearing the child produced a neurotic man full of fear and with an oversevere conscience. How then does one cure such an unconscious illness? By unconscious means, of course!

The neurotic, in the course of treatment, develops a "positive transference" and begins to attribute to the analyst celestial powers. The patient then attends to the interpretations of this "deified" analyst and purportedly gets well. The analyst, to whom he unconsciously has attributed celestial powers, absolves him from his unconscious conflict. And so the Freudian story of neurosis is one in which the neurotic unconsciously is victimized into health, just as he was victimized into illness. I can see no freedom here.

The psychoanalytic method of treatment has been challenged many times, but, until recently, Freud's basic theory has been endorsed almost wholeheartedly, *especially in its de-emphasis on free will*. Fortunately, the past few years have brought a reinterpretation of the origin of neurosis, through the work of Mowrer. In Mowrer's terms, the neurotic is guilty for his wishful impulses. Naturally, the neurotic feels guilty. He also feels himself a social outcast because *privately* he fails to live up to the standards that he endorses *publicly*. The conflict inherent in his hypocritical behavior aggravates his neurosis.

Some evidence for this point of view comes from a University of Tennessee study in which the backgrounds of twenty-five women seeking therapy at the University of Tennessee were compared with the case histories of a control group. The women with the most troubling emotional problems were those who indulged in sexual practices they actually believed were wrong.

If Mowrer's view of neurosis continues to be upheld,

the individual soon may be able to know the risks he takes with his mental health, just as he now knows some of the risks he takes with his bodily health. If he violates his "principles," his chances of falling victim to neurosis are increased significantly, just as his chances of coming down with pneumonia are increased if he walks bare-chested through Central Park in late December.

Recalling my Mr. A, who so wanted to be reassured that his failures were not his fault, I wonder if the more rigorous and more realistic practice of psychotherapy as outlined by Mowrer ever will be as popular as the Freudian school. A neurotic by the very nature of his illness is quite pleased to shuck off responsibility for whatever personality traits disturb him or upset those close to him. The psychoanalyzed neurotic has purchased an anesthesia called peace of mind, which allows him to act out his life while at crucial moments refusing all responsibility for his actions and their consequences. Such a man is not free. But his situation brings us to a universal problem and to a question for the future of psychotherapy: Can a man live with the knowledge that he and he alone is responsible for his decisions?

What Makes Men Feel Free?

According to sociologist Karl Mannheim, it is entirely unrealistic to expect that man can exist in the context of unlimited choice; a certain degree of conformity is necessary. Probably quite true, but what degree? And where should man exercise his freedom? These well may be areas for psychology to define. Psychology can play a vital role in securing an empirical basis that permits man to exercise his freedom effectively. To do so, psychological knowledge must free man from ignorance and warn him of some of the dangers implicit in his free choice of how he is to live his life. As a physician would warn a youth against heroin by giving information about addiction, so could the psychologist warn man of the addictive (and therefore enslaving) nature of certain mental stimuli. We all have heard, of course, of the big-lie technique, perfected by the man whom I introduced at the beginning of this article. The big lie, if repeated often enough, becomes a soporific on the critical powers of the mind. A subject who thus has been desensitized to reality ceases to be able to make free decisions, but rather he reacts involuntarily to the big lie.

An example of how psychological knowledge brings freedom is in the role it has played in effecting the freedom of women. Psychological knowledge has allowed women to admit to pleasure in sexual love and to make more of their own decisions about sexual love. Also, in hand with medical science, it has allowed women to determine how many children they will have.

Within the Freudian perspective, man cannot determine the strength and magnitude of his sexual motives; at best he only decides on their manner of expression. Freud construed man as having to express behaviorally some optimal quota of his sexuality or suffer from psychic consequences. Thus Freudian man is the victim of his own uncontrolled and scarcely known sexual forces. Actually, there is evidence that, rather than circumscribing fixed needs, man's sexual constitution exhibits considerable malleability. Kenneth Hardy has advanced an appetitive theory of sexual motivation that argues that mere exercise of sexuality increases one's subsequent sexual appetite. Should the appetite theory of sexual motivation continue to be consistent with accumulating empirical evidence, psychology soon may advance to a point where decision making and freedom of choice will affect an area long regarded as a closed system. That is, man will neither fear his sexual drives as somehow sinful, nor will he resign himself to a sexual life predestined for him from the cradle. Rather, he may decide for himself how, and how much, to use his sexual drive, somewhat as he decides how and how much to indulge his appetite for food. In all of this we have an increase of knowledge and of free choice, and hence of responsibility.

Since I seem to have employed Freud for a whipping boy in discussing free will, I should explain that the choice hardly was arbitrary. Freud's heavy emphasis on the "irrational" factors governing human behavior has been the major influence in twentieth-century psychology. In the *Psychopathology of Everyday Life*, published in 1904, Freud discusses the very issue of free will. But the principal goal of that investigation was to show that even the seemingly trivial, unmotivated, "accidental" behaviors of everyday life were "determined" by unconscious "causes." In 1904, psychoanalysis seemed upon the threshold of predicting what had been regarded as unpredictable—accidents. Unfortunately, Freud's slim volume today remains the most definitive statement yet made on the subject. We have ventured little beyond the threshold.

But if psychology would investigate what makes men feel free, I am convinced the findings would not contradict the view that behavior is lawful and predictable. The motivational conditions that make men feel free clearly represent another line of study from scientific causality. The latter can reveal what man actually does, while the former dwells upon what he thinks he does. Certainly the realm of man's thought is truly the area of human life that should be peculiarly his own.

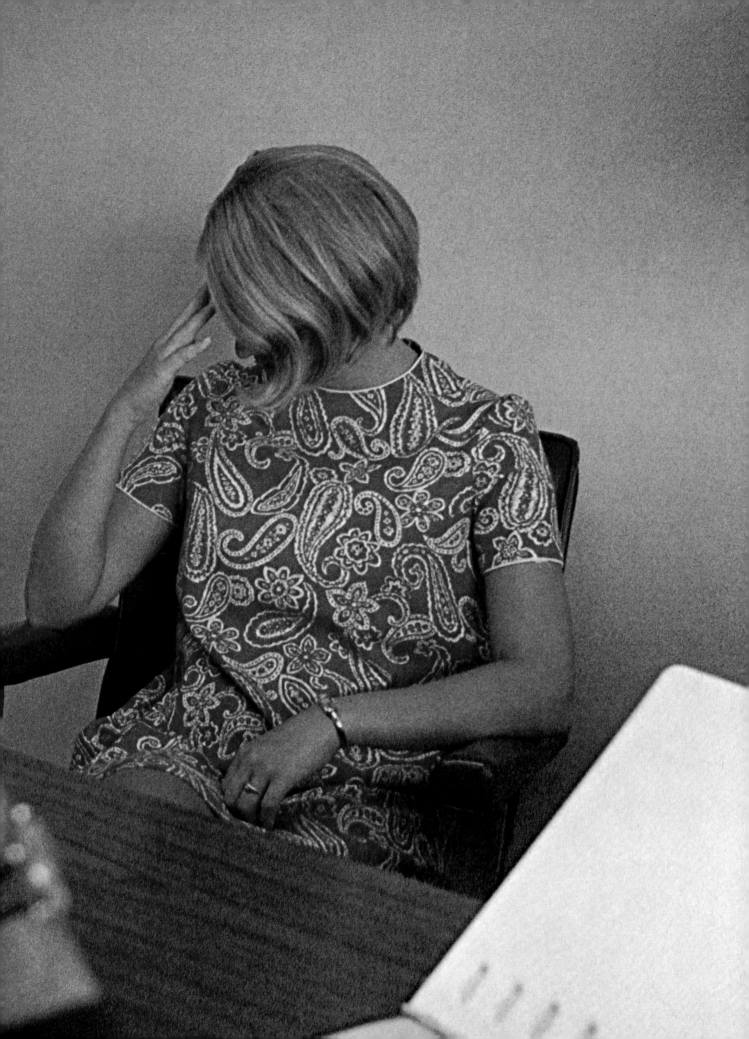

Inside Psychotherapy
David E. Orlinsky and Kenneth I. Howard

What do patients think of their therapy sessions? Do they find them pleasant? Unpleasant but helpful? Do people enter therapy with well-defined attitudes and expectations? Do they expect the therapist to behave in a prescribed manner? Are the goals of the patient congruent with those of the therapist? David Orlinsky and Kenneth Howard attempted to answer such inquiries into the subjective experience of psychotherapy by having patients and therapists complete questionnaires immediately after therapy sessions. They found three different patterns of patient-therapist encounter, so they caution against the conventional one theory–one treatment approach to psychotherapy.

How a person's internal expectancies influence his external behaviors is of high interest. For instance, individuals led to believe that a certain drug will make them euphoric indeed report euphoria after taking it, whereas in persons expecting the opposite, the same drug creates anxiety. Similarly, children expected by teachers to show gains in IQ scores actually do show gains. Such findings imply that in the case of psychotherapy, both the therapist's and the patient's expectancies may significantly affect therapeutic outcome. The method used by Orlinsky and Howard could also be turned to measuring the presence and effects of such expectancies, which might then be harnessed in aid of therapeutic change.

Psychotherapy has been described by some as the confessional of the secular man, and as the weekday solace of the overeducated and underemployed suburban housewife. It has also been presented as the individual's best hope for attaining self-knowledge and personal authenticity in a confused and troubled society.

Because of its important place in our culture, psychotherapy has been put on frequent display in novels, films, and plays—sometimes humorously and sometimes with serious intent. Yet with all this publicity, what do we actually know about psychotherapy? What takes place after patient and therapist disappear behind the closed office door? What is the experience of psychotherapy really like?

The theories and case histories of psychotherapists offer some answers, and so do the observations and evaluations of scientific researchers. But each of these sources has limitations. The clinical literature, though often suggestive and sometimes brilliant, is almost always impressionistic and purely qualitative. The re-search literature, though more systematic and quantitative, comprises chiefly objective observations by nonparticipants and after-the-fact evaluations. Such studies provide valuable knowledge, but they give no information about what the patients and therapists see, hear, and feel during their sessions; about what they want from therapy; or about what they think of their psychotherapy.

Our desire to obtain reliable, precise information about psychotherapy as a subjective experience—to find out, in a precise, systematic, and quantitative way, how the people who participate in psychotherapy see and feel it—led us to develop the Psychotherapy Session Project, based on reports from patients and therapists themselves.

For subjects, we turned to a group of patients and therapists at the Katharine Wright Mental Health Clinic in Chicago. During the first six months of the study, sixty patients filled out reports on a total of 890 sessions, and seventeen therapists completed questionnaires on a total of 470 sessions. All patients were being seen in individual outpatient psychotherapy, and almost all had sessions once a week. All the patients were women between twenty and sixty years of age, but most were on the younger side—their average age was twenty-eight. In general, the patients were well educated: 90 percent had finished high school, and a third had completed college or graduate studies. More than 80 percent were employed, and 25 percent were currently married.

The therapists who participated were both men and women. They had been trained in psychiatry, clinical psychology, or psychiatric social work, with an average of six years' experience in the practice of psychotherapy. Most of them acknowledged some influence of Freud on their thinking and practice, but few would consider themselves psychoanalytically oriented in a strict sense. Like most clinicians, they draw upon a variety of approaches.

The reports were made independently by each patient and therapist as soon as possible after the session was over, while the experience was still fresh in their minds. We used two parallel questionnaires, one for patients and one for therapists, to survey various aspects of the therapy experience (see Table 1).

The questionnaires took only ten or fifteen minutes to complete because they called for simple descriptions and evaluations rather than lengthy analyses. Before the first study, the questionnaires were trial-tested with a substantial number of therapists and patients, and modified where necessary. We tried to avoid the terminology of any special theoretical school or orientation but to include issues that are meaningful to most of them. The confidentiality of each person's answers was strictly assured so he could feel free to give his honest reactions to the questions.

The Typical Session

To gain a composite picture of the typical therapy experience, we tabulated the most frequently endorsed responses of patients and therapists to the items on the questionnaires (see Table 2). What patients seemed to want most in coming to therapy was to deepen their understanding of personal problems that they have difficulty talking about and, presumably, difficulty dealing with. This deepened understanding might be expected to alleviate the problems, or at least to help the patient deal with them more comfortably and more effectively. As they tried to move toward these goals, patients talked most frequently about themselves as they are in their present intimate social relations and vocational settings.

This contradicts the expectations based on clinical theory, which call for talk about relations with parents or siblings, memories of childhood experiences, and dreams or fantasies.

Though patients might find their sessions helpful,

TABLE 1
Patient Questionnaire*

1. **How do you feel about the therapy session which you have just completed?** [Alternatives from "one of the best" to "really poor session"]

2. **What did you talk about during this session?** [Checklist of 18 topics representing basic areas of life concerns]

3. **What did you want or hope to get out of this therapy session?** [Checklist of 20 potential patient goals]

4. **How did you act towards your therapist during this session?** [Checklist of 16 types of interpersonal behavior]

5. **How did you feel during this session?** [Checklist of 45 feelings]

6. **To what extent were you looking forward to coming to this session?** [Alternatives from "could hardly wait" to "had to make myself come"]

7. **How freely were you able to talk with your therapist during this session?** [Alternatives from "a great deal of difficulty" to "didn't have any difficulty in talking"]

8. **How clearly did you know what you wanted to talk about during this session?** [Alternatives from "knew clearly" to "my mind was blank"]

9. **How well did your therapist seem to understand how you were feeling and what was really on your mind during this session?** [Alternatives from "understood very well" to "misunderstood"]

10. **Do you feel that what your therapist said and did this session was helpful to you?** [Alternatives from "very helpful" to "made me worse off than I was"]

11. **Do you feel that you made progress in this session in dealing with the problems for which you are in therapy?** [Alternatives from "considerable progress" to "my problems got worse"]

12. **How well do you feel that you are getting along, emotionally and psychologically, at this time?** [Alternatives from "the way I would like" to "I can barely manage"]

13. **What do you feel that you got out of this session?** [Checklist of nine possible satisfactions]

14. **To what extent are you looking forward to your next session?** [Alternatives from "wish it were sooner" to "not so sure I will want to come"]

15. **How did your therapist act towards you during this session?** [Checklist of 16 types of interpersonal behavior]

16. **How did your therapist seem to feel during this session?** [Checklist of 34 feelings]

The only major difference between patient and therapist questionnaires was question 13. Therapists were asked, "In what direction were you working with your patient during this session?"

they did not, as a rule, find them pleasant. They tended to feel anxious and tense during interviews—understandably, perhaps, since they were trying to discuss and work out their most difficult personal problems. However, patients did appear to be actively and positively involved in the therapy relationship. This contrasts somewhat with their problematic concerns and felt distress. Patients come to a therapist for help but do not seem particularly helpless, at least in relating to him.

Inspection of the therapists' responses showed that patient and therapist generally worked toward the same

TABLE 2
The Typical Therapy Experience
(Collated from questionnaire data)

Patient wants to:	Get a better understanding of my feelings and behavior. Get help in talking about what is really troubling me. Work out a problem that I have. Work together with my therapist on a person-to-person basis. Get advice on how to deal with my life and with other people.
Patient talks about:	Feelings and attitudes toward myself. Social activities and relationships, friends and acquaintances. Relationship with spouse, boyfriend or girlfriend.
Patient feels:	Anxious Tense
Patient relates by:	Initiating topics. Engaging in a give-and-take relationship. Being friendly. Being emotional or stirred up.
Therapist tries to:	Increase my patient's insight and self-understanding. Move my patient closer to experiencing her real feelings, what she really is. Engage my patient in an honest person-to-person relationship, work together authentically.
Therapist feels:	Interested Calm Involved Alert Confident Sympathetic
Therapist relates by:	Interacting, working together. Engaging in give-and-take relationship. Being friendly. Being emotionally responsive, stirred.
Patient gets:	A sense of having an honest person-to-person relationship with my therapist, of working together. Help in being able to talk about what was troubling to me and really important. Better insight and self-understanding.

goals, with some difference in nuance and detail. Patients, for example, were inclined to seek advice about their problems; therapists were less inclined to offer advice and wanted their patients to experience feelings rather than merely talk about them.

As one might expect, therapists generally felt comfortable with and positively responsive to their patients. (The joke that is told to beginning therapists, optimistically describing a therapist as the *less* anxious of the two persons in the room, seems to be borne out by the facts.) Our research showed that the popular image of the therapist as a reserved, neutral, unresponsive person seems to be a mistaken view. Therapists related to their patients the same way patients related to them: collaboratively, positively, and feelingly.

Returning to the patients, what benefits did they find in their sessions? The most frequently reported satisfactions were a sense of honestly working together with the therapist, help in talking about important troubling matters, and better self-understanding. Thus patients typically did find what they sought in coming to therapy, and what their therapists hoped to give them. The process was often emotionally trying but, with their therapists' active support, the patients seemed to achieve helpful self-understanding.

The Ideal Session

Psychotherapy as it occurs in the typical session is undoubtedly a mixture of better and worse experiences. In order to deepen our understanding of essential therapeutic processes and to develop more effective practices, we felt it was desirable to isolate the better elements of the experience—to portray psychotherapy at its best (see Table 3). A composite picture of the "ideal" experience—the aims, feelings, and so forth that *distinguish* the ideal session—was drawn from our

TABLE 3
The Ideal Therapy Experience
(Collated from questionnaire data)

Patient wants to:	Get a better understanding of my feelings and behavior. Let my therapist see how I've improved. Work together with my therapist on a person-to-person basis.		
Patient talks about:	Relationship with spouse, boyfriend or girlfriend. Dreams, fantasies. Social activities and relationships, friends and acquaintances. Childhood experiences with family members and feelings about them.		
Patient feels:	Relieved Trusting Accepted Optimistic Alert	Interested Likeable Calm Relaxed Secure	Confident Satisfied Effective Energetic
Patient relates by:	Initiating topics. Interacting, working together. Engaging in give-and-take relationship. Being friendly. Being emotional.		
Therapist tries to:	Increase my patient's insight and self-understanding. Move my patient closer to experiencing her real feelings, what she really is. Support my patient's self-esteem.		
Therapist feels:	Optimistic Satisfied Close Involved Effective	Alert Pleased Interested Sympathetic	Confident Intimate Tender Attracted
Therapist relates by:	Interacting, working together. Engaging in give-and-take relationship. Being emotionally responsive, stirred.		
Patient gets:	All listed satisfactions.		

data by noting the responses that correlated most highly with patients' and therapists' evaluations of the overall quality of their sessions.

Both the ideal and the average therapy experience included a desire on the patient's part for self-understanding and collaborative involvement with the therapist. The wish for insight and collaboration, present in the typical experience, was simply *more intense* in the ideal experience. And in the ideal experience, patients wanted to display their gains and successes to the therapist rather than to present their problems or solicit help and advice. The accent was on the positive, perhaps because some real gains were being made.

The better the session, the less emphasis patients placed on discussing immediate feelings about themselves. Instead, they stressed dreams or fantasies and memories of childhood experiences with family members, subjects that theoretically reflect underlying or unconscious patterns of motivation. The ideal session came closer than the typical one to clinical expectations of what is most profitable to discuss in therapy.

The patients' feelings during the ideal session were quite different from those reported for the typical session. Instead of feeling anxious and tense, patients felt confident and pleased. On the other hand, the way patients acted toward their therapists was essentially the same in the ideal and the typical experiences. They were, presumably, *more* friendly, *more* interactive, and so forth in the ideal case than in the typical one. As might be expected, in the ideal session patients reported getting *all* the satisfactions listed on the questionnaire. This finding strengthens our confidence in the validity of their overall evaluations.

Therapists' goals in the ideal and typical sessions were essentially the same. These goals corresponded, in general, to what is prescribed by theories of psychotherapy. However, in the ideal session the therapists' goals also included support for the self-esteem of their patients. (The tendency to be rewarding or encouraging, like the patients' concern to show improvement, may be greater once real gains are at hand.)

In the ideal session, therapists felt more alert and effective, but also warmer and more personally involved, than in the typical session. Their way of relating to patients was essentially the same in the ideal as in the typical session, only more so. Patients and therapists approached each other in much the same way, except that patients generally took more initiative in determining what was discussed in the session.

The typical session and the ideal session have many features in common, suggesting that by and large the average experience is a good one—or at least that the typical experience is considerably closer to the best than it is to the worst. But we must remember, too, that the ideal therapy experience is an abstraction, a composite of positive tendencies within the many real experiences of different patients and different therapists. It is not safe to assume that there is only one type of good therapy experience, or only one way to achieve it.

Indeed, we are warned against any such conclusion by other analyses of the questionnaires, which revealed at least three distinct positive patterns in the relationship between patient and therapist. Because these patterns emerge, independently or together, in any relationship, we have called them "therapeutic potentials." A brief description of what they are and how they were found should help illuminate the more complex connections between the typical and ideal patterns of therapy experience.

In the Psychotherapy Session Project, we have been interested in how the experiences of individual patients and therapists differed from one another, as well as in average or composite patterns. To study these differences, and to define empirically the dimensions along which individual variation occurs, we applied the statistical technique of factor analysis. We analyzed the experiences of patients and of therapists separately, and then combined the results of these and analyzed the experiences of patient-therapist pairs together in order to determine the patterns of "conjoint experience" within the relationship. Three therapeutic potentials—"collaborative analytic progress," "healing magic," and "mutual personal openness"—were defined.

"Collaborative analytic progress" is the type of good therapy relationship described in the psychoanalytic literature. It is marked by an effective "therapeutic alliance," or task-oriented collaboration, between patient and therapist; by an emotionally involving but basically cognitive ("analytic") exploration of the patient's significant problems and relationships; and by a sense of forward movement or progress in understanding. The role of the therapist in this pattern of good therapy experience is that of a "head shrinker," or as younger and more hip patients sometimes say with affection, a "shrink." The image of head shrinking appears to refer both to the characteristic *reduction* of emotional problems through their verbal intellectual formulation, and to the *deflating* effect that recognition of one's less attractive unconscious desires has on the patient's ego.

"Healing magic," on the other hand, is marked by a very positive, enthusiastic, happy response on the part of the patient, who feels greatly helped by the effective power and benevolent acceptance of the therapist. In this type of good therapy experience it seems that it is not so much what the therapist does that counts as it is the personal qualities that the patient perceives in him. The therapist appears to enter the patient's experience as a "good parent" whose concern and acceptance are a balm to hurt feelings. This pattern, known in the psychoanalytic literature as "positive transference," has been likened to a kind of therapeutic honeymoon. Patients sometimes refer to their therapists in this type of positive experience as the "Wizard" (or simply as

"Wiz") because of the power he seems to have to make them feel better. (Both the Wizard of Oz and Gandalf, the good wizard in Tolkien's *Lord of the Rings,* come to mind as possible prototypes.) One's tendency in this rationalistic age is to disbelieve in the potency of magic. But only those who have never experienced charismatic influence (or who have never been in love) can doubt that it has real effects in the realm of interpersonal relations.

"Mutual personal openness" is the type of good therapy experience that has been most fully described and advocated in existential, experiential, and recent client-centered writings on psychotherapy. In our sampling this pattern was marked by a sense of equality, trust, and personal openness between patient and therapist. The therapist did not appear as a superior or as an impersonal being whose private reactions are hidden from view. Each participant had confidence in himself and confidence in the other, which permitted mutual sharing of "confidences" in a more intimate manner than had been the custom in a "professional" relationship. Mutual personal openness included, on the therapist's part, a willingness to be frankly evaluative and confronting with the patient: to let the patient know what was on his mind. This honest availability of the therapist's personal reactions to the patient was matched, on the patient's part, by a greater willingness or capacity to make inner feelings and fantasies known to the therapist. The patient and therapist appeared to esteem and to treat each other as adult persons who can "take it." Because of the personal nature of the encounter, the patient is frequently on a first-name basis with the therapist: the patient calls the therapist "Carl," for example, rather than "Doctor So-and-so."

Each of the three therapeutic potentials was reflected in the composite ideal therapy experience. The influ-ence of "collaborative analytic progress" is seen in the desire of both patient and therapist to work together to deepen the patient's insight and self-understanding. It can also be seen in the topical focus on dreams and on memories of childhood experiences with important family members.

The influence of "healing magic," on the other hand, is found in the euphoric quality of the patients' feelings and in their reports that, in the ideal therapy experi-ence, they received all the satisfactions listed on the questionnaire.

The effect of "mutual personal openness" can be traced in the sharing, give-and-take, emotionally respon-sive manner in which both patients and therapists related to each other, and in the heightened personal involvement shown in the therapists' reports of their own feelings.

Thus the evidence now available indicates at least three paths toward an experience that has therapeutic value. And this evidence may suggest a "three-factor theory" of therapeutic efficacy. The three types of experience are independent but not mutually exclusive, and they seem to be rooted in the potentials of the psychotherapy relationship as a helping and helpful experience. Further exploration along these lines may resolve some of the current differences between the various theoretical orientations to psychotherapy, each of which appears to stress one or another of these therapeutic potentials and to neglect the rest of them.

What we have learned from the Psychotherapy Ses-sion Project thus far is particularly exciting to us be-cause it is based on a scientific analysis of the subjective experience of psychotherapy. It has given us an impor-tant glimpse "inside psychotherapy." As results come in from other studies now in progress, we hope this glimpse will become a much broader view.

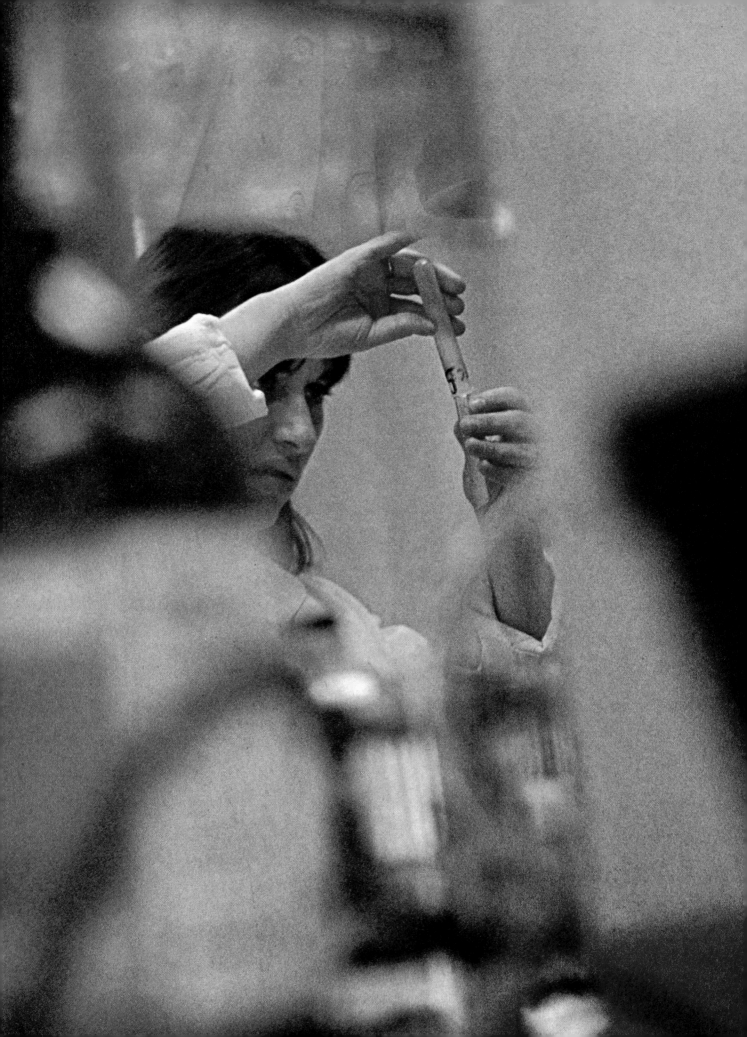

The Psychopharmacological Revolution

Murray E. Jarvik

Psychopharmacology is a relatively new scientific discipline; in the past fifteen years many new chemical agents have been developed to treat anxiety, depression, and even psychosis. In this area, biochemists, experimental psychologists, and clinical psychologists must work closely together for therapeutic success. Murray Jarvik here presents a brief history of drug use—including use of such nontherapeutic agents as hashish, marijuana, and LSD, which are the subject of so much current public concern. He also presents the results of recent studies into chemical agents prescribed for treatment. He outlines the chemical structure of groups of drugs, their clinical effects, and the known or hypothesized biochemical mechanisms by which they work.

Drug use in psychological treatment is widespread; although we may not yet have entered the "Brave New World," tranquilizers and "pep pills" are prescribed for millions throughout the world. This fact alone makes the study of psychopharmacology a vital one—for the now generation and their posterity.

One hot August evening in 1955, Helen Burney sat listlessly on her bed in the violent ward of the large Texas hospital where she had been confined for the past four months. During most of that unhappy time, Helen had been highly vocal, abusive, and overactive. Only the day before she had tried to strike a ward aide, but immediately several burly attendants had grabbed her, roughly tying her into a straitjacket and pinioning her arms against her chest. But today Helen's behavior was very different. Her incessant talking and shouting had stopped; all day long she spoke only when spoken to; most of the time she lay on her bed with her eyes half closed, moving little, and looking rather pale. However, she was unusually cooperative with the nursing personnel, got out of bed when told to, and went to the dining room without resisting. What had happened to bring about this remarkable change?

That morning she had received an injection of a new synthetic drug, chlorpromazine, which had been discovered a few years earlier in France. On the same day thousands of mental patients throughout the world were receiving the same drug, many of them for the first time. News of the drug's usefulness had spread rapidly in the preceding months, and it was being tried in mental hospitals throughout the world. Few of those taking or administering the drug realized that they were participating in a revolution in psychiatric treatment. In fact, many psychiatrists felt that this drug would be no more effective in treating schizophrenia than the other drugs that had previously been tried with little success. But they were wrong—and luckily, too—for there was little else they could offer the masses of impoverished patients who clogged the mental institutions all over the world. Soon it would be difficult to find a psychotic patient who was not receiving a drug of some kind for the treatment of his illness. The era of clinical psychopharmacology had begun, and the new drugs were hailed as the first real breakthrough in the treatment of one of man's most serious and mysterious afflictions—psychosis.

Until it was discovered that drugs could help the severely disturbed, almost the only recourse in the management of such patients was physical restraint. Philippe Pinel, the famous French psychiatrist, campaigning for humane treatment of the insane at the end of the eighteenth century, freed the inmates of the grim

Bicêtre mental hospital from their iron chains. Unfortunately, other physical restraints had to be substituted when patients became assaultive or destructive, and though the padded cell and the camisole, or straitjacket, may have been softer than chains, they allowed no greater freedom. Not until the mid-1950s did drugs finally promise total emancipation from physical restraint for most patients. Despite the fears of some psychiatrists, psychologists, and social workers that the social and psychological factors contributing to mental illness would be ignored, the use of psychopharmaceuticals radically improved the treatment of the mentally ill within and without the hospital. Indeed, only with their use has it been possible for some families to be held together, for some individuals to be gainfully employed, and for some patients to be reached by psychotherapy.

Since 1955, psychopharmacology has burgeoned as an important scientific discipline in its own right. In the past fifteen years, many new chemical agents have been developed for the treatment of each major category of mental illness. These drugs include phenothiazines, rauwolfia alkaloids, butyrophenones, propanediol and benzodiazepine compounds, monoamine oxidase (MAO) inhibitors, dibenzazepine derivatives, and many more. They have been found useful in the treatment of psychoses, neuroses, and depressions. Even autistic behavior, psychopathy, sexual deviation, and mental retardation have been attacked with drugs, but clinical psychopharmacologists feel that the surface has only been scratched in these areas. The search continues, though presently on a smaller scale than in the past, for more effective agents.

Folk Psychopharmacology

Although as a full-fledged scientific discipline, psychopharmacology is less than fifteen years old, the psychological effects of drugs have piqued the curiosity of occasional researchers for almost a hundred years. Indeed, it is surprising that interest was so slow in developing, for man's empirical knowledge of the effects of drugs on behavior is both ancient and widespread.

The records of mankind, going back thousands of years, are filled with anecdotal and clinical reports of the psychological action of drugs obtained from plants. Though we can be sure that most of these folk remedies were merely placebos, a few have demonstrable medicinal properties and are still in use today. The cuneiform tablets of ancient Assyria contain numerous references to medicinal preparations with psychological effects. For more than 5,000 years, the Chinese have used the herb Ma Huang (yellow astringent), which contains the potent stimulant, ephedrine, and in the earliest writings of China, Egypt, and the Middle East there are references to the influence of various drugs on behavior.

In the first century before Christ, the Roman poet Horace wrote lyrically of the psychological effects of alcohol: "What wonders does not wine! It discloses secrets; ratifies and confirms our hopes; thrusts the coward forth to battle; eases the anxious mind of its burthen; instructs in arts. Whom has not a cheerful glass made eloquent! Whom not quite free and easy from pinching poverty!" And "In vino veritas" was already a familiar Roman adage when it was cited by Pliny.

Opium, an effective folk remedy, is mentioned in the Ebers papyrus, and Homer tells us that Helen of Troy took a "sorrow-easing drug" obtained from Egypt— probably opium. Although the analgesic and sedative properties of opium were extensively described in classical literature, little was said about its addictive properties until Thomas de Quincey hinted at them, early in the nineteenth century, in his Confessions of an English Opium Eater. And while the chemical isolation of morphine and the invention of the hypodermic needle, in the middle of the nineteenth century, made profound addiction truly feasible, morphine is still considered by many physicians the most essential drug they use— "God's own remedy."

Morphine and its derivatives and analogues (for example, heroin) are self-administered by countless thousands of people throughout the world, although in many countries, especially in the West, such use is illegal. The practice persists, nevertheless, perhaps for the reasons given by the French poet, Jean Cocteau, who was himself an addict: "Everything that we do in life, including love, is done in an express train traveling towards death. To smoke opium is to leave the train while in motion; it is to be interested in something other than life and death."

Like morphine, cocaine is another vegetable product discovered by primitive man. It is clearly not a placebo, and its use is illegal. The Indians of Peru have chewed coca leaves for centuries, and still do, to relieve hunger, fatigue, and the general burdens of a miserable life. The alkaloid cocaine was isolated in 1859, and its systematic use was not only practiced but advocated by such respected figures as Sigmund Freud and William Halsted, as well as by the legendary Sherlock Holmes. It is highly doubtful that the continued use of cocaine produces a physiological dependence. Today, cocaine-taking is relatively uncommon in the northern hemisphere.

On the other hand, an ancient drug that remains exceedingly popular, though its medical uses today are nil, is marijuana, the dried leaves of the hemp plant Cannabis sativa. Cannabis is so ubiquitous, and grows so easily, that its widespread use is not surprising. Marco Polo is credited with bringing the "Green Goddess" to the Occident, although Herodotus tells us that the Scythians inhaled the vapor, obtained by heating hemp seeds on red-hot stones, and then "shouted for joy." To this day, cannabis is almost always smoked; this allows its active ingredients to be absorbed into the pulmonary blood circulation and, avoiding the liver, to be promptly carried to the brain. Similarly, the active ingredients of opium and tobacco are usually self-administered by inhalation of the vapors from heated plant products.

Hashish, derived from *cannabis*, and smoked, chewed, or drunk, has been widely used for centuries throughout the Middle East. The Arabic term for a devotee of hashish is "hashshash"; from the plural, "hashshashin," comes the English word "assassin," for at the time of the Crusades, the Hashshashin were a fanatical secret Moslem sect who terrorized the Christians by swift and secret murder, after having taken hashish to give themselves courage. Richard Burton, the famous traveler, adventurer, and writer, described his experiences with hashish during a pilgrimage to Mecca at the end of the nineteenth century. About fifty years earlier, Moreau de Tours suggested that physicians should take hashish in order to experience mental illness and thereby understand it better. Claude Bernard, the great French physiologist, is said to have declared that "hashish is the curare of the mind." Today we know a great deal about the mode of action of curare and almost nothing about that of hashish, but Bernard suggested a working hypothesis. Perhaps *cannabis*, like curare, blocks some vital neurohumor in the brain.

Quantitative, objective studies of *cannabis* are rare, even today. However, a recent report by Carlini indicates that *cannabis* facilitates maze-learning in rats. In the absence of comparative studies, it is difficult to say how *cannabis* resembles or differs from other drugs; anecdotal reports suggest that it resembles lysergic acid diethylamide (LSD).

Another drug with a long history of use is *mescaline* or *peyote*, which the Aztecs are credited with having used five centuries ago, and which has been and still is used by certain Indians of Central America and the southwest United States. Its effects resemble those of marijuana and LSD; they have also been compared with those of *psilocybin*, a drug that the Aztecs derived from a psychotogenic mushroom they called "teonanacatl," or "God's flesh."

The Chemical Era

Until the nineteenth century, the only drugs known to affect behavior were those derived from plants and long familiar to mankind. With advances in chemistry during the first half of the nineteenth century, however, the general anesthetics, including nitrous oxide, diethyl ether, and chloroform were discovered and brought into widespread use; and by the time Emil Kraepelin began his psychopharmacological investigations in the 1880s, a few new sedatives, including the bromides and chloral hydrate, were available.

Nitrous oxide, an artificially prepared inhalation anesthetic, was investigated by Sir Humphrey Davy, who described its effects thus in 1799: "I lost all connections with external things; trains of vivid images rapidly passed through my mind and even connected with words in such a manner as to produce perceptions perfectly novel. I existed in a world of newly connected and newly modified ideas."

Inhaling nitrous oxide soon became a favorite student diversion, and enterprising showmen charged admission for public demonstrations of its effects; the popular interest in this gas reminds one very much of the current preoccupation with LSD. But though nitrous oxide was beguiling to thrill seekers, it never became as popular as LSD, perhaps because the gas is difficult to transport.

Although *diethyl ether* was originally prepared in 1543 by Valerius Cordus when he distilled alcohol with sulfuric acid, its potential as an anesthetic remained unknown for 300 years until Crawford Long and William Morton first used it clinically in the 1840s. Ether parties subsequently became popular among students, although the drug's extreme flammability probably discouraged more widespread popular use. *Chloroform* was introduced about the same time as ether, but its toxic effects upon the heart, recognized almost immediately, discouraged its nonmedical use. It was not known for many years that the liver, also, is severely damaged by this drug.

Chloral hydrate, a powerful sleep-producing drug, was introduced into medicine in 1869 but has been generally ignored by experimental psychologists—though not by the underworld where, in the form of "knockout drops" mixed with alcohol, it has been the active ingredient of the "Mickey Finn." *Paraldehyde*, first used in 1882, has similarly been eschewed by psychological investigators, perhaps because of its extremely unpleasant odor; nevertheless, it has been used extensively for many years in mental institutions for producing temporary narcosis in dangerously violent patients, especially those with delirium tremens from alcohol withdrawal.

Bromides, particularly potassium bromide, slowly gained popularity during the nineteenth century to the point where millions of people were taking them as sedatives. Unlike the barbiturates however, the bromides produce psychoses involving delirium, delusions, or hallucinations, as well as a variety of neurological and dermatological disturbances. For a time, chronic toxicity resulting from continued use of these compounds became a leading cause of admission to mental hospitals. Bromide is still a common ingredient in headache remedies, "nerve tonics," and over-the-counter sleeping medications.

The Antipsychotic Drugs

With the antipsychotic drugs, as happens more often than is supposed, use preceded research. The ancient preparation, Indian snakeroot powder, mentioned more than 2,500 years ago in the Hindu Ayurvedic writings, deserves at least as much credit for ushering in the era of clinical psychopharmacology as does the modern synthetic drug, chlorpromazine. According to the ancient doctrine of signs, since the roots of the plant *Rauwolfia serpentina* were snakelike, they were administered for snakebite. Snakeroot was also used for insomnia and insanity—quite rational uses, in view of modern findings—as well as for epilepsy and dysentery, which it actually aggravates, and for a host of other conditions for which its value is questionable.

The first scientific intimation that Indian snakeroot might be useful in mental illness came in 1931 when Sen and Bose published an article in the *Indian Medical World* entitled "*Rauwolfia serpentina*, a New Indian Drug for Insanity and High Blood Pressure." But this suggestion was not confirmed for almost a quarter of a century. *Rauwolfia* began to attract the attention of the Western world only in 1949, when Rustom Valkil advocated it for hypertension, and the Swiss pharmaceutical firm, Ciba, subsequently isolated the active ingredient, which they named *reserpine*. In 1953 a Boston physician, Robert Wilkins, confirmed that reserpine was effective in the treatment of hypertension, and a year later a New York psychiatrist, Nathan Kline, announced that he had found reserpine useful in the treatment of psychotic disorders. Soon numerous psychiatrists in other parts of the world corroborated Kline's results, and the use of reserpine spread with amazing speed. When Frederick Yonkman at Ciba used the term "tranquilizing" to describe the calming effect of reserpine, the word "tranquilizer" entered all modern languages to designate a drug that quiets hyperactive or anxious patients.

The subsequent clinical history of reserpine is a strange one. Reserpine and chlorpromazine were twin heralds of the dawn of psychopharmacological treatment, but the popularity of reserpine in the treatment of mental disease has dwindled until today, a decade and a half later, its use has been practically abandoned for such therapy while chlorpromazine is still the leading antipsychotic drug. Yet there are many studies that attest to the efficacy of *rauwolfia* and its derivatives in the treatment of psychiatric disorders; probably its tendency to produce depression was one of the chief reasons for its near demise. Furthermore, chlorpromazine has spawned scores of offspring-phenothiazines, widely used for the mentally ill.

Like reserpine, *chlorpromazine*'s usefulness as an antipsychotic drug was discovered more or less by accident. In the early 1950s the French surgeon, Henri Laborit, introduced chlorpromazine into clinical anesthesia as a successor to promethazine, known to be a sedative antihistamine capable of heightening the effect of other drugs. It was noticed that chlorpromazine reduced anxiety in surgical patients and enabled them to face their ordeal with indifference. This led to its trial with agitated psychotics, whom it calmed with dramatic effectiveness. In 1954 the drug was released

commercially in North America by Smith, Kline and French as an antiemetic, but shortly thereafter it was tried with psychiatric patients. Large-scale controlled studies by the United States Veterans' Administration and by the Psychopharmacology Service Center of the National Institute of Mental Health showed chlorpromazine and the related phenothiazines to be useful in the treatment of acute schizophrenia. Other studies show that phenothiazines help discharged mental patients to stay out of the hospital. A drug with ubiquitous actions on all body systems, chlorpromazine has been used in the treatment of anxiety and tension, depression, mental retardation, senility, drug addiction, pain, nausea and vomiting, and spasticity. Since its mechanisms of action are still not known, it is difficult to delimit the validity of these applications.

Antianxiety Drugs

Anxiety is such a common experience that everyone reading this article has a subjective understanding of the term. It may be defined as an unpleasant state associated with a threatening situation, and is closely allied to fear. Sedative hypnotic drugs including alcohol, barbiturates, bromides, and chloral hydrate, have frequently been employed for the treatment of anxiety. In 1955 a number of new drugs with properties common to the sedative hypnotics were introduced for the treatment of anxiety, but the most successful of these, by far, was *meprobamate*, popularly known as Miltown or Equanil. Many of the arguments concerning the uniqueness of meprobamate revolve around its similarity or dissimilarity to the barbiturates. But since the properties of the various barbiturates differ from one another, it is not easy to compare the whole class to meprobamate. All, however, tend to produce sleep when used in large doses, to produce effects reported as pleasant, and to produce convulsive seizures as a consequence of sudden withdrawal after the prolonged administration of large doses. Giving meprobamate to a patient suffering from neurotic anxiety is not quite the same as inserting a nail into a broken bone to hold it together, or giving insulin to a diabetic. In giving meprobamate, we are employing a drug with a poorly defined action to treat a poorly defined condition. But the condition is widespread and demands action, and the drug seems to help.

In any case, meprobamate's standing as the most popular tranquilizer was soon usurped by *chlordiazepoxide* (Librium). This compound strongly resembles meprobamate and the barbiturates, but there do appear to be differences the experimentalist can measure. For example, Leonard Cook and Roger Kelleher recently reported an experiment in which rats could postpone a punishing shock by pressing a lever. Cook and Kelleher found that at some doses chlordiazepoxide will produce an increase in the rate of lever pressing whereas meprobamate does not. Also it has been shown with a Lashley jumping stand that rats will sometimes become "fixated" if the discrimination problem is made insoluble. Chlordiazepoxide seems to eliminate this fixated behavior whereas meprobamate does not. The possible differences in the behavioral effects of sedative hypnotic drugs have not yet been fully explored, and the study of these differences should tell us a great deal about the drugs themselves.

Antidepression Drugs

While depression, at least in a mild form, is an experience perhaps as common as anxiety, it can also constitute a severe disease (formerly called melancholia), which sometimes leads to suicide. Psychiatrists are far from unanimous in their definitions of this complicated entity, but during the past decade they have found two classes of drugs helpful in combating it—the *monoamine oxidase* (MAO) *inhibitors*, and their successors, the *dibenzazepine* compounds. As with reserpine and chlorpromazine, their usefulness as antidepressants was discovered by accident when iproniazid (a MAO inhibitor) was given to tubercular patients and found to elevate their mood, and when imipramine (a dibenzazepine derivative related to chlorpromazine) was found to relieve depressed psychotics.

In attempting to understand the etiology of depression, it is ironic that biochemists have not hesitated to rush in where experimental psychologists fear to tread. What has emerged, based on a combination of clinical observations and animal studies, is the *catecholamine theory* of depression. Broadly interpreted, the theory says that a state of well-being is maintained by continuous adrenergic stimulation of certain receptors in the brain by catecholamines like norepinephrine and dopamine (hormones produced in the brain). For example, reserpine's so-called tranquilizing effect—indifference to surroundings, lack of appetite, and apparent lassitude—is attributed to depletion of catechola-

mines. Another compound, alphamethyltyrosine, which decreases the synthesis of catecholamines, has been found to produce "depression" in animals. On the other hand, some compounds have been found that produce an increase in the level of brain catecholamines. Administration of MAO inhibitors, which inactivate MAO and thus prevent catecholamine from being destroyed, produce increased levels of catecholamines and greater alertness, activity, and degree of electrical self-stimulation (in animals implanted with electrodes in "reward" areas of the brain). Administering the precursors of catecholamines—for example, dihydroxyphenylalanine (DOPA)—or MAO inhibitors will prevent or reverse the depression caused by reserpine (see Figure 1).

The dibenzazepine compounds, typified by *imipramine* (Tofranil), do not change the level of brain catecholamines in animals, yet they are effective antidepressants. However, the mode of action of these compounds may be compatible with the theory. Studies show that the catecholamine level in the brain is reduced, not only by enzymatic destruction, (for example, by MAO), but also by reabsorption of the catecholamines into the neurons. It has been hypothesized that the dibenzazapine compounds potentiate the action of normally present catecholamines by preventing this reabsorption.

LSD

LSD shares the responsibility with reserpine and chlorpromazine for ushering in the psychopharmacology era. Albert Hofmann's accidental discovery of this substance at Sandoz Pharmaceuticals in Basel, Switzerland in 1943 is now well known. LSD is a semisynthetic compound of plant origin, a derivative of ergot (a fungus that infects rye). Although its effects are similar to those of marijuana and mescaline, its outstanding characteristic is its extreme potency and its ability to pro-

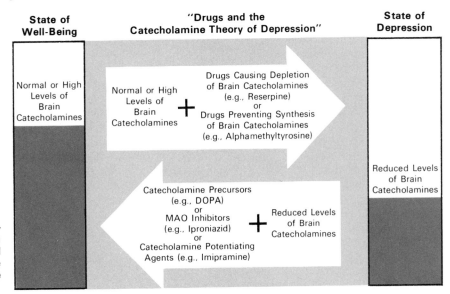

Figure 1. The relationships between drug-produced changes in brain catecholamine levels and changes in mental states provide evidence for the "catecholamine theory of depression."

duce bizarre mental states picturesquely described by Humphrey Osmond as psychedelic or "mind-expanding." The ability of LSD to block 5-hydroxytryptamine (another amine resembling the catecholamines in some respects, abbreviated 5HT) and thus to change brain levels of 5HT, has excited interest. More recently Maimon Cohen has reported the frightening finding that LSD can damage chromosomes. The role of LSD in producing a psychotic state has not been established. Despite thousands of papers dealing with this substance, we have very little idea of what LSD does, and we don't know how it does it. It is unfortunate that legal restrictions and the manufacturers' understandable diffidence make this fascinating chemical inaccessible for research.

There is something in the use or action of psychotogenic or "hallucinogenic" drugs that appeals to certain towering if unconventional figures in literature and the arts. From the time of Toulouse-Lautrec through the era of the expatriates (Gertrude Stein, James Joyce, Ernest Hemingway), bohemian Paris was not exactly abstemious, nor did it restrict itself to alcohol for thrills or new sensations. Though the virtues of illicit drugs do not appear in paid advertisements in the public press, nevertheless very talented "copywriters" have turned out glowing testimonials to promote the use of these drugs. Thomas de Quincey and Samuel Coleridge, at the beginning of the nineteenth century, recommended opium, and Paolo Mantegazza in 1859 gave highly colored accounts of the beatific effects of coca. Freud also approved of cocaine and advised his fiancée to take it. Charles Baudelaire, called the "De Quincey of hashish," was supported by Arthur Rimbaud and Paul Verlaine in acclaiming the beneficence of this drug; more recently Aldous Huxley declared that the "doors of perception" could be opened by mescaline and LSD. Many jazz, swing, bop, and other musicians claim that marijuana and other stimulant drugs enhance their playing or composing.

Whether drugs truly enhance creativity is a moot point. Artists, poets, scientists, and inventors will testify that LSD or marijuana or amphetamine inspired them to produce works of value, but controlled experiments to test these claims are lacking. Who would not like to find a magic drug that would turn an ugly frog into a handsome prince, or a Cinderella into a princess? Drugs can sometimes seem to have magic powers, but they do not ordinarily instill beauty, wisdom, and virtue into the taker. Yet estrogens can change a skinny, adolescent girl into a beauty queen and, if one can extrapolate from cases of precocious puberty (or infant Hercules), super-androgens must be responsible for Clark Kent's transformation into Superman.

Drugs do change our perception of the world, and when this perception becomes unbearable, as in terminal cancer, drug use is clearly justified. The question is whether it is justified for the relief of unhappiness, dissatisfaction, or boredom. The religious uses of wine and peyote for sacramental purposes have, in part, inspired Timothy Leary to found a new religion, the League for Spiritual Discovery (LSD), which advocates the use of LSD and other so-called psychedelic drugs. The legal difficulties of this organization have spurred city, state, and federal legislative and enforcement bodies to enter the field of psychopharmacology in order to control the distribution and use of behavior-affecting drugs. But the government is trying to make rules about substances that are still poorly understood, and it rests with psychopharmacologists to clarify the action of psychotogenic drugs so that such rules can be made on a more rational basis.

The Birth of Scientific Psychopharmacology

Without the spur of clinical success, it is doubtful that basic research in the effects of drugs on behavior could have advanced very rapidly. During the first half of the twentieth century, drugs were seldom used in the treatment of mental illness, since morphine, cocaine, barbiturates, and other sedative hypnotics had already been tried and proven generally ineffective. Other more physical approaches to therapy, including hydrotherapy, occupational therapy, and psychosurgery had been employed with varying results. Only electroconvulsive shock (ECS) seemed to be very successful, but its administration required considerable skill. Psychiatrists depended chiefly, therefore, on psychological methods (primarily communicative interactions), which, unfortunately, were usually inefficient and ineffective for the majority of severely psychotic individuals.

Experimental psychologists showed only an intermittent and desultory interest in the effects of drugs on behavior. A handful of drugs had already been investigated, but the results were of very little interest to the most influential psychologists, who were busy, in the 1930s and 1940s, building their own psychological systems or attacking rival systems.

In fact, however, psychopharmacology had already been born more than half a century earlier. In 1879 the first laboratory of experimental psychology had been established at Leipzig by Wilhelm Wundt. One of Wundt's most famous students was Emil Kraepelin, sometimes called the father of modern psychiatry because he invented a widely used system for classifying mental disorders. Kraepelin might also be called the father of scientific psychopharmacology, for he applied Wundt's new experimental methods to investigate the influence of drugs on psychological functions. Kraepelin studied pharmacology at Tartu in Estonia, then a center of research in this field. During his stay there he demonstrated that alcohol, morphine, and other drugs impair reaction time and the mental processes involved in associational learning. It is an ironic coincidence that Kraepelin was interested in the two areas that finally

Drug Group	Example	Trade or Common Name	Natural or Synthetic	Usage	How Taken	First Used	Evidence of Addiction?
PSYCHOTHERAPEUTICS							
Antipsychotic							
Rauwolfia alkaloids	reserpine	Serpasil	natural	greatly diminished	injected, ingested	1949	no
Phenothiazines	chlorpromazine	Thorazine	synthetic	widespread	injected, ingested	1950	no
Antianxiety							
Propanediols	meprobamate	Miltown	synthetic	widespread	ingested	1954	yes
Benzodiazepines	chlordiazepoxide	Librium	synthetic	widespread	ingested	1933	yes
Barbiturates	phenobarbital	see SEDATIVES					
Antidepressant							
Monoamine oxidase inhibitors	tranylcypromine	Parnate	synthetic	diminished	ingested	1958	no
Dibenzazepines	imipramine	Tofranil	synthetic	widespread	ingested, injected	1948	no
Stimulant	amphetamine	see STIMULANTS					
PSYCHOTOGENICS							
Ergot derivative	lysergic acid diethylamide	LSD, Lysergide	synthetic	widespread?	ingested	1943	no
Cannabis sativa	marijuana	hemp, hashish	natural	widespread	smoked	?	no
Lophophora williamsii	mescaline	peyote button	natural	localized	ingested	?	no
Psilocybe mexicana	psilocybin		natural	rare	ingested	?	no
STIMULANTS							
Sympathomimetics	amphetamine	Benzedrine	synthetic	widespread	ingested, injected	1935	yes
Analeptics	pentylenetetrazol	Metrazol	synthetic	rare	ingested, injected	1935	no
Psychotogenics	lysergic acid diethylamide	see PSYCHOTOGENICS					
Nicotinics	nicotine		natural	widespread	smoked, ingested	?	yes
Xanthines	caffeine		natural	widespread	ingested	?	yes
SEDATIVES AND HYPNOTICS							
Bromides	potassium bromide		synthetic	widespread	ingested	1857	no
Barbiturates	phenobarbital	Luminal	synthetic	widespread	ingested, injected	1912	yes
Chloral derivatives	chloral hydrate		synthetic	rare	ingested	1875	yes
General	alcohol		natural	widespread	ingested	?	yes
ANESTHETICS, ANALGESICS, AND PARALYTICS							
General anesthetics	nitrous oxide	laughing gas	synthetic	rare	inhaled	1799	no
	diethyl ether		synthetic	greatly diminished	inhaled	1846	no
	chloroform		synthetic	rare	inhaled	1831	no
Local anesthetics	cocaine	coca	natural	widespread	applied, ingested	?	yes
Analgesics	procaine	Novocaine	synthetic	widespread	injected	1905	no
	opium derivatives	morphine, heroin	natural	widespread	injected, smoked	?	yes
Paralytics	d-tubocurarine	curare	natural	widespread	injected	?	no
NEUROHUMORS (NEUROTRANSMITTERS)							
Cholinergic	acetylcholine		natural synthetic	laboratory	injected	1926	no
Adrenergic	norepinephrine		natural synthetic	laboratory	injected	1946	no
Others (?)	5-hydroxytryptamine	5-HT, serotonin	natural synthetic	laboratory	injected	1948	no

coalesced seventy-five years later—basic, quantitative, experimental psychopharmacology, and the treatment of mental disease.

Though psychopharmacology had little scientific status at the beginning of the twentieth century, Kraepelin's early work was continued by a few psychologists who studied the effects of alcohol, caffeine, cocaine, strychnine, and nicotine. In 1908 the Englishman W. H. R. Rivers reported on the influence of drugs on fatigue; in 1915 the Americans Raymond Dodge and Francis Benedict, and Harry Hollingsworth examined the effects of drugs on motor and mental efficiency. In 1924 even Clark Hull, one of the most influential psychologists of the mid-twentieth century, studied the effect of pipe smoking and coffee drinking on mental efficiency, before he turned his attention to building theoretical systems.

Psychopharmacological research was spurred in the 1930s and 1940s by the imminence and advent of World War II, which aroused military interest in the applications of drugs, particularly the amphetamines, and concern about the psychological consequences of anoxia, severe oxygen deficiency. Both allied and German soldiers were given amphetamines to combat sleeplessness and fatigue; these drugs were found to diminish fatigue, but whether they could raise performance above normal levels was an open question that is still not fully answered. Insufficient supply of oxygen to the brain was shown to adversely affect reasoning, memory, and sensory functioning; for example, it renders the subject less sensitive to visual stimuli and prolongs the time needed for the eyes to adapt to the dark. Such impairment was particularly serious in military pilots for whom the loss of judgment and sensory function resulting from lack of oxygen at high altitudes could be disastrous.

More recently a number of factors have converged to make psychopharmacology a popular field for research. During the mid-1950s, Europe and the United States were prospering, and governmental support for health services and medical research began to expand at an unprecedented rate. Spurred by therapeutic success and the possibilities of large profits, and as yet unencumbered by severe governmental restrictions concerning drug safety and efficacy, pharmaceutical companies were eager to discover new drugs prescribable to millions of waiting patients. Support for research on new psychotherapeutic drugs became big business. In addition, the Psychopharmacology Service Center, established within the National Institute of Mental Health, contributed millions of dollars for research on the psychological effects of drugs.

With the rise of psychopharmacology, clinical psychologists immediately began to devise methods, such as rating scales and questionnaires, to evaluate the effects of the new drug therapies. However, some of the psychotherapeutic achievements credited to the action of drugs may also be attributed to reforms in mental hospitals and better programs of community mental hygiene.

Psychological Methods in Psychopharmacological Research

To screen potentially useful drugs and characterize their action, psychopharmacologists have used a variety of procedures in studies carried out with rats and mice. Measures of spontaneous motor activity are widely employed, as are other observational and rating techniques. Among the most favored procedures are those based on operant conditioning, because they are objective, automatic, generally quite reliable, and permit extended investigation of a single animal. The chief apparatus is the Skinner box, a cage containing a lever-pressing mechanism. Depending on the experimental conditions, depression of this lever can produce either a positive reinforcement (food) or a negative reinforcement (electrical shock). Some investigators feel that the schedule, and not the kind or amount of reinforcement, determines a particular drug susceptibility. Some schedules require that the animal respond quickly, or slowly, or in certain patterns, in order to obtain food or avoid shock. On the other hand, even before the phenothiazines and reserpine appeared on the market, it was shown that these drugs seemed to selectively impair conditioned responses controlled by aversive consequences (that is, punishing shock) but had less effect upon unconditioned responses. It appears that the strength of the stimulus and the nature of the motor response required are vital factors determining the relative susceptibility to different drugs.

Many psychopharmacologists not trained in the Skinnerian approach use discrimination boxes and mazes to study the effects of drugs, and a number also use classical conditioning procedures; maze-learning was used in a recent study, which demonstrated that analeptics (such as strychnine) facilitate learning. Similarly, work on the amnesia produced by intracerebral antibiotics was based on results obtained with mazes and shuttle-boxes. Even single-trial learning procedures are being increasingly used to study the effects of drugs. Psychological research has not yet reached a point at which any one method of measuring behavior can be considered superior to any other.

Chemistry and the Brain

Psychologists have subdivided behavior in different ways, but they are in general agreement about certain broad categories of functions. If different psychological functions depend upon discrete chemical substances, then we might expect to find specificity of drug action—that is, that certain drugs selectively affect certain functions. If the localization of psychological functions involves a grosser type of organization—if it depends, say, on complex neural connections—then we would not necessarily expect to find such specific relations between drug action and psychological function.

Certain sensory structures are clearly chemically coded. Taste and smell receptors obviously are, and respond to specific drugs. Sodium dehydrochlorate and saccharin, even when injected into an antecubital vein, respectively produce a characteristic bitter or sweet taste on reaching the tongue and are used for measuring blood circulation time. Streptomycin and dihydrostreptomycin selectively, though not exclusively, attack the eighth nerve; visual effects are produced by santonin, digitalis, and LSD. Haptic sensations are said to be produced by cocaine ("cocaine bug"), but there is no good evidence that somesthetic sensory pathways are selectively affected by any chemical substance. Histamine and polypeptides, such as substance P or bradykinin, will at times produce itch or pain, and hint that sensory chemical specificity is a possibility.

Motor structures are also chemically coded and enable curariform drugs to have a selective paralyzing action. Similarly, autonomic ganglia can be affected selectively by different drugs, and the vast field of peripheral neuropharmacology rests on such specificity.

We are beginning to learn how the central nervous system is organized neuropharmacologically. Histochemical, radioautographic, and fluorescent techniques are making such mapping possible. For example, it is known that the central nervous system pathways that control motivational mechanisms such as hunger, thirst, and sex are susceptible to cholinergic, adrenergic, and hormonal substances. Further mapping of this kind is bound to result in better understanding of the relationship between drug action and functional localization in the central nervous system.

One can inhibit activity with a wide variety of depressant drugs or activate animals with stimulant drugs. No simple role can be ascribed to acetylcholine, norepinephrine, or 5-hydroxytryptamine (serotonin) in the control of behavior. What part, if any, these substances play in learning is even more mysterious. Some theorists have proposed an inhibitory cholinergic system balanced by an excitatory adrenergic system, and the facts seem to fit thus far. Of course, the brain is full of all species of chemicals that are waiting to be investigated by psychologists. Nucleic acids and particularly ribonucleic acid (RNA) have been assigned a special role in learning by some, but evidence is conflicting. Proteins seem a more likely candidate, and such inhibitors of protein synthesis as puromycin and cyclohexamide do interfere with both memory and learning. The production of retrograde amnesia and the posttrial facilitation of learning by drugs provide evidence for a consolidation process. But the experiments are difficult to perform, and many unspecified sources of variability will have to be identified before general mechanisms can be revealed.

The Future of Psychopharmacology

Ever since Loewenhoek's invention of the microscope, scientists have tended to believe that in the "ultrafine structure" of an organism lie the explanations for its functioning. Hence it is not surprising that attempts to explain drug action are couched in terms of chemical binding to specific molecular receptors. However, behavior can no more be seen in a test tube full of brain homogenate than can the theme of a mosaic be determined from an analysis of its stones. The Gestalt principle that the whole is something more than the sum of its parts is not always recognized by physical scientists who tend to be very analytical, to look at "parts" in their approach to explanation. The psychologist has an increasingly important role to play in psychopharmacology, for he must determine whether the particular sedative, antidepressant, psychotogenic, or facilitating drug that the biochemists and neurophysiologists want to study really has the behavioral properties they think it does.

In the future it should be possible to say in what ways each important psychopharmaceutical influences behavior, and thus to characterize it by a behavioral profile, just as we can now describe a chemical in terms of its chromatographic pattern. Ultimately, it ought to be possible to look at the chemical structure of any new drug and predict whether it will be useful as an antipsychotic, an antifatigue agent, an appetite stimulant, and so forth. By the same token, the physiological determinants of behavior will be so well worked out that we will understand why a drug that causes alertness also depresses hunger, or why one that causes difficulty in doing arithmetic also causes peculiar sensations in the skin. One can envisage the day when drugs may be employed not only to treat pathological conditions (reduce pain, suffering, agitation, and anxiety) but also to enhance the normal state of man—increase pleasure, facilitate learning and memory, reduce jealousy and aggressiveness. Hopefully such pharmacological developments will come about as an accompaniment of, and not as a substitute for, a more ideal society.

III
Psychotherapy and
Behavioral Change–Approaches

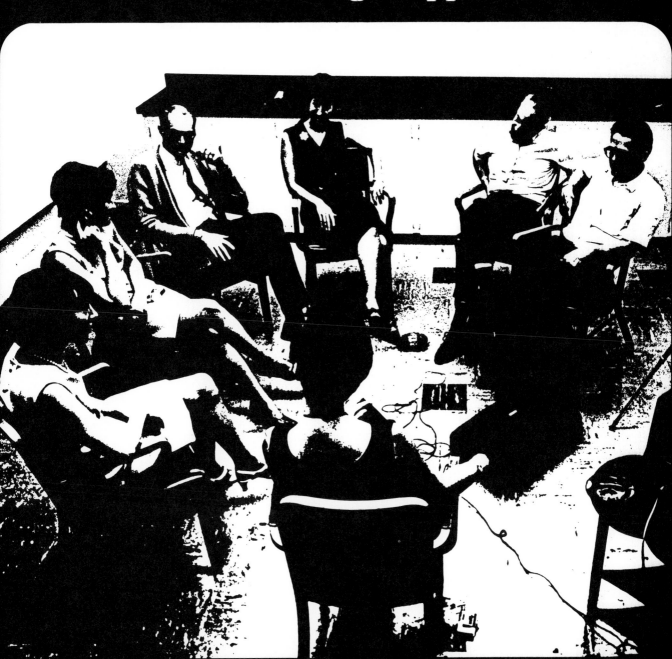

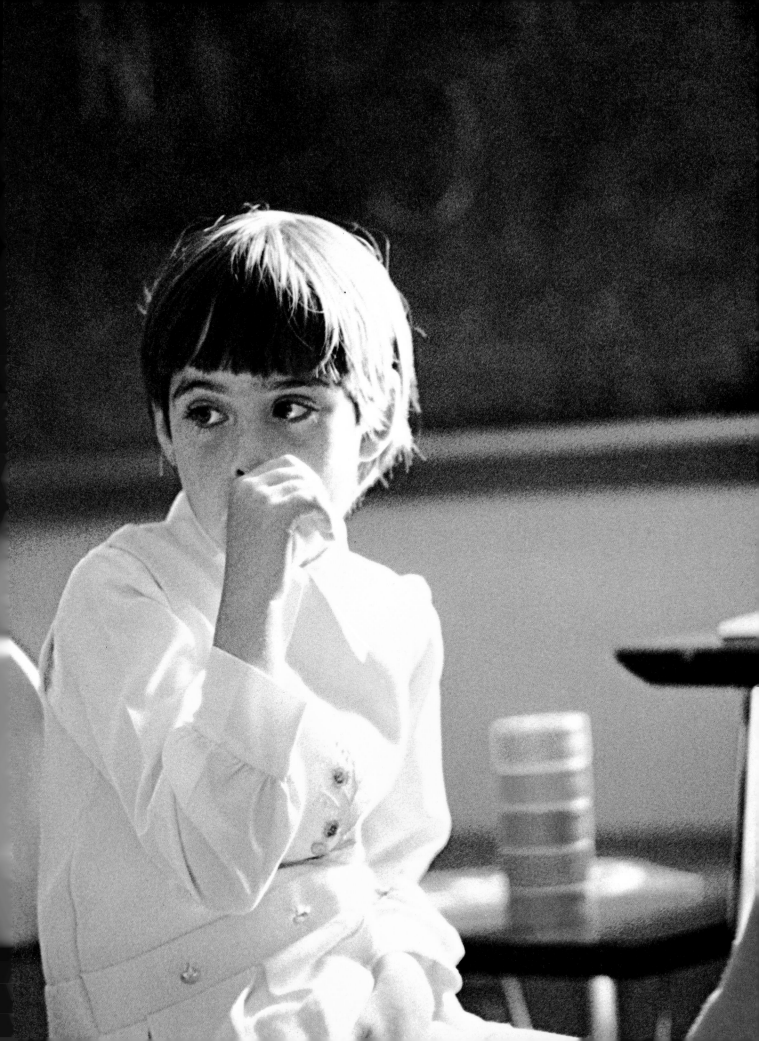

The Autistic Child

C. B. Ferster

We have no idea whether the initial causes of autism are biological or psychological, but we do know that early learning has a grave influence in its development. Parents soon stop lavishing affection on a child who does not return it. They reduce their efforts to teach new things to a child who has such difficulty learning them. And when these things happen, the child learns even less; the autism becomes more pronounced.

How can such a child be helped? Operant reinforcement, says C. B. Ferster, is one hopeful method. Many of the autistic child's unusual behaviors were learned, perhaps inadvertently. In the same way, through training him to respond to cues and dispensing clear-cut rewards, the autistic child can learn more normal responses.

Ferster illustrates this approach with a vivid incident that occurred at Linwood Children's Center, a collaborative effort between experimentalists and clinicians, and thereby also reveals the way in which learning theory can clarify and refine techniques that have a nontheoretical, more intuitive genesis. The complex, delicate encounter between the autistic little girl and Jeanne Simons, the Center's director, followed all the principles of operant reinforcement, yet Miss Simons moved sheerly with the sensitivity and insight given by long experience and intimate observation. By applying the systematic analysis of learning theory to Miss Simons' intuitive working methods, Ferster shows how a synthesis of clinical experience and theoretical principles can generate a treatment approach that promises help for many autistic children.

The autistic child lives in a world apart from others. He cannot reach out, and no one can reach in. A good part of the time the child does nothing but sit quietly in a chair, or sleep, or lie huddled in a corner. At other times he is active, sometimes violently so, but his activity affects only himself. He may spend hours compulsively rubbing a rough spot on the floor, moving his fingers in front of his face, babbling to himself, licking his body like a cat, or flipping sand to produce a visual pattern. He may beat his head against the wall, hit himself until he is covered with bruises, or use his fingernails and teeth to tear his own flesh.

Some autistic children are mute. Others make inarticulate sounds or echo bits of the speech they hear around them. But they do not talk to or with other people. When an autistic child does try to communicate, it is by biting, kicking, screaming, having tantrums—primitive forms of behavior, called *atavisms*, which create a situation others will go to almost any lengths to eliminate.

If one were to watch an autistic child for a day and then watch a normal child for a month, one would see much of the autistic child's behavior reproduced by the normal child. Almost any child, on occasion, will gaze out the window for an hour or more, make bizarre faces, or have severe tantrums. Any child may run sticks over picket fences, step on (or over) all the cracks in the sidewalk, or chew a piece of rubber balloon to shreds.

But normal children are only out of touch with their surroundings once in a while, and primitivisms are not their only form of behavior. They interact with their physical and social environment in many different ways. The autistic child's behavior is far more restricted. He has very few ways of changing and being changed by the world around him.

Since his behavioral repertoire is so small, what there is of it is used over and over again. It is the *frequency* of withdrawn, self-stimulatory, or atavistic behavior, not simply the fact that it occurs, that distinguishes the autistic child from the normal one.

Autism is a very rare disorder, affecting only one child out of 50,000 or 100,000. We need to know how autism comes about and how it may be treated not only because these few children desperately need help but because the study of autism contributes to our understanding of other forms of behavior. There are parallels, for example, between the development of autism in young children and the development of schizophrenia in adolescents. In addition, the past experiences of the autistic child, like his present behavior, differ from those of the normal child not so much in *kind* as in *intensity* and *frequency*.

We do not know yet whether the causes of autism are biological or environmental, or both. Parents of autistic children sometimes report that the child seemed "different" from birth, that he stiffened each time he was picked up. Some autistic children have shown neurological anomalies such as abnormal EEG patterns. So far, however, the evidence for an inborn biological deficiency is meager.

A child's environment can have very dramatic effects on his behavioral development. This has been shown repeatedly. There have been infants who spent most of their early lives locked in closets and became primitive, animallike children. There also have been primitive, animallike children who have learned new forms of behavior when a new environment was arranged for them. Thus, it makes sense to examine the surroundings of the autistic child for circumstances that might explain the gross deficiencies in his behavior.

The major processes by which behavior is acquired and lost are *reinforcement* and *extinction*. If a rat receives a pellet of food when it presses a bar, the rat will press the bar more and more often. When the pellets are no longer delivered, bar pressing decreases in frequency and finally stops. Similarly, a person's ordinary speech usually is reinforced by the reply it gets, and a speaker who gets no reply soon stops talking. Behavioral processes are harder to observe in a natural social environment than in an experimental laboratory, but they operate similarly.

Lack of Reinforcement

The very limited repertoire of the autistic child may come about because his behavior is not successful. Ted is an example of an autistic child whose behavioral development was thwarted because little of his behavior was reinforced. At first this was hard to see because Ted's mother did not seem unresponsive. She was a very active woman who moved busily around the house, accomplishing many tasks and talking a great deal.

The child, however, was prevented from completing any action he happened to begin. When he reached for a lamp, his mother appeared as if by magic to seize his hand and hold it back. When he reached for the doorknob, again she intercepted him. When he approached his brothers and sisters, his mother separated them. When he held out a receipt he had gotten from the newsboy, she walked past and left him standing with the slip of paper in his hand.

Even the mother's speech did not make contact with the boy. While the boy was in the living room, his mother called him from the kitchen. "Ted, come over here," she said. "I want to read you a story. Ted, Ted, don't you want to read a story? Ted, come over here and read a story, TED, where are you?"

Ted paid no attention. After five minutes of calling, the mother came into the living room and picked up the book. She continued to call, "TED, TED, TED. . . . Come on and read your book." When he happened to wander near enough, she took hold of him, sat him down next to her, and began to read.

The boy did not object and seemed happy to sit with his head against his mother's shoulder. But it was obvious that the physical contact was what kept him there. The reading was irrelevant, as was most of the mother's speech.

In short, only a tiny part of the mother's behavior had a reinforcing effect on the child. Furthermore, by interrupting or ignoring his attempts to do things for himself she was preventing him from successfully completing an action—any action—of his own.

Sometimes a child's behavior succeeds only under very specific conditions—with one particular person, for example. If the circumstances suddenly change, a great deal of behavior can be lost. This happened to a little girl of four who spent a year in the care of a teen-age baby-sitter.

The girl's mother was a very disturbed, nearly psychotic, woman. She remained in the home while the baby-sitter was there, but she had nothing whatever to do with the child. If the child said, "Mom, can I have a cookie?" there was no answer. If she said, "Janet, can I have a cookie?" Janet said yes and gave her a cookie. If the girl said, "Let's go out," the mother did not answer. Janet might reply and take the child outside.

This situation might be compared to that of a laboratory pigeon being trained to peck a green key instead of a red key. If the pigeon pecks the green key, a piece of grain appears, but if it pecks the red key, nothing happens. After a while the pigeon doesn't bother pecking the red key at all.

When the baby-sitter left at the end of the year, this child lost almost her whole behavioral repertoire. She became incontinent, she talked less and less, she could not be kept in nursery school. Eventually she needed chronic care at a state home for the retarded. The reason for this massive loss of behavior was not just the sudden switch in caretakers but the fact that the mother had been present at the *same time* as the baby-sitter. If the mother had been away for the year and had been able to respond normally to the child when she returned, there probably would have been only a slight, temporary break in behavior. If the mother had been away but had *not* been able to treat the child normally when she came back, the same severe loss probably would have occurred, much more slowly.

Punishment and Primitive Behavior

Parents and children constantly influence each other's behavior. Even punishment is usually more productive than no reaction to the child at all.

This is not to say that punishment is a desirable form of behavioral control. Although its main effect is to *strengthen* behavior that avoids or ends the punishment, punishment can weaken behavior if all positive reinforcement is withdrawn. If a parent not only spanks a child but refuses to speak to him for the rest of the day, he may reduce the frequency of parts of the child's repertoire that he did not intend to affect.

In addition, punishment can promote less advanced forms of behavior. Punishment is most likely to be dispensed when a child is doing something fairly active, such as finger-painting on the wall or trying to drive his parents' car. A child who sits on the kitchen floor studying his fingers will probably be left alone. If a child is consistently punished when he tries to have a strong effect on the environment, such attempts will begin to produce considerable anxiety. So the child may substitute simpler activities, such as rubbing a spot on the floor.

He may also resort to primitive controlling behavior, like screaming and tantrums. If he finds that he *can* affect his environment in this way, he is likely to keep on using atavisms in preference to other behavior.

When one sees the amount of control some autistic children exert over their parents by means of tantrums and other atavisms, it is hardly surprising that the behavior is so durable. One child's parents told us that they took turns standing guard all night at the door of his room because a tantrum started if they left and ceased only when they moved back. Another mother slept with her arm over her child every night for five months, so that she could stop him when he woke and clawed at his face.

Possible Causes of Autism

Everything described so far—lack of reinforcement, sudden changes in its source, the withdrawal of approval, and practices that encourage primitive behavior—also occurs in the lives of children who do not become autistic. Accounting for the autistic child's massive failure of development therefore presents a problem. The explanation seems to be that the autistic child has faced more severely damaging situations more often than the normal or nearly normal child. Most of the evidence that this is true is anecdotal, but compelling.

One often finds, for instance, that autistic children have parents who are completely unable to respond to the child's behavior. A parent who is a drug addict, an alcoholic, chronically ill, or severely depressed may not even acknowledge the child's existence for days on end. One also finds parents who have beaten, tortured, starved, or incarcerated their children for long periods of time. One woman kept her child in a dog run.

When we look at the child rather than at the parents, we often discover a history of serious or chronic illness during infancy. In such cases, the child's standard way of communicating with the parents usually has been to cry and fret. After the child recovers, the crying may persist, and the parents may very well keep on reacting. So the child deals with the parents through primitive behavior, and the parent responds in order to end the behavior. The child's development, already retarded by his illness, may progress no farther.

A child is not usually identified as autistic until some complex form of behavior (such as speech) fails to develop—that is, until the child is two, three, or even four years old. Although this does not prove that autism was not present earlier (indeed, parents occasionally report deviant behavior in very young infants), it does suggest a careful examination of that period in the child's life when the disorder may express itself.

A two-year-old is at a stage of development when his behavior is especially vulnerable to disruption. For one thing, he is more likely than a younger child to provoke a negative reaction from his parents. The activities of a baby are simple and relatively unobtrusive. But when a child begins to crawl, walk, reach for ashtrays and lamps, and cry loudly when crossed, he may also begin to frighten and upset his parents and thus to invite the kind of treatment that weakens behavior.

Furthermore, the child's new behavior is not at all firmly established. New behavior develops fastest when it has a consistent, reliable effect on the environment. Since the child can only approximate what he is trying to do at first, his efforts succeed only part of the time. If an enthusiastic parental response is lacking too, the child may very well abandon the behavior.

Sometimes a parent will praise the child's first nonsense syllables but become angry a month later when the child still cannot speak in complete, intelligible sentences. This sudden shift in the performance required for reinforcement can have the same effect on the child as suddenly requiring a laboratory pigeon to peck 300 times instead of 25 for a piece of grain: the behavior stops.

Adolescence

However, sudden changes in the kind and amount of behavior required for reinforcement are more likely to occur in adolescence than in early childhood. A ten-year-old may need do no more than hold out his hand for his allowance or run next door to find a playmate. A sixteen-year-old is expected to work for his money and to master an elaborate courtship ritual. At school, where assignments used to be frequent and short, the teen-age student may have to work for weeks or months before he finds out from the teacher how he is doing. In general, the adolescent must perform a substantial number of specific acts before his behavior is reinforced, often without benefit of a complete series of intermediate, transitional experiences.

If the change in kind or amount of behavior an adolescent must deliver is too sudden or too large, the effect on his development can be disastrous. One cannot build the Empire State Building if there is only a toothpick holding up the twentieth floor. One schizophrenic boy had a job as a truck driver before he was hospitalized; he would not stop at the restaurant where the other drivers ate because he did not know how to order food from the waitress. Another young man in the ward had frequent and violent temper tantrums; their source turned out to be his inability to tie his shoelaces.

Treatment

Autistic children are very difficult to treat. Until recently, they were considered virtually hopeless. So much of the normal repertoire is missing; a long history of experiences must be re-created; dealing with a six-year-old child as if he were one or two years old presents innumerable problems. Some therapists have succeeded with prolonged residential treatment. In addition, recent experimental attempts have sometimes produced dramatic changes in the children's behavior. Even when these experiments are not entirely successful from a therapeutic point of view—when, for example, the changes do not last—they represent progress because they show the child's potential for development.

One promising approach to rehabilitation is illustrated by a project that I am participating in at the Linwood Children's Center for autistic children, located between Washington, D.C., and Baltimore. The Director of the Center, Jeanne Simons, is chiefly a clinician, and I am chiefly an experimentalist. What we are trying to do is produce a kind of model for cooperative work between the two fields.

During our collaboration we found that our methods are a great deal alike. I tend to approach an experiment, even in the animal laboratory, from a clinical point of view; Miss Simons manipulates the environment in her clinic much as I do in the laboratory. I might be called a sheep in wolf's clothing, and she a wolf in sheep's clothing.

Miss Simons is an unusually gifted therapist. Like many gifted therapists, she has trouble explaining to other workers how she gets her results. Her metaphors —"Walk behind the child so that you can see where he is going"—describe the principles of operant reinforcement very well, but they helped the staff little in everyday dealings with the children.

Here was an area where an experimentalist could help. A functional analysis of Miss Simons' methods, in objective language, would make it easier for the staff to understand and evaluate them. It would also give Miss Simons a new perspective on her own work.

As I watched Miss Simons deal with the children, I saw the application of every principle of behavior that I know. But I did not always recognize them at first. There was one boy who teased Miss Simons by pulling her hair. When she continued to give him her full attention, I wondered why. It seemed clear that her attention was reinforcing the annoying behavior. But when I looked more closely, I saw that Miss Simons was

holding the boy's wrist close to her hair so that he couldn't pull it. She released her grip only when he made a move toward some more desirable kind of behavior.

To illustrate the kind of thing Miss Simons does (and the way behavioral language can clarify it), I will describe an encounter she had with an autistic girl named Karen. Karen was mute and had very little contact with her environment. She cried continuously and softly, and she had a doll that she always carried with her.

The encounter took place only a short time after Karen arrived at Linwood, and it was the child's first sustained interaction with another person. It lasted for about half an hour. During that time, there were perhaps 200 instances in which Miss Simons' behavior was clearly contingent on that of the child. The general therapeutic goals were to diminish Karen's crying, weaken the compulsive control of the doll, and begin developing more constructive forms of behavior that Karen could use to manipulate the environment herself. The third goal was the most important, and during the encounter it became clear that the extinction of the crying and the weakened control of the doll were by-products of the reinforcement of other behavior.

Miss Simons placed Karen on a rocking horse in the playroom and began to rock her and sing to her. The rocking and singing stopped the child's crying. Then, for brief periods, Miss Simons kept on singing but stopped rocking. She sensed very accurately how long the pause could be without the child's beginning to cry again.

After a few minutes of this, the therapist took the doll from the child and placed it on a table. But she moved the table very close to Karen so that the child could easily take the doll back again. When she leaned over to do so, Karen rocked *herself* slightly. From then on, Miss Simons sang only when Karen rocked herself, which Karen did more and more frequently.

Miss Simons placed the doll on the table several times and the child calmly took it back. Then Karen *herself* put the doll on the table. Miss Simons began to rock the horse vigorously. The intensity of her voice as she sang kept pace with the rocking.

Up to this time, Miss Simons sang whenever the child rocked herself, but now she occasionally did not sing even though the child rocked. As this new situation began, Karen took the doll back off the table—having been without it for more than a full minute for the first time since her arrival at Linwood.

As she picked up the doll, it accidentally dropped to the floor. Karen began to cry. "Do you want to pick it up?" Miss Simons asked. "I'll help you." She lifted Karen off the horse and the *child* picked up the doll. When Miss Simons asked if she wanted to get up again, Karen raised her hands and Miss Simons helped her climb back into the saddle.

Karen dropped the doll again, and again Miss Simons helped her pick it up and get back on the horse. This time Karen came closer to mounting by herself, though Miss Simons still provided some support. The therapist rocked the horse vigorously and moved the doll to a couch, not far away but out of reach, and she stopped the rocking for a moment. Karen glanced at the doll and then withdrew her attention. Miss Simons picked up the doll and tapped it rhythmically; Karen looked at her, made a sound, and began to rock in time with the tapping. Miss Simons gave her the doll.

The next time the therapist took the doll away, Karen cried but kept on rocking. Miss Simons began to sing, which stopped the crying. Then she took the child off the horse so that Karen could get the doll from the couch. They sat together on the couch for a few moments, the child on the therapist's lap. When Karen tried to persuade Miss Simons to go back to the horse by pulling her arm in that direction, Miss Simons smiled and picked the child up but carried her in another direction.

Here there seemed to be a deliberate switch in contingencies. Miss Simons had developed a repertoire of performances in Karen that involved the rocking horse. Now she had shifted to a new set of reinforcers, picking Karen up and interacting with her through body contact and singing. She did not reinforce any attempts to go back to the horse. I don't know what Miss Simons would have done if Karen had struggled in her arms and continued gesturing toward the horse, but I suspect she knew this was improbable before she made the shift.

Even though the behavioral processes that operated here were the same ones I knew from laboratory experience, I would not have been able to put them into practice as Miss Simons did. For example, I might have kept Karen on the horse, without the doll, until her crying stopped. What Miss Simons did instead was wait until Karen's behavior was strongly controlled by rocking and singing before she took the doll away. Later, when Karen dropped the doll and began to cry, Miss Simons reacted at once and used the doll itself to reward the girl for picking it up.

Observation of Jeanne Simons' therapy has taught me many new ways in which the behavior of autistic children can be developed. As for her, she says she is more aware of her own actions. She sees more clearly the individual elements in her complex interchange with a child and has a better understanding of the specific effect of each small act. This helps her refine and modify her procedures and also allows her to describe them more clearly for the staff.

"I think I can explain little step-by-step procedures now so that people don't just look blindly at me with awe," she says. "I'm not even sure intuition is so mysterious. I think it's having eyes all over the place and seeing the tiny little things that children are doing. . . . And I am able to see the tiny little steps and explain much better what I am doing with the children. So the magic is out of Linwood—which I think is wonderful!"

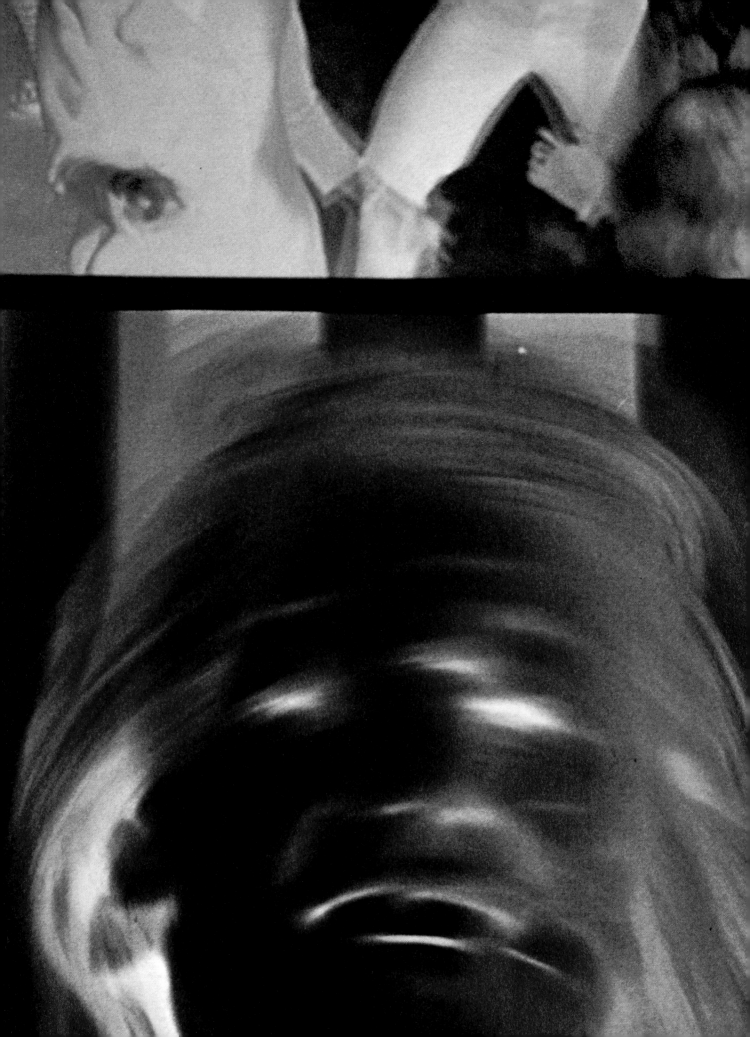

Hypnotherapeutic Conditioning
John M. Coyne

Hypnosis has always worn an aura of mystery. The very word evokes images of a psychoanalyst probing his patient's early memories or of a public performer revealing the power of suggestion. Hypnosis is now an acknowledged therapy that, as John Coyne explains, is widely used for rapid treatment of such problems as migraine headache or impotence-frigidity.

Coyne's article, in itself, is almost an operational definition of psychotherapy's new eclecticism. Coyne uses the neo-Freudian, psychodynamic model in his description of emotional tensions; he regards psychosomatic disorders as symptoms of underlying conflicts. His techniques for hypnosis and explanations of conditioning stem from behaviorism and learning theory. The rationale behind it all comes from neurophysiology. The end product is a creative synthesis of three diverse viewpoints into an integral theory of hypnosis.

What is said here about the physiological side of hypnosis and conditioning principles qualifies as a very fruitful set of hypotheses but not—at least yet—as a set of established principles or facts. For example, Coyne draws a parallel between induced hypnosis and the effect of such drugs as phenothiazines. When we know more about both hypnosis and drugs, the two may not seem so similar. Also to be taken with caution are statements such as "hypnotic reconditioning can eliminate psychosomatic disorders in any organ governed by the autonomic nervous system."

Harry is thirty-four, an intelligent, articulate, likeable man with a just slightly belligerent manner. He is active and aggressive, works hard at his job and enjoys it, though he claims no illusions as to its social worth. At twenty-five, he married; at twenty-nine, he was divorced for what he describes as "the usual reasons." Since his divorce he has had several affairs, some of them "on the convenient side."

He eats too much, drinks too much, smokes too much—but he tries to keep himself under control. He likes things to work properly. If they don't, he wants them fixed. "If my car doesn't run, I take it to the garage. If I can't sleep, I take a pill. I don't really care what the trouble is, I just want it stopped." Harry smiles, issuing a challenge of sorts. He has become impotent. He is a candidate for hypnosis. Hypnotic reconditioning can eliminate psychosomatic disorders in any organ governed by the autonomic nervous system.

Autogenic or "self-produced" conditioning of the integrated nervous system under hypnosis will eliminate or arrest the symptomatic distress of most psychosomatic disorders in six brief sessions.

Harry is, of course, entirely fictional. His disability, and his attitude toward it, are not. His kind of impotence belongs to that large and perhaps even growing group of functional or organic disorders that originate from psychological tensions.

Psychosomatic disorders are often placed in one of three reasonably distinct categories. The first category covers *organ-system malfunctions* like migraine headaches, asthma, hypertension, constipation, urinary urgency, and impotence or frigidity, in which the *function*, rather than the actual structure of the organ system, is primarily affected. The second category contains *induced diseases*, in which pathology occurs in an organ or organ system: inflammation, ulceration, hemorrhage, thrombi, constrictes. The third category includes disorders in which the *symptoms* of primary organic disease are present although the relevant organ system is functionally and structurally intact.

The demand has grown for relatively quick, efficient techniques to eliminate these disorders. Psychologists, psychiatrists, and laymen become increasingly impatient with therapy that depends upon lengthy analysis. In practical terms, the problem is reinforcement; six months of traditional psychotherapy is unlikely to eliminate or even alleviate the severe and chronic emotional tensions of which migraine is a symptom. But if a man who has suffered migraine headaches for most of his adult life is suddenly relieved of the physical discomfort of those headaches, he is much more likely to go on to bigger and better things in therapy. Psychosomatic symptoms of severe tension, such as asthma, ulcers, migraine, and impotence-frigidity, can be made to disappear, in most cases permanently, under hypnosis. When major emotional tensions remain unresolved, however, another disorder will sooner or later pop up as a symptom or signal of distress. Patients understand this, and the majority of them—between 70 and 80 percent—go on eagerly, or at least with a good will, to depth psychotherapy.

Much resistance to the clinical application of hypnosis comes from people who really do not know what hypnosis is. They object to hypnosis as sinister hocus-pocus. And there are many who believe that hypnosis is a form of unwarranted meddling with delicately balanced human functions about which little is known, and place hypnosis on a danger list likely to include the more powerful hallucinogens.

Psychologically, hypnosis can best be described as an induced state of selectively altered sensory awareness. Sensory awareness is mediated by three sets of receptors: *exteroceptors*, which provide the organism with information on the environment outside the body; *interoceptors*, which provide information on internal body processes; and *proprioceptors*, which provide information on the position of the body in relation to the environment. In hypnosis, certain types of awareness are selected for focus and amplification, while the awareness of other sensations is obscured and subdued. The sensations chosen for amplification are those conducive to progressive muscular or visceral relaxation; the distracting or noncontributing awareness is selectively tuned out.

All psychosomatic disorders come from more or less conscious mental interference with the reflex programs generated and controlled by the autonomic nervous system. We could call this interference static from the central nervous system. Under hypnosis, the static can be blocked or translated by subconscious reconditioning, so that normal reflex patterns are allowed to reassert themselves.

There is an old misconception that the operations of the autonomic nervous system are not subject to external modification or to internal voluntary influence. It is true that the autonomic nervous system normally functions independently of conscious regulation. The routine instructions that govern the operations of the blood vessels, heart, stomach, smooth muscles, glands, intestines, and so on do not emanate from the centers of conscious control.

A man cannot instruct his heart to stop beating in the same way he can willfully order major (though temporary) changes in respiration. But the reactions effected by the autonomic nervous system are developmentally patterned by conditioning or learning—which is, of course, mediated by the central or conscious nervous system. With certain limited exceptions, identification of emotion-producing stimuli and the appropriate behavioral responses to them are learned—they are culturally, socially, and individually conditioned. Through conditioning, the autonomic nervous system is programmed for emotional or visceral reactions in the presence of sensory or cognitive cues.

Under normal circumstances, reaction patterns, once triggered, fulfill themselves automatically. Severe or chronic emotional tension results when these reaction patterns of approach or avoidance are never allowed to fulfill themselves, or when their sequence is permanently disturbed in some way, usually by the continual presence of contradictory or inconsistent cues.

If a man is presented with a set of sensory or mental cues that enrage him, the autonomic nervous system automatically prepares the body for an expression of anger. But, if that same sensory or cognitive cue-pattern also includes a powerful stimulus that says anger must *not* be expressed—as, for example, when the anger is directed at one's boss—a psychophysiological storm rages. It usually translates itself into an atypical, self-punishing somatic response.

If the storm, or neurological tempest, is fairly permanent, a quite durable or chronic expression of the disturbance emerges—migraine headaches or ulcers are likely. What autogenic conditioning does, in essence, is allow the hypnotized subject to relearn selectively or rearrange certain stimulus-response cues so that they do not produce contradictory or undesirable autonomic reaction patterns.

The Battleground

Both neurological and psychological evidence indicates that the principal site of interaction between the central and autonomic nervous systems is the hypothalamus, which also marks the junction between the brain stem and cerebral hemispheres or cerebrum.

If we include the pituitary gland, this location becomes a three-way junction that integrates and coordinates the functions of the central nervous system, the autonomic nervous system, and the endocrine-gland or hormonal system. The brain stem, which originates at the medulla oblongata (the base of the brain and the top of the spinal cord), contains several programmed reflex centers that regulate such vital body functions as respiration, heart rate, blood pressure, and elimination, as well as certain protective reflexes including eye-blinking, swallowing, coughing, sneezing, and vomiting.

In addition to holding these vital and protective reflex centers, the brain stem has a function of even greater significance to general psychosomatic interactions. The core of the brain stem from the medulla oblongata up through the hypothalamus is composed of a network of loosely knit neural fibers. This network functions as a preamplifier for the sensory (awareness) and motor (responsive) areas of the cerebral cortex, a thin sheath of neural grey matter that completely covers each cerebral hemisphere and is the site of all conscious, volitional mental activity.

This brain-stem core, known as the *reticular activating system*, performs two significant functions in conscious awareness. First, the constant-pulse signal it generates keeps the cerebral cortex alerted for incoming impulses, both from the cranial nerves and from the nerve tracts of the spinal cord, which collect and send up all other incoming sensory signals. Second, the reticular activating system operates as a "tunable amplifier" for the cortex, which selectively facilitates or amplifies some incoming sensory impulses while inhibiting or suppressing others. This latter discriminatory function is primarily under conscious control and permits a selective or voluntary shift of attention or sensory focus.

The reticular activating system, which is the principal site of action for the major (phenothiazine) nonsedating, tranquilizing drugs, is also the location of the most significant neuroelectrical activity change under the deeper stages of induced hypnosis.

As a whole, the autonomic nervous system incorporates two separate but interactive neural networks. Thus it functions as a two-phase governor, regulating the expenditure and conservation of emotional energy. The first of these neural networks is the sympathetic (or thoracicolumbar) division. It consists of a pair of twenty-two ganglion chains paralleling each side of the spinal column. This sympathetic network *energizes* the activities of the vital and visceral systems of the organism by the postganglionic release of epinephrine (adrenaline). The other neural network forms the parasympathetic (or craniosacral) division. It is a bilateral network of certain cranial and sacral nerves, and it connects diffusely with the same visceral systems energized by the sympathetic division. The parasympathetic division serves to relax or tranquilize the various visceral reactions in quiescent emotional states by a localized release of acetylcholine.

All sympathetic or alerted states are not, of course, subjectively related to anything that might be called avoidance or "fight-or-flight" responses. Many alerted states are subjectively pleasurable, being equivalent to agreeable thrills of one sort or another. And not all

parasympathetic or relaxed states are related in a positive or pleasurable way to approach; some of these emotionally inactive states are regarded as negative, unpleasant experiences that are perceived as apathy or depression.

Clinical hypnosis can be used to connect or associate sensory or cognitive stimuli with either sympathetic or parasympathetic reactions and effects (see Table 1).

TABLE 1
Effects of the Sympathetic and Parasympathetic Divisions of the Autonomic Nervous System on the Body's Organs

Sympathetic Reaction	Organ System	Parasympathetic Reaction
	Visual	
dilation	iris	constriction
relaxation (far vision)	lens (muscles)	contraction (near vision)
	lacrimal gland	secretion of tears
	Respiratory	
constriction, dryness	trachea	dilation, secretion
dilation	bronchi	constriction
rapid, shallow breathing	diaphragm	slow, deep breathing
	Cardiac (heart)	
acceleration	rhythm (rate)	inhibition
dilation	arteries	constriction
	Vascular	
constriction	cerebral vessels	dilation
constriction	respiratory vessels	dilation
dilation	heart vessels	constriction
constriction	visceral vessels	dilation
constriction	genital vessels	dilation
constriction	peripheral vessels	dilation
	Gastric	
inhibition of motility	stomach wall	increased tone, motility
contraction	stomach sphincter	relaxation
inhibition	stomach glands	secretion
inhibition of glycogen release		stimulation of glycogen release
secretion of bile	liver	
inhibition of enzyme secretion	pancreas	stimulation of enzyme and hormone secretion
	Intestinal	
inhibition of motility	wall	increased tone, motility
contraction	sphincters	relaxation
inhibition	glands	secretion
	Urinary	
relaxation	bladder wall	contraction
contraction	bladder sphincter	relaxation
	Adrenal Gland	
secretion of adrenalin	medulla (core)	no effect
	Genital	
constriction	penis vessels	dilation
constriction	vaginal vessels	dilation
constriction	clitoral vessels	dilation
constriction	uterus (pregnant)	no effect
relaxation	uterus (unpregnant)	no effect
	Skin	
secretion	sweat glands	no effect
constriction	blood vessels	dilation
contraction	hair erector muscles	no effect
	Salivary Glands	
limited secretion		heavy secretion
thick saliva		watery saliva

Selective Concentration

The key psychological factor in hypnosis is selective concentration, or directed attention. It involves a *preoccupation* or saturation of one or more of the primary exteroceptor systems (auditory, visual, or tactile) combined with a directed *inhibition* of the normal proprio-ceptor sensations and interoceptor awareness of visceral activity.

It is important to differentiate psychologically in-duced hypnosis from other states of altered sensory awareness, such as sleep, intoxication, sedation, and tranquilization. In sleep, for example, *all* channels of sensory input are equally inhibited from conscious or cortical awareness. During sleep, all the sensory inputs are heavily subdued by the inhibitory activity of the reticular activating system. In states of intoxication in-duced by drugs or alcohol, the depression of neural activity occurs at the level of the cerebral cortex. The main effect of moderate intoxication is a discoordina-tion between sensory awareness and motor response to it; in heavier intoxication, loss of consciousness is the eventual result. In chemical sedation, sensory blocking is generalized (as in normal sleep), while most of this inhibition occurs at the cortical level (as in heavy in-toxication).

The heavier tranquilizing agents, such as phenothia-zine derivates, show the greatest similarity to induced hypnosis. Like hypnosis, these tranquilizers have their principal effects in the hypothalamus and the brain-stem reticulum, and serve to diminish anxiety, muscular tension, and behavioral hyperactivity without depressing cortical activity. The principal difference between these tranquilizers and hypnosis is that under hypnosis, *selec-tive reconditioning is possible*, so that alteration of posthypnotic or waking-state behavior occurs. In the tranquilized state, such reconditioning takes place tem-porarily or not at all.

This altered awareness under hypnosis is achieved by selectively directing the subject's attention to sensory awarenesses that are conducive to progressive muscular and visceral relaxation, and thus to the reduction of *critical* conscious control. The increasing comfort of this progressive relaxation shifts the subject's attention away from awareness that might be distracting or disruptive. In such a relaxed, noncritical state, the subject responds to the conditioning and posthypnotic programming, which are the goals of the hypnotic experience.

Hypnotic induction actually begins during an ex-ploratory interview that provides the hypnotist with in-formation on the way his subject usually responds. We are all aware of the methods used to induce a hypnotic state. As the subject begins to respond to sensations of increasing heaviness and warmth or tingling, he is directed to amplify his own awareness of these sensa-tions by focusing progressively more attention on them. The eye-muscle fatigue associated with the visual fixa-tion is usually intensified by this developing awareness of body heaviness and warmth, and the onset of invol-untary eye closure and eye-muscle catalepsy is accel-erated.

As the eyes close and the subject approaches maxi-mum awareness of body heaviness and warmth, the first *associative* suggestion is introduced. The induced con-ditions of heavy muscular relaxation, body-surface warmth, and toned-down visceral processes are those normally associated with the beginning of sleep. Since the hypnotist wishes to preclude sleep, or generalized sensory blocking, he suggests that the subject feel a light, increasingly pleasant drowsiness—a suggestion that serves to intensify the subject's awareness of the pleasurable conditions or sensations. At this point the subject is instructed to use the exhalation phase of his breathing cycles to set his own pace in the progressive deepening of the hypnotic state.

Induced deepening of the hypnotic state is effected through a directed reinterpretation of the established body sensations of heaviness and warmth. This deepen-ing is initiated by directing the subject to shift his focus of attention, gradually but steadily, from a saturated awareness of body heaviness to the equally pleasurable warm, fluid, and loose sensations from the internal organs. As he does, the subject is informed that he will experience an accelerated deepening of the drowsiness, accompanied by increasing awareness of lightness or floating sensations from the body, and a pleasant sensa-tion of numbness over the body surface.

The physiological basis for this perceptual translation is quite valid. First, the induced parasympathetic domi-nance of the visceral systems does produce increased blood flow (warmth), increased gastrointestinal motility (fluidity), and increased smooth-muscle tonus (fre-quently experienced as a sensation of "controlled" looseness). Second, the atonic relaxation of the skeletal muscles cancels out the information from the Golgi receptor (a sort of "strain gauge"), causing a feeling of weightlessness or floating that is often accompanied by the sensation of numbness.

As the subject's awareness becomes more and more saturated with generalized sensations of drowsiness, fluidity, and numbness, his attention can more and more easily be focused on specific cognitive processes. Such processes include association, vivid memory recall, positive or negative hallucination, programmed recogni-tion of waking-state cues, and sensory blocking, shifting, or masking—all of which are essential to the selective autogenic conditioning of the autonomic nervous system.

Programmed Reconditioning

Because hypnotic reconditioning can eliminate psycho-somatic disorders, hypnotherapy is effective in alleviat-ing many kinds of functional or structural damage in the respiratory, cardiac, vascular, gastric, intestinal, urinary, and genital organ systems.

Because of the increasing incidence of impotence and frigidity, both as prime symptoms of severe personal tensions and as a frequently cited reason for interper-sonal breakdowns, let us examine hypnosis in relation to these malfunctions.

Sexual adequacy is a blend of abilities: the ability to

respond and to satisfy one's self and the ability to satisfy the sexual expectations of one's partner. If either of these abilities is jeopardized or lapses, the resulting anxiety can result in self-imposed sexual impotence or frigidity.

By sociocultural tradition, the man has been placed in the role of sexual pursuer, and the woman assigned a passive, receptive role.

In affluent, post-pill societies, however, the sexual initiative has tended to shift from the man to the woman. Sharing the initiative with the woman implies more "on demand" sexual responsiveness than the man is used to traditionally. For the woman, the more explicit possibility of on-call male sexual responsiveness causes a reexamination of herself as an active participant rather than as a passive recipient.

Functionally, impotence can be defined as the inability to attain an erection sufficient for adequate penetration of the vagina, the inability to maintain such an erection, inability to prevent premature ejaculation, or inability to attain ejaculation.

Psychologically, impotence can be either a cause or an effect of a man's loss of prestige and self-respect. In either case, the onset of impotence gives rise to a generalized anxiety that not only perpetuates and aggravates the condition itself but causes deterioration in other dimensions of the male personality. A loss of sexual potency frequently poses either a challenge or a threat to the femininity of his partner. If the woman sees it as a challenge, she often becomes more aggressively seductive, which only intensifies the man's feelings of inadequacy. If the man's impotence is seen as a rejection, an already insecure female may become hostile and accusing, and thus arouse greater guilt and anxiety in the male. The emotional problems most frequently associated with impotence are depression, castration anxiety, homosexual panic, and generalized hypochondriasis.

The patterns of female frigidity include vaginal muscular spasticity and inhibition of vaginal secretion; the inability to respond to clitoral excitation; the inability to attain vaginal or totally satisfying orgasm; and psychological aversion to sexual contact of any sort. As with impotence, frigidity can be the cause or the effect of deterioration in other aspects of femininity.

Further, because of the traditionally passive nature of the woman's sexual role, her frigidity is often a catalyst for the development of impotence in an insecure male. If this frigidity is perceived by the man as a manipulation or a rejection, it may drive him to outside sexual involvements. From the wife's point of view, this may excuse the frigidity but at the same time it increases her anxiety about her general adequacy. The emotional ramifications of frigidity include involutional depression, abandonment anxiety, hypochondriasis, and neurotic overdependency.

The neurology of sexual arousal and responsiveness plays a significant role in both impotence and frigidity.

The term "responsiveness" designates a state of excitement—that is, sympathetic dominance—and this is an accurate description of the increasing stimulation leading to ejaculation or climax, the *second* phase of the sexual experience. What is omitted from this description is the first phase, the preparatory "arousal," or cognitive awareness, of sexual stimulation and the preparatory visceral relaxation, a vital parasympathetic response that is essential to adequate sexual arousal in male or female.

For the man, the primary physiological index of sexual arousal is the attainment of erection.

The most critical point in the human sexual arousal sequence is the parasympathetic relaxation phase of responsive preparation. It is in this phase than any apprehension or anxiety about one's sexual adequacy can trigger a premature sympathetic alerting reaction that *inhibits* rather than facilitates preparation for sexual contact. Cognitive *awareness* of this inhibition increases the anxiety, intensifying the inhibitory sympathetic dominance. The most disruptive effect of this self-intensifying anxiety reaction is that it stimulates an increased *conscious* effort to respond—an effort that has the same disastrous effect as a centipede's becoming conscious of his feet.

Now that some of the general cultural, psychological, and neurological scenery has been sketched in, let us return to our mythical—but typical—Harry and put him through a mockup of an actual hypnotherapeutic sequence.

| SESSION 1: | General exploratory interview. Harry confesses to general fears of declining sexual attractiveness and advancing age. These fears intensify and coalesce in the presence of certain visual and auditory cues, principally the sight of female breasts and the sound of certain bed noises. Whether these fears are the basic causal ones or not is unimportant; they are real enough to Harry, and they are instrumentally responsible for the inhibition of the crucial preliminary parasympathetic relaxation.

| SESSION 2: | Preliminary induction of hypnosis. (Not only can most people be hypnotized, but recent studies have shown that most people *have been* hypnotized; they have been in a state of selectively altered sensory awareness that is, technically, hypnotic.) Harry alternately tries too hard and resists, but a mild or shallow state of hypnosis is finally induced. Posthypnotic cues are introduced that will allow easier reinduction.

| SESSION 3: | Deeper levels of the hypnotic state are achieved. Cues are inserted that will permit a rapid induction of a very deep or somnambulistic state. (Sometimes cues are introduced that will allow the subject to self-induce the hypnotic state so that he can recapitulate and hence reinforce a particular hypnotic experience.)

| SESSION 4: | The crucial session, in which reconditioning takes place. Deep hypnosis is induced. The subject is directed to dwell upon his fears and vividly to imagine

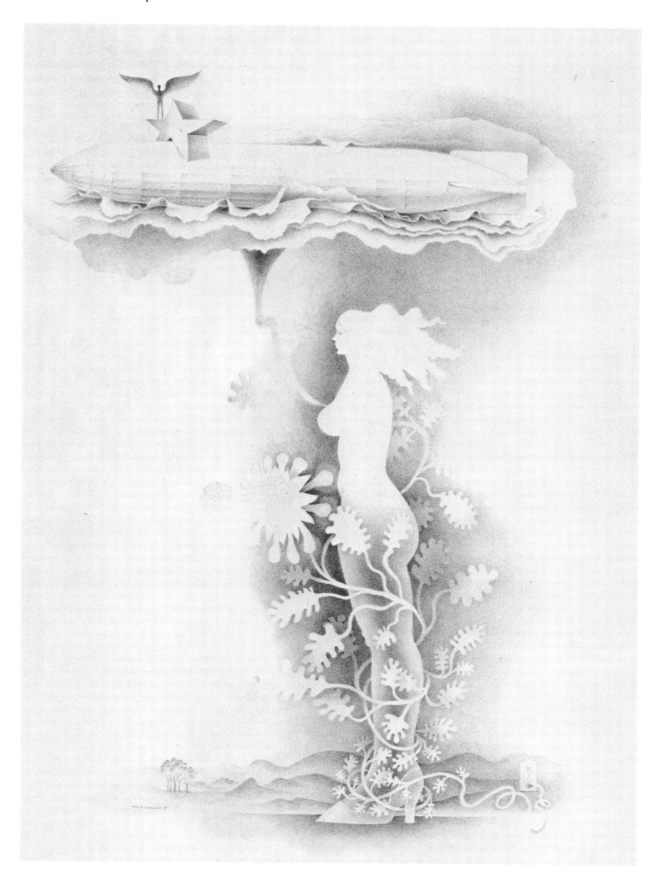

the sensory cues that trigger acute anxiety—in Harry's case a darkened bedroom, and so forth. (In the case of migraine sufferers, not only the sensory cue pattern but the migraine itself is generated, although the actual pain is dampened and translated into a different, less harmful set of sensations.) Harry is then led through a step-by-step autoerotic reenactment of a particularly memorable and pleasurable sexual success, emphasizing the initial parasympathetic visceral reactions. These reactions are then directly associated with the sensory cues or stimuli that formerly inhibited the agreeable reactions.

| SESSION 5: | The reassociation or deconditioning of the

inhibiting stimuli is further reinforced in this session.

| SESSION 6: | Further probing of the strength of the re-conditioned response. (These fifth and sixth sessions are not always necessary; sometimes seven or eight or more are needed. Six is the average.)

A genial posthypnotic chat follows, in which Harry grudgingly agrees to try more thoroughgoing therapy. He expresses enthusiasm about hypnotherapy and wonders about its applications in the restructuring or elimination of habit patterns—weight control, cigarette smoking. Wonders why *all* reeducative psychotherapy cannot take place in the hypnotic state. I warn him not to get carried away. Although . . .

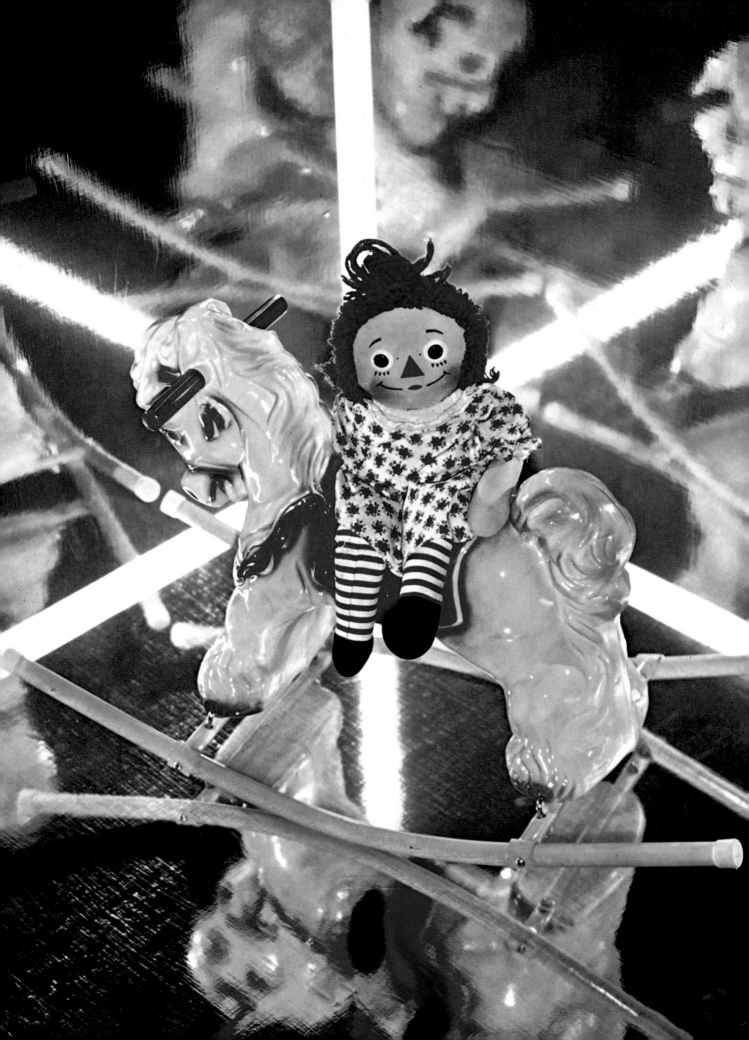

Mimosa Cottage: Experiment in Hope

James R. Lent

Parents who have a retarded child must often face an agonizing decision—whether or not to institutionalize their child, to place him in a residential treatment center. For the child, such placement means protective custody and good care but little treatment, in the psychological sense, and little challenge.

At Mimosa Cottage, life has quite another nature. The girls are patiently taught basic skills and energetically encouraged to do things on their own. The goal is to make life at the cottage resemble, as closely as possible, life in an actual community.

The root of Mimosa Cottage treatment is the same underlying the work with autistic children described by Ferster: operant conditioning. The operant approach often brooks criticism because it relies on external, tangible rewards and ignores the "internal" reasons a person may have for doing (or not doing) something. James Lent's description of the Mimosa Cottage project presents one of the least controversial uses of operant conditioning: In this case, the internal reason that is overlooked is the mental retardation itself.

Parsons, Kansas, is an unremarkable town inhabited, for the most part, by unremarkable people. One of them is a girl named Ellen, who helps care for the elderly patients in the community nursing home, where she works as a nurse's aide. At home, Ellen does her share of the housework; she prepares and serves the meals and babysits with the youngest member of the family, her six-year-old foster brother.

Today, Ellen's life is not very different from the lives of millions of unskilled and semiskilled workers in the United States, but that has not always been so. Five years ago, Ellen entered Mimosa Cottage at Parson's State Hospital and Training Center, a school for mentally retarded girls with measured IQs from 25 to 55. When she arrived, at the age of fourteen, Ellen was unable to tell time, count money, or find her way from the dormitory to the dining room alone. Now, at nineteen, she is almost a self-sufficient member of the community.

The Mimosa Cottage Demonstration Project, conducted since 1965 by the Parsons State Hospital and Training Center and the University of Kansas Bureau of Child Research, is a program designed to modify the behavior of mentally retarded girls between the ages of eight and twenty-one. Its overall goal is to train the Mimosa girls to behave as much like nonretarded members of the community as possible. Many girls, like Ellen, will eventually be able to live in the community. Others will continue to require care in an institution, but their adjustment to institutional life should be smoother as a result of the training they have received.

There are seventy-one "trainable" mentally retarded girls living in Mimosa Cottage. They are housed on three floors, according to age. On the bottom floor, Mimosa A, the girls are eight to twelve years old. Mimosa B, the middle floor, includes girls from twelve to sixteen. On the top floor, Mimosa C, are the older girls, aged sixteen to twenty-one. The overall goals are the same for all three groups. However, the reinforcement systems and the training programs differ in difficulty and complexity to reflect the different developmental levels of the three groups of children.

The basic method of the program is operant conditioning (see the preceding article), which is based on the premise that the receipt of a reward or reinforcer for specific behavior increases the probability that similar behavior will occur in the future. During the initial stages of the project, research assistants observed the dress and behavior of the people in the community, and the specific aims of the program were formulated from those observations.

The program includes four general training categories: personal appearance, occupational skills, social behavior, and functional academic subjects. Each of these is broken down into small and carefully defined behavioral components. These small components are the first objects of training. As the program proceeds, they are built into increasingly complex units of behavior.

As reinforcers to support the training, we use tokens

—generalized rewards that can be exchanged for items and privileges ranging from food and cosmetics to movies and dances. To serve its purpose, a reinforcer must have value for the person who receives it. Thus, our first task with each group of girls is to teach them that the tokens have value.

At first, we do not reinforce with tokens at all. Instead we offer such nontoken rewards as candy for desired behavior. Gradually, we substitute tokens for food. When the tokens are first used, we allow the girls to exchange them for food immediately. Then we increase the time between token exchanges. Eventually, we are even able to introduce saving by requiring several tokens for certain purchases.

Like the token system itself, the behavior for which tokens are given becomes more and more complex as training proceeds. It might be necessary at first, for example, to reward a girl for taking the smallest step toward painting a picture—for approaching the easel, say, or for touching the paintbrush. Later, the girl receives tokens only when she has painted for some time. Still later, the activity itself may become desirable and therefore reinforcing, and we can *require* tokens for the privilege of participating.

The tokens we give the younger girls (on Mimosa B) are coins—British half-pennies—which they keep in a bank attached to a wall of the cottage. They may spend the tokens for privileges, such as the use of a record player, or for items stocked at the cottage store. The cottage store, which resembles a small variety store, is an excellent place to teach the girls the behavior appropriate for shopping downtown. They must dress suitably, for instance, and they must communicate to the adult in charge what it is they want to buy. Depending on a girl's abilities, she is required to point to an item, to imitate its name after the adult in charge has said it, or to ask for it in a complete sentence.

The older girls on Mimosa C use a somewhat more abstract token-and-banking system. Their tokens take the form of marks on a gridded point card. The points on one side of the card can be redeemed for money; those on the reverse are "privilege points" that permit certain activities. Once a week, on Bank Day, the girls receive the amount of money shown on the financial side of their cards, money that they may keep themselves or, if they prefer, bank under lock and key. At the same time, their privilege points are recorded for use later on.

The money the older girls earn is spent in downtown Parsons—experience that helps shift the control of their behavior from extrinsic reinforcers to the normal reinforcers found in the community. To be eligible for a trip downtown, a girl must have privilege points, and to make purchases, she must use her own money. Thus she must have accumulated both kinds of tokens in order to "afford" an outing.

When a girl refuses to do a specific task or displays extremely deviant behavior, tokens may be taken away from her. Behavior that leads to the removal of tokens is called "costly behavior." One advantage of this system is that there is no need for emotionalism on the part of the staff. Without reprimands, nagging, or scolding, the adult simply removes the tokens.

It is important to keep the cost of goods and privileges realistic in comparison to community standards, and to accustom the girls to no more purchasing power for recreation than unskilled workers ordinarily have. Daily records of tokens received and spent allow us to make changes to meet the needs of individual children and, if necessary, to shift the level of the entire economy to offset depressions and inflations. This can be done by changing the quotas on token delivery, by changing the prices of articles stocked in the cottage store, and by changing the cost of activities.

The training itself includes personal skills such as cleanliness, grooming, and sitting and walking in ways that are appropriate to a noninstitutional community; domestic and occupational skills such as those needed to care for a house and to do simple repetitive work like that required in a sheltered workshop; social skills such as interpersonal relations and attitudes; and educational skills such as time-telling, arithmetic, vocabulary, and reading. A few examples will show how the training is done, and with what results.

Many of the Mimosa girls wear clothing that does not fit and is in poor condition. In part, the reason is the circumstances of institutional living—budget limitations, clothes sent by parents or issued by the institution without an opportunity for the girls to try them on. In addition, however, the girls do not know how to match colors and patterns or how to select styles that are appropriate for different occasions. These skills can be improved by training.

We begin by taking baseline data on each girl's level of skill without training. A test movie is shown of girls wearing various outfits. As each picture appears on the screen, the adult in charge describes the clothes ("This is a plain white blouse and a plaid skirt") and asks, "Do they match?" Then training begins. The staff member shows the girl different-colored cards and swatches of material and gives her a token when she matches them correctly. More complex matters follow, such as the proper use of checks and plaids and the choice of clothing appropriate to the season. At the end of the training, the test movie is shown again.

The results of the clothing program as a whole show some improvement in all areas. In three of the categories, color matching, type matching, and appropriateness to the occasion, our test showed significantly fewer errors after training than before. In the categories of figure matching and proper fit, however, the distribution of scores indicates that the program needs improvement. It is being revised this year.

Another fairly obvious deficiency in the personal

appearance of the Mimosa girls is their hair, which is often poorly combed, inappropriately styled, and dirty. Part of the problem is poor habits, but almost all the girls also lack skill in setting and combing, and they cannot identify hair styles that are suitable for them or for different social occasions.

One evening a week, a beautician from the community comes to the cottage and shows the girls how to style, set, and care for their hair. At first, the girls receive tokens each time they groom their own hair. Once they learn to do this regularly, the tokens are faded out and replaced with more natural consequences, such as beauty contests, Polaroid pictures, and praise from an adult or from another girl.

Townspeople from Parsons can often tell the Mimosa children from other children in the community simply by the way they walk. So we devised specific corrective programs for each small motor movement involved in walking. Many of the girls, for example, walk with their heads forward and down. To correct this, we use the following procedure. A piece of tape is attached to the wall at the exact height of the girl's chin, and the girl is asked to walk toward the spot from twenty feet away, keeping her eyes focused on it and pointing her chin at it. If necessary, the instructor places the girl's head in the proper position manually. Later, the girl walks toward the instructor instead of the spot of tape, maintaining eye contact and aiming her chin at the instructor's. When the girl holds her chin too low, the instructor signals that fact by raising his own chin. At the same time, an audio signal sounds. Finally, the girl walks twenty feet toward a mirror, maintaining eye contact with her own reflection and using the mirror to determine whether she needs to raise her chin. If her self-evaluation is faulty, the audio signal is used.

In addition to head position, the walking training includes five other components. Data taken at the end of 1966 showed considerable improvement in all six areas.

Not too surprisingly, good results obtained in training sessions do not always generalize to other life settings. Currently, we conduct the sessions on walking with a background auditory stimulus presented at a tempo of 116 beats per minute. Later, outside the training sessions, the auditory stimulus will be presented intermittently for short periods of time in the hope that the walking patterns established in training will be evoked. In the meantime, we have received a bonus: Performance during training has improved simply because the girls must always walk at the selected tempo; 116 beats per minute is an average walking speed, and walking and posture errors apparently are exaggerated when the pace is noticeably slower or faster.

Domestic skills such as sewing, ironing, housekeeping, and cooking are built up in the same gradual way as motor skills like walking. Sewing, for instance, begins with needle threading and button sewing and progresses through straight-line sewing to, for many girls, machine sewing. Several girls have been able with little help to make shifts, dresses, jumpers, and slacks. They choose and buy their own patterns, lay them out, cut the material, and sew the garments on the machine.

In the writing of all such training programs, the most useful rule we have discovered is: Do not assume that the subject will be able to generalize. This means that training programs must be written in far greater detail and much more explicitly than teaching plans for children of higher mental ability. It also means that what the girls learn to do in the cottage they may not do outside the cottage—in a home, in a job, or in a community store. Some problems with generalization can be foreseen and prevented. For example, housekeeping training begins in the model living area at the cottage and continues in more intensive and more complex form in homes in the community.

Other problems with generalization must be taken up individually as they occur, which may not be until after the girl has left Mimosa Cottage to live in the community. A girl who has been trained to recognize stewed tomatoes in a certain kind of can and to read prices marked in a certain numbering style may have trouble when she confronts the array of tomato products stocked by the usual grocery store. If she cannot generalize, she must be retrained—not only on tomatoes, but on beans, corn, and a variety of other products.

Like most institutionalized retarded persons, the girls at Mimosa have limitations, often severe, in such behavior as speech, social attitudes, and heterosexual interaction. For this reason, training in social skills is an important concern of the cottage program.

Leisure-time activities, some individual and some group, show the children how to entertain themselves and teach them to get along with one another. The games and activities must have absolute carry-over value, that is, they must be the same things many people in the community do to occupy their time—puzzles, card games such as canasta and solitaire, dominoes and checkers, jacks.

Dances are organized for the girls from Mimosa Cottage and retarded boys from a nearby cottage. The dances offer an opportunity for instruction in social manners and in posture. Many of the girls show poor posture when sitting or standing, and they do not really know how to begin or end a dance. Training includes nine steps, beginning when the girl is asked to dance and ending when she tells her partner she enjoyed the dance. The instructor tells the children the behavior expected of them and uses marks on their reinforcer cards to indicate that they have performed satisfactorily. At the end of the dance session, the children can use the marks they have earned to attend a special party, where cookies and punch are served.

Our experience with this program taught us something about the selection of target behavior. All the children in the first two classes attained criterion behavior, and we were pleased that the program was serving its purpose. However, in reviewing a movie of a training session, we suddenly noticed that the session did not look like a teen-age dance. The children's manners and movements were more similar to those of middle-class, middle-aged persons. At this point, the middle-aged author designed a new program on the basis of actual observations of teen-age dances held in the community.

Instruction in heterosexual association and sex hygiene is a regular part of the social training. It is frank and to the point. An illustrated program covers the fundamentals of reproduction; in addition, again with boys from another cottage, the girls are taught what is proper and what is not and what is proper in some places but improper in others.

Although the measured IQs of the Mimosa girls classify them as trainable rather than educable, many of them are able to acquire basic academic skills. Instruction in arithmetic, time-telling, phonics and reading has been initiated with individuals and small groups, and the procedures are being analyzed and improved as we gain experience.

All programs, with one exception, have been developed by the project staff, since published materials have not proved useful with trainable (as opposed to educable) children. The Rainier Reading Program developed by Sidney W. Bijou and his colleagues is the one available program that we have been able to use with the Mimosa girls.

The development of speech and language skills in the Mimosa girls is one of our most important goals. The articulation improvement program carried out with ten girls on Mimosa C for the past year will illustrate.

The method of therapy was such that learning was acquired gradually and surely. A set of ten words was presented to each girl by means of picture cards. Her verbal responses to the cards were our baseline data. Then we evoked responses by means of simple, concrete stimuli and gradually shifted to more abstract, more natural means of evoking responses. The sequence was (1) auditory-visual (word and picture); (2) visual stimuli (picture card); (3) grapheme (printed word); (4) intraverbal stimuli (a sentence with a missing word to be supplied by the girl). As a final test, we presented words that contained the same sound elements as those used in training, but had not themselves been used. This was a partial measure of generalization.

Nine of the ten girls did significantly better on the post-test than on the pre-test for each set of ten words and were able to generalize the effects of training to new words with considerable success. The tenth girl made few errors to begin with, and therefore did not make significant gains.

One final type of training that should be mentioned is that used to remedy the specific behavioral problems of individual girls. For instance, one fourteen-year-old

resident of Mimosa Cottage made a practice of placing rocks, beads, and other small objects in her ear canal. She did so with such force that the objects could not be removed except by medical specialists. We tried to find out just what circumstances preceded and followed the girl's behavior, but it was not possible to identify a pattern. We did discover, though, that the doctors and nurses at the hospital where she was taken for treatment took care of her almost immediately and expressed great sympathy and concern. It seemed that this process might well be maintaining the behavior.

Since irreparable damage had already been done to the child's eardrum and ear canal, the hospital agreed to try anything that might reduce further damage. The next time the child placed an object in her ear, the cottage aide said, "All right, see me about it tomorrow. I'm busy now." The next day the child was sent by herself to the outpatient clinic, where the only attention paid to her was that her name was taken down by a nurse. Three hours later she was seen by the doctor, who treated her in a very matter-of-fact manner and assigned her to a recovery room. She stayed there for two weeks, by herself; her only contact with the staff was at meals, bed change, and clean-up time, and these encounters were brief.

After the behavior modification procedure began, there was one further incident and then an abrupt cessation for eight months. At that time, the child was called for a hearing examination. She prepared herself for the occasion by placing a bead in her ear. Since then there have been no further incidents.

Using the same principles of behavior modification and similar techniques, several other individual behavior problems have been successfully modified. Many of these problems are quite ordinary, such as tantruming and loud talking. Others are more bizarre—a girl who smeared butter over her face and clothing at meal time; a girl who stole food from other children's trays; a girl who tore her shoes at the seams; a girl who talked incessantly and incoherently to herself and to others. In many instances it was possible to discover events that typically followed the child's behavior and maintained it. Modification then involved manipulating the environment in such a way that reinforcement was no longer provided. In addition, we tried to arrange for the child to develop an alternative—a desirable response that was incompatible with the undesirable one. For instance, there are children who only get attention from adults when they are screaming or yelling. Training adults to ignore the tantrum is half the job; training the child to get attention in desirable ways is the other half.

People who hear about the Mimosa project often have questions to ask, some about its design and some about its "ethics." Here are a few of the ones we hear most often, and the answers we give.

"Couldn't time rather than training be responsible

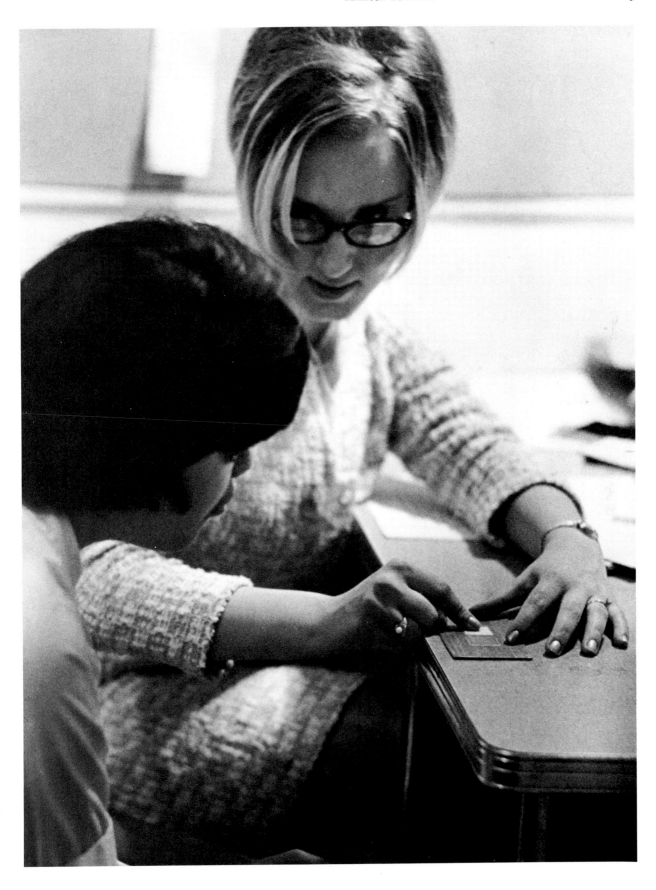

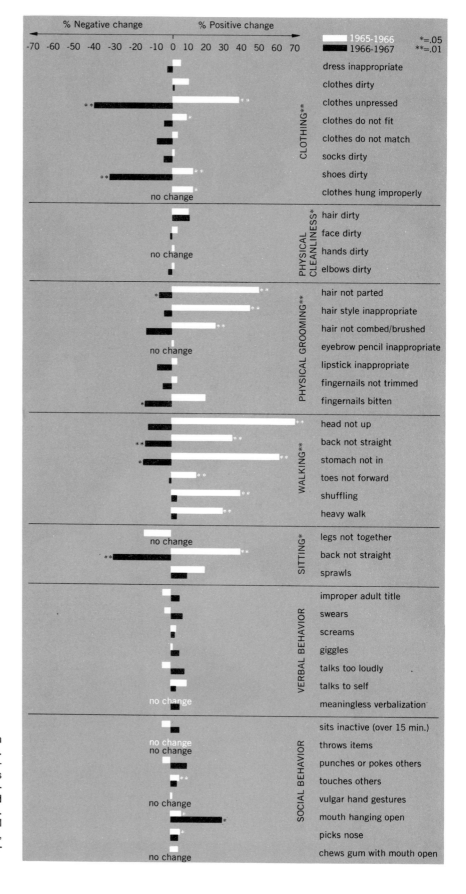

Figure 1. Behavior modification as a result of the girls' training. Note that in 1965–1966, improvement in personal skills was stressed, with noticeable improvement, whereas their verbal and social behavior had not improved. In 1966–1967, training in verbal and social skills was stressed, and these areas showed improvement.

for changes in the girls' behavior?" Several studies, conducted in this country and abroad, have shown that institutionalization has a crippling effect on the behavior of retarded children. Their behavior tends to deteriorate with time, not to improve. For example, L. F. Cain and S. Levine of San Francisco State College gave a social competency test to trainable retarded children living in institutions and to similar children living at home. They found that the scores of the children living at home rose with the passage of time, while those of the institutionalized children decreased significantly.

"Isn't it hard for aides to act natural, spontaneous, and 'happy' with the children when so much behavior is prescribed?" When aides first start reinforcing on a schedule, their behavior is somewhat mechanistic and stilted. However, they soon become accustomed to giving reinforcement and they are, after all, pleased when a child behaves appropriately. As the training takes effect, the children behave appropriately more and more often, which reinforces the staff and makes them "happy." The children, in turn, are reinforced by the quiet, predictable, pleasant behavior of the adults in charge.

"Doesn't it seem *wrong* to pay a girl to do something she should do for nothing, like comb her hair?" Well, the alternative is to *punish* the girl when she does *not* comb her hair, which seems wronger and is also less effective. Positive reinforcement is the best way we have to establish new forms of behavior. Once the behavior is established, tokens can be phased out and natural reinforcers substituted.

"Are you sure you chose the right goals for the girls?" Behavioral principles themselves are amoral. They can be used to prepare a child to vegetate in an institution, or to prepare him for life in the community. What we do is use them to reach goals on which most members of the community agree. For example, most people in Parsons agree that it is better for an adolescent girl to know how to cook and sew than not to know how to cook and sew. Most agree that it is better for a girl to say "please" when she requests something than not to say "please."

"Isn't the program terribly expensive?" Yes, the program is expensive. It costs about $35,000 per year more than regular hospital treatment. However, if it trains a girl to support herself outside an institution for the rest of her life, it will save the taxpayer about $100,000.

The final question, of course, is "How well does the program work?" The answer is that it works fairly well, and we keep trying to make it work better. During 1965–1966, the girls improved considerably in such personal skills as care of clothing, physical cleanliness, physical grooming, walking and sitting. However, there was no overall improvement in verbal or social behavior. This meant that the training procedures, or the reinforcement system, or perhaps both, needed revision.

In 1966–1967, we shifted the emphasis of training away from personal skills and toward verbal and social ones. The space for verbal and social tokens on reinforcement cards was more than tripled, and aides were told to give more points for appropriate responses in these areas than they had the last year. In addition, aides and research assistants received supplementary training to develop their sensitivity to social behavior.

The change in emphasis worked almost too well: the pattern for 1965–1966 reversed itself in 1966–1967. Social and verbal behavior improved significantly, while personal skills held steady and even, in some cases, declined. The decline suggested that we had overreacted to the preceding year's results—although, since personal skills had already reached a high level, the decrease was not as serious as it might have been (see Figure 1).

Twelve of the Mimosa girls have now returned to the community. Five are too young to work and are living with their natural families. Seven are older and they are all working, full- or part-time. These older girls range from 20 to 69 in IQ and from seventeen to twenty-two in age. They have spent between four and one-half and twelve years in institutions.

Some of these girls have rejoined their natural families; others have been placed in foster homes. They are not fully independent, but they are able to take care of most of their personal needs and to move about the community alone. One of them is Ellen and, like Ellen, all of them lead simple but productive lives. Those around them may even forget, at times, that they were ever labeled "mentally retarded."

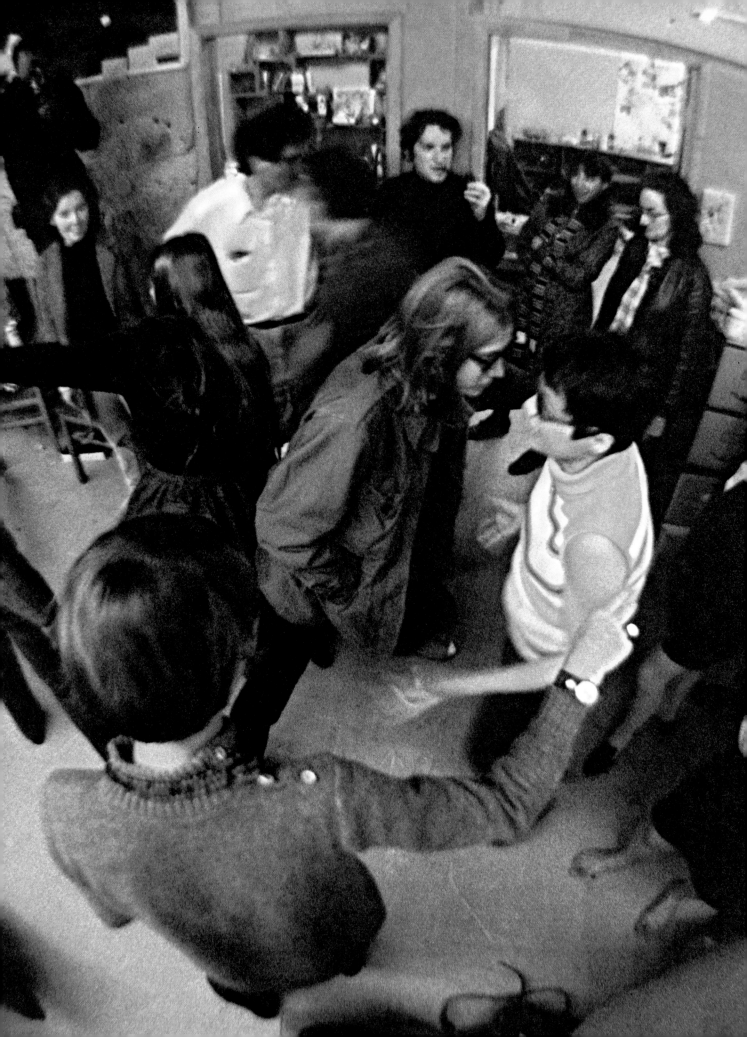

Daytop Village

Alexander Bassin

A *few years ago, several investigators surveying narcotic treatment centers happened into Synanon, a California community for drug addicts modeled on a strong patriarchal family structure. The startling success of Synanon dwellers in enjoying a creative, communal life, healthy and drug-free, impelled these investigators to develop an extensive program for drug addicts on probation along the same lines; hence, the halfway house of Daytop Village. Alexander Bassin, one of the initiators of this project, here reviews Daytop's brief and ruffled history, and presents in simple, graphic terms the rationale and methods that so markedly set the Daytop experiment apart from conventional drug treatments.*

The core at which Daytop workers hack away is the addict's motivation for change. From the junkie's first tentative inquiry throughout the calendar of interviews and encounters informing Daytop existence, fellow addicts challenge his will to get rid of drugs and the wasting way of life in which they submerge him.

The Daytop methods are not limited to dealing with drug addicts and are being adopted eagerly by many who see in the techniques and sanctions of this therapeutic community the seeds for revitalization in a number of fields. Evaluation of this and other revolutionary approaches flourishing in psychology today will have to await time's arbitration.

A pretty coed from nearby Wagner College, fulfilling a class requirement for *Sociology 416*, "Social Problems in Modern America," visits Daytop Village on New York's Staten Island during a Saturday night open house party. Soon she is in deep conversation with a young man who might pass as a college senior—except that he is neatly dressed, wears coat and necktie, and his hair is short and combed.

"What is Daytop all about? What do you do?"

"I'll tell you right up front. We take a guy, say twenty-five years old, who's been a waste all his life. He's been stealing and robbing, and is in and out of jail. He's a thief and a parasite who would con his own mother out of her food money to buy some crap to shoot into his veins. And do you know what we do with him?"

"No, what? What do you do?"

"In a matter of a year and a half to two years, we transform him into an honest, decent, responsible human being who has a new set of values, who has some interests beyond the bang-bang on the boob tube, who knows a little something about art, music, literature, and the war in Vietnam. In other words, we, like, take

an order of scrambled eggs that has been spoiled and smells, and we change it into a sweet and cool lime Jello pudding."

"Gosh," murmurs the collegiate miss, "you Daytop people are wonderful."

The message gets through to the coed very well indeed. As well it might. The drug addict the young man is talking about is *himself*.

The psychological basis for treating drug addicts at Daytop Village differs radically from conventional methods. Neither punishing the addict by jailing him for extended periods nor slobbering over him with sympathy and pity has shown any great rehabilitative value. Nor has it helped to regard the addict as a sick person, a "medical problem," as some well-meaning folk put it. The Daytop philosophy is to consider the addict as an adult acting like a baby: childishly immature, full of demands, empty of offerings.

The addict sees nothing as his fault—not his addiction, not his degradation, nor his desperation. He is convinced he has been thrown into life without the armor and weapons that others have. Heroin enables him to escape from the unfair battle. It deadens his desire for friends, for achievement, for wealth, for strength, for sex, and even for food. The satisfactions sought so relentlessly by other people, the junkie obtains, for a short time anyway, with a five-dollar deck of heroin.

In pursuit of heroin, the addict is able to muster extraordinary cunning, shrewdness, gall, and acting ability. Usually, he is untouched by normal psychotherapeutic approaches. For him treatment is a game of upmanship, an arena for practicing his confidence-man skills.

Conventional methods of treating drug addicts have been grossly ineffective. For example, follow-up studies of addicts treated in the U.S. Public Health Service hospitals in Lexington, Kentucky, and in Fort Worth, Texas, reveal that more than 90 percent of released patients relapse into drug addiction within a few years. And many of the addicts treated at these excellent medical facilities do not show even the simple respect for their $50-per-day treatment of waiting forty-eight hours after release before taking a shot of heroin.

The change agent most likely to be effective with the junkie is another addict who has made a commitment to change himself, one who is prepared to use himself as a role model and become *involved* with his "brother." When a professional therapist attempts to communicate with the addict, he is simply turned off with: "This dumb bastard doesn't know what he's talking about. He doesn't know the scene. He's never been there."

Who Gets In

The Daytop intake process is organized to challenge the applicant's sincerity in wanting to break his habit. Thus, when a kind-hearted social worker, psychologist, psychiatrist, judge, probation or parole officer telephones Daytop in an effort to smooth the admission of a "worthy" case, he is politely advised it would be best if the addict applied for himself or herself. The applicant should be over sixteen years of age and not a pillhead. When withdrawal takes place outside the hospital, Daytop personnel consider the barbiturate, amphetamine, and methadrine addict to be in far greater danger than the heroin addict. In any case, the addict himself must telephone to arrange for admission to Daytop.

When the addict does call he is told that Daytop is crowded, many addicts are clamoring to get in, and space is limited. But if he is really interested in getting in, if he wants to make an "investment to save your life," he may call again tomorrow at 2:30 sharp. If he "forgets" and calls a day late, he is told, "I guess you're not very serious about helping yourself. So we are putting you at the bottom of the list." When he calls at the designated time, he is commended for his interest and told to call again a day later. If this commitment is kept, he is invited to present himself at Daytop Village, clean of drugs for at least twenty-four hours, with his

parents and family if possible. Some applicants go through a half-dozen telephone calls before they receive an invitation.

What is the rationale for this apparently heartless system?

Few addicts are motivated for therapy and change. Treatment is usually the lesser of two evils to the junkie. He comes to Daytop because he thinks it is "easier time" than jail, or because there is a panic in the streets and no drugs are around anyway, or because the heat is on and he needs a hideout, because he has been kicked out of the house by his wife, because he wants to dry out for a while and is tired of finding ways to pay for his expensive habit. But permanently give up the use of junk? Impossible! Once a junkie, always a junkie. So the addict reasons with himself about the prospect of going straight.

Every step of the Daytop intake procedure is designed to shock the addict into realizing that this place is basically different from the social agencies he has learned how to manipulate. Here he will not be indulged like a spoiled child, here his usual con games will not work.

When the addict arrives at Daytop on the scheduled date and on time, he is admitted to the reception area and told to sit on the "prospect's chair" and wait until he is called. Meanwhile, his parents and relatives are ushered next door and given counsel that makes their jaws drop as tears come to their eyes.

"Mama, here at Daytop we don't blame parents for the misdeeds of their children. We know you never encouraged him to use dope but he's always tried to make you think it was all your fault. He's stolen money from you, lied to you, abused and cursed you, made your life a hell on earth. How do we know all this? Did we read it in some book or in *Life* magazine? No, mama, we are all ex-junkies, just like your Johnny, and that is what we did to our own parents."

Members of the interviewing team then give the relatives thumbnail autobiographical sketches of themselves. Next, each extols the near-miraculous benefits of a year or two at Daytop.

Finally, the parents are given some astonishing advice: Make yourselves as cold, as hostile, and rejecting as you can toward Johnny. If he telephones, hang up! If he sneaks out a letter, return it unopened to Daytop. And if he suddenly turns up at home and turns on the woebegone, contrite mannerisms the addict puts on so well, if he tries to melt your hearts with tales of the abuse he suffered at the Village, then grit your teeth and tell him, "Go back to Daytop, get lost." And slam the door in his face.

Meantime, back at the reception desk, the prospect has been going through a nerve-shattering experience. He sits facing a wall. Behind him is the open door—and freedom. By now, he has cased the setup and notes that there are no bars anywhere, that the windows are at ground level—and wide open. All about him is the hustle and bustle of a happy family household rather than the aseptic silence of a hospital or of a prison. Nobody is walking around in hospital pajamas or prison uniforms; there are no doctors with stethoscopes hanging out of their pockets, no nurses in white uniforms, no uniformed security personnel.

Then he sees a blood brother, a crony with whom he had shot up only a short time ago in alleyways and public toilets—sharing the same spike. But instead of the warm welcome he would have received in any prison or hospital in the country, his former pal looks through him as though he were invisible and doesn't respond to Johnny's big hello.

Momentarily uneasy, Johnny relaxes with the thought that junkies will be junkies. They must have a supply stashed away someplace, and once he gets into the swing of things, he will be able to cut himself into the action. For the third time in twenty minutes, he asks when he will be interviewed. His frustration tolerance is low, and he has never willingly waited for anyone.

"We are very busy here, as you can see, and you will have to wait until the interviewers can see you," the receptionist answers coldly. The implication is clear; if he doesn't like it, he can beat it. No one is keeping him. He may wait from forty-five minutes to four hours before being called for the interview. If he does not flee through the open door, he passes another initiation rite for admission to the Daytop fraternity.

The interview room is cozy, homelike, a room without desk, or diplomas, or any of the accouterments of the professional office. Three clean-cut, conventionally dressed young men politely ask Johnny to come in, apologize for the delay, and start questioning him in a kindly, sympathetic manner. What did he want from Daytop? What was the problem? What neighborhood did he come from?

Within a few minutes, Johnny has sized up the situation. These cats are obviously social workers and he can con them out of their bank accounts if he really tries. He talks to them about his hard and sad life, about his fears and anxieties, his unresolved conflicts, his determination to be cured of the horrors of drug addiction and to make himself over into something better.

Suddenly, one of the interviewers jolts Johnny:

"Hey, stop this garbage! Who the hell do you think you're talking to?"

Two of the interviewers talk to each other: "Did you ever hear such bullshit in your life?"

"This crazy dope fiend thinks he's inside another joint."

"Maybe he didn't get enough luff from his mudder and fodder!"

The interviewers curl up with laughter and poke one another in the ribs as they mimic the addict's words and expressions. After a few minutes, they turn serious and begin a "cleanup" operation. No, they are not social workers, psychologists, intake workers, or whatever he thought they were, but street junkies just like him.

Right now they can tell him just what is going through his mind because junkies are pretty much alike. They are under the impression the world owes them a living because they are hooked on dope, and they dare anybody to cure them. But here at Daytop you learn "there ain't no free lunch."

They tell Johnny that despite his physical size and age, he is a baby in terms of maturity, responsibility, and judgment. So he will be treated like a three-year-old who is told what to do because at this point he simply does not have enough sense to keep from getting killed.

"You'll see a lot of things you don't understand. Don't waste time asking a lot of fool questions. Your brain is not strong enough for that kind of exercise just yet. Maybe in a few weeks or months you will understand. But for the time being, you must *act as if* you understood, *act as if* you are a man, *act as if* you want to do the right thing, *act as if* you care about other people, *act as if* you are a mature human being."

At Daytop, Johnny is told, we don't spend valuable time trying to find the essential *cause* of his addiction. That whole process would be exploited by the addict to avoid the responsibility for his behavior. At Daytop we *know* why somebody is a dope fiend—because he chooses to act STUPID! That's the only acceptable explanation for addiction: stupidity.

At the end of the interview, the "noodle-head" is told there are only two cardinal rules of the house:

1. No chemicals or drugs or alcohol may be used.
2. No violence or even the threat of violence.

No excuse is accepted for breaking either of these two basic rules. If he does, he will be kicked out, exiled.

Daytop Methods

The interviewers now become affable. They say that Daytop is one place where the people really care for one another, treat each other like brother and sister. Everybody tries to live as openly and honestly as possible. No con games, manipulations, lying, or cheating. Everybody in the house, from the director to that girl at the reception desk, is a junkie. There's no "we versus they" business here. Everybody is a member of the staff, and there's no job he can't aim for—even director.

Johnny is assigned a low-status job at once. He cleans the toilets, washes pots and pans, or mops floors. He is introduced to his three roommates, who have been trained to welcome him to their midst and to assume responsibility for the welfare of their new brother.

If he is experiencing any withdrawal symptoms, no big fuss is made about it. He goes through the withdrawal on a couch in the living room with residents all about him, laughing, playing cards, listening to music, dancing. He is too ashamed to put on the expected exhibition of wall climbing and swinging from chandeliers. He knows that these people will not be impressed by his performance. He knows there will be no payoff for his histrionics from these wise, hard-nosed critics. And somewhat to his own surprise, he kicks the remnants of his habit in record time with no more discomfort than the average guy with a mild case of flu.

One of the principal methods for achieving self-image and behavioral change at Daytop is the three times a week *group encounter* therapy.

During the encounter, at which attendance is compulsory, the building echoes with ear-piercing screams, curses, oaths, blasphemy, shouts, tears, and laughter. The vehemence is hard to believe. Gutter language and four-letter epithets explode from the rooms. One member after another is assigned to the "hot seat," where he is attacked and criticized for failing to adhere to the basic precepts of Daytop, for being less than 100 percent honest and open, for being insensitive to the feelings of others.

The encounter is called a *pressure cooker* by David Deitch, the thirty-five-year-old director of Daytop Village. "It is a safety valve to relieve the tensions that have built up during the previous day. The Daytop resident cannot use profanity at any time except during the encounter. He cannot act moody or irritable or be overcome with self-pity between encounters. He has to *act as if* and wait until the encounter to get the garbage out of his system. The encounter is a gut-level teaching device that speeds up personality alteration, just as a pressure cooker speeds the preparation of food."

Many professionals are abashed and frightened by the fierceness of the attack therapy. But Dr. Lewis Yablonsky, research consultant to Synanon, after his first twenty-five sessions, found that the group "attack" was an act of love in which was entwined the assumption: "If we did not care about you or have concern for you, we would not bother to point out something that might reduce your psychic pain or clarify something for you that might save your life."

Every day but Sunday, at one o'clock, the Daytop membership assembles in the auditorium. Before them, on a blackboard, they see a quotation, perhaps from Emerson, or from Einstein. It may be a Biblical quotation or a poem by Emily Dickinson.

A different leader is appointed for each seminar. He asks: "Who wants to say something about this?" Before the words are out of his mouth, a dozen hands are waving in the air. The leader points and a member rises, nervous and uneasy. He mumbles a few words, and sits down to a broadside of friendly applause. For an hour, the performance is repeated with speakers of differing degrees of fluency.

Other seminars feature free choice sessions, in which residents talk spontaneously about a designated topic, or mock speaking engagements, in which members act as if they are appearing before an outside community group.

A visitor to Daytop sees signs and slogans promi-
nently hung in the kitchen, dining room, offices, and hallways. Typical slogans are:

There is no free lunch.
Honesty *is* the best policy.
Hang tough! (Don't give up.)
Seek and assume responsibility!
Be careful of what you ask for.
You may just get it!

Every resident seems to incorporate these shorthand behavioral prescriptions into his speech repertoire. You hear them spoken at encounters, seminars, and while "rapping with the squares" (talking to nonaddicts) at the Saturday night open house party.

If a Daytop resident commits the heinous offense of "splitting" (leaving without permission), an emergency Fireplace meeting might be called when he returns, even if it requires routing everybody out of bed at three in the morning. He is placed on the hot seat and must beg at the top of his voice to be readmitted into the house. Sometimes he is subjected to a "haircut," a severe verbal reprimand. And if his offense is serious, his hair is actually cropped to the skull while house members boo and jeer.

John Ruocco, director of Daytop at Staten Island, once told me: "An errant member submits to a haircut to show he is sincerely sorry for the stupid thing he did and that he wants to make a solid investment in his recovery. His bald head helps him remember not to act stupid and irresponsible in the future."

Banishment is the most serious sanction at Daytop Village. But it is reserved for a flagrant violation of the house rules. Exile is considered equivalent to a death sentence—an all too frequent fate of the junkie, who can end up at the city morgue, dead of an overdose.

The greatest number of dropouts in the Daytop program occur during the first thirty days. About 8 percent of the addicts who come through the front door leave immediately or within a month. The great majority remain for three months, when another critical period is reached. Approximately 17 percent will split after ninety days. According to Dr. Daniel Casriel, medical psychiatric director of Daytop, the addict who remains three months has better than a 75 percent chance of completing the program and emerging as a new vibrant human being.

Dave Deitch, on the other hand, adamantly refuses to become involved in a numbers game about the success rate of Daytop. He notes that besides the several hundred residents of Daytop who are leading lives free of drugs and crime, there are more than sixty who have met Daytop's extraordinarily high standards for personal transformation and are leading active and self-supporting lives in outside communities.

Every three months or so, a marathon encounter led by specially trained staff members is held. Basically, the

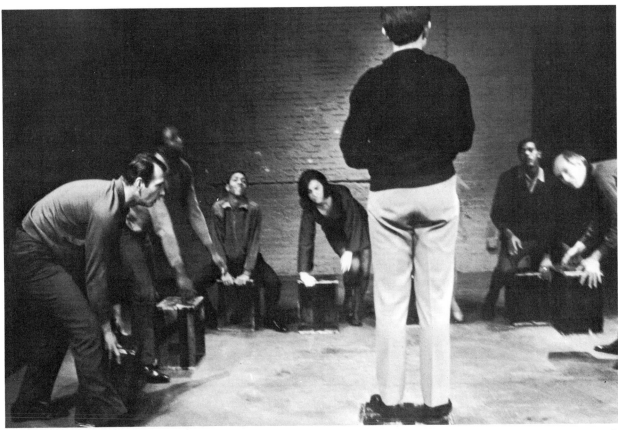

The Concept, a hit off-Broadway play, is one of Daytop's proudest achievements. Hailed by drama critics as truly outstanding theater, the play is an improvisation by ex-narcotic addicts from Daytop about one person's drug addiction and recovery. This photograph and the one on page 132 are from a performance of the play.

marathon is an extension of the floor encounter for a period of twenty-four to forty-eight hours. The meeting is continuous except for a few hours of sleep. In many cases, there are experiences of rebirth and personality alteration that have no exact parallel in psychiatric literature.

Twice a year, Daytop closes its doors, unhooks the telephone, calls in all members, and engages in a week-long retreat. It is a time of self-criticism, meditation, institutional assessment, and charting new directions.

On Saturday night, Daytop Village is open to visitors. A phone call will reserve a place but frequently every opening is filled weeks in advance. This open house has become a favorite field-trip assignment for professors of psychology, sociology, and education. There are some speeches followed by music and dancing, but the best part, most visitors agree, is the opportunity to talk with a remarkable group of intelligent, alert, healthy minded young people.

History of the Approach

About seven years ago, a team consisting of the late Professor Herbert Bloch, criminologist at Brooklyn College, Dr. Daniel Casriel, a psychiatrist with many years' experience in treating addicts, Joseph A. Shelly, chief probation officer of the Brooklyn Supreme Court, and myself visited and evaluated the leading narcotic treatment centers in all parts of the United States. Nothing very exciting turned up until we came to a little-known converted armory located on the beach at Santa Monica, California. Here our psychiatrist was surprised to find several former patients of his whom he had dismissed as being hopeless. But here they were healthy and happy, and most important of all, they were free of drugs!

The place was Synanon, and its founder, Chuck Dederich, assured us that it was destined to become one of the most significant developments in treating not only drug addicts but all forms of deviant behavior, even chronic criminals and the so-called psychopath.

In a gravel-tone voice, our bull-necked host explained his approach in anthropological terms: "We attempt to create an extended family of the type found in preliterate tribes which usually have a strong, almost autocratic, father-figure, who dispenses firm justice combined with warm concern, who is a model extolling inner-directed convictions about the old-fashioned virtues of honesty, sobriety, education and hard work."

Our mission experience resulted in a proposal to the National Institute of Mental Health for the establishment of a halfway house for drug addicts on probation, who would be treated along the lines we observed at Synanon, except that they would be regularly tested for traces of heroin. On April 15, 1963, we were informed that NIMH had awarded us $390,000 for a five-year study.

For a name we selected the acronym *Daytop* (Drug Addicts Treated on Probation) and *Lodge*, to avoid the unfortunate semantic associations with orthodox treatment centers.

Our first manager was driven to the verge of a nervous breakdown by the antics of the residents and the problems of setting up a pioneering experiment

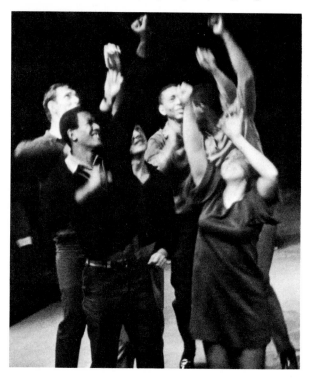

under the aegis of a court bureaucracy. In the first year the project chewed up half a dozen managers. At the same time, residents of the local community protested against the presence of Daytop with picket lines, law suits, and angry letters in the local newspaper.

The turbulent development of Daytop was stabilized with the acquisition of a new manager, David Deitch, a native of Chicago with a history of some fourteen years of addiction. He curbed his habit at Synanon, rose to a position of leadership there, but left after two years because of some differences with Dederich.

Although conditions at Daytop improved under Deitch's leadership, a plateau was reached that called for a reevaluation of methods and goals. Up to this time, only male addicts had been admitted. It was decided that the small initial group of thirty males did not provide the diversity of personality types required to operate the dynamics of a therapeutic community. Ac-

cording to Deitch, "The junkie needs new faces on whom to try out his recently acquired skills. It is necessary to create a community of men, women and children who live and work and love together if our people are to grow into mature responsible citizens."

NIMH agreed to permit the original research plan to be expanded and the inclusion of females. The name of the project was changed from Daytop Lodge to Daytop Village.

Its Present and Future

Today, Daytop is operating a 100-residence facility at Staten Island, and another with a capacity of 200 at Swan Lake in the Catskill Mountains, about 120 miles from New York City, and a third at New Haven, Connecticut, in joint sponsorship with Yale University.

Methods developed at Daytop are being applied to new fields. For professionals, such as psychologists, social workers, and clergymen, Daytop has conducted several hundred Intensive Training Institutes at its center in the Catskill Mountains. Participants become members of the Daytop community and experience the encounter process. They come to grips with their own emotional and social problems. Almost all emerge with the comment: "This has been one of the most meaningful experiences of my life."

Daytop has established three storefront centers called SPAN, which are designed to induce the street addict to sample the Daytop approach. These centers also work directly with people in the ghettos to improve their community.

Abraham Maslow, president of the American Psychological Association, and O. Hobart Mowrer, a former president, both have proclaimed Daytop as one of the great therapeutic community developments of our time. Mowrer is now writing a book on Daytop, *The Daytop Dynamic*.

Daytop is optimistic about its future. The leading force in the organization of Daytop, Monsignor William B. O'Brien, sees the principles and methods developed there as useful not only for the rehabilitation of narcotic addicts but also for the training and revitalization of teachers, psychologists, psychiatrists, social workers, businessmen, and government officials.

"The Daytop approach can be used in prisons, penitentiaries and reform schools," he says. "As a fellow priest once remarked to me after spending a month at the Village: 'God is not dead, He lives at Daytop!' People in all helping professions can learn from Daytop how man can be taught to help himself."

Epilogue

After five years of exciting existence, Daytop reached the ultimate crisis of its being when the Board of Directors recommended that David Deitch be retired. The stormy events leading to this decision are difficult to chronicle in an altogether dispassionate manner, but in essence the Board felt that Deitch was establishing a cult of personality and infallibility. He flatly refused to consider a relaxation of his rule excommunicating any member who "split," regardless of extenuating circumstances or subsequent patent success of the Daytopper in dealing with the strains and stresses of the outside community. He also refused to consider the proposal that Daytop affirm the goal (set at the time of its establishment under NIMH and Brooklyn Supreme Court auspices) of returning the residents to their homes and communities after one to one and a half years. In trying to dissuade Dave, board members pointed to the evidence that most of the splittees were making it reasonably well in the street, so why not recognize the remarkable impact of the Daytop experience in changing basic attitudes and behavior and strive to become a short-term therapeutic center rather than an institution requiring a lifetime of residence and a monastic type of existence? But Dave would not be moved.

Many members of the board were convinced that it was Deitch's personality, the force of his leadership, that accounted for Daytop's success, and they were afraid that without him, the institution would disintegrate. The board's dilemma was resolved by those who argued that if Daytop was primarily interested in establishing a *treatment methodology,* a philosophy, and set of techniques with interchangeable parts, it could not depend on one person for its viability.

After the decision, Deitch threatened to barricade the premises and fight eviction with force. But at the last moment he heeded a court order and departed, taking with him almost the entire leadership corps and the majority of residents. Board members Monsignor O'Brien, Dr. Casriel, and Mortimer Levitt promptly reorganized the management of Daytop and stepped back to see whether the Daytop approach possessed the inner vitality and creative force to survive as an institution and treatment procedure. Eight months after the departure of Deitch the verdict is in. *Daytop is alive and doing better than ever.*

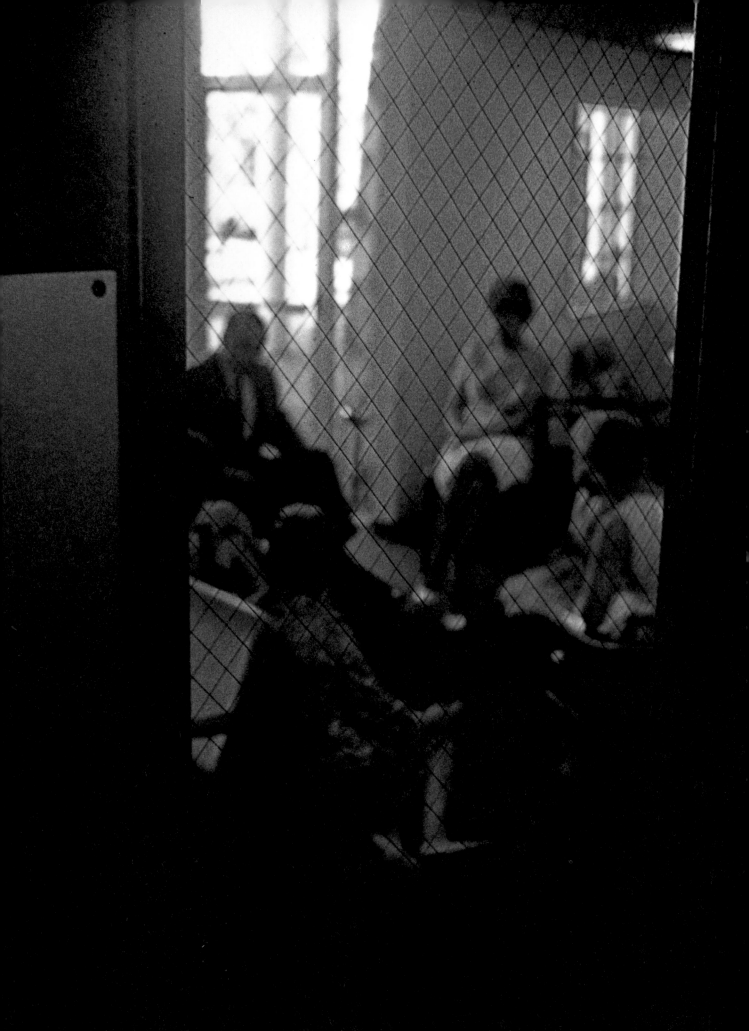

The Long Weekend

Frederick H. Stoller

Conventional psychotherapy is based on the disease model. The doctor is an expert who attempts to cure the patient's illness by probing his childhood and his unconscious. The two participants have precisely delimited roles. The patient talks about himself; the doctor listens and comments but reveals little about himself.

In the following selection, Frederick Stoller describes a group approach based on quite another model. The patient, or group member, seeks not cure but new experiences and self-exploration. The doctor, or group leader, becomes not the controlling expert but a cooperative member of the group. At various times each group member plays the roles of patient, therapist, and silent observer.

The theory and techniques of the encounter group are very different from those of behavior therapy as detailed by Eysenck earlier. Nevertheless, the two approaches have some things in common: The disease model is discarded for an emphasis on unlearning or relearning. The therapeutic targets are immediate behaviors rather than childhood memories. Technological innovations are freely incorporated. The participants are not restricted to chairs or couches, nor limited to verbal communication.

Quick, substantial, and often dramatic gains have been reported by participants in encounter groups. How lasting these changes are is an important question, yet to receive the answer that only further research and the course of time can give.

A young Mexican-American, imprisoned for drug addiction, inarticulate, fearful, and sullen, becomes a forceful dormitory leader.

A Greek-Jewish survivor of a Nazi concentration camp, having vegetated for seven silent and inactive years in a state mental hospital, suddenly decides he wants to leave, begins work in the hospital laboratory, and earns his discharge within a few months.

A clinical psychologist whose sole aim has been competence as a technician begins to function as a recognized innovator in his field.

The drug addict, the concentration camp survivor, and the psychologist are linked by a common bond. Each, within a relatively brief time, made use of personal resources whose existence had been totally unrecognized by himself and by others. And each participated in an intense group experience that changed his view of himself, his world, and his future.

These three people did not undergo traditional group therapy. They were members of a different kind of group, one of the new intense encounter groups whose goal was exploration rather than cure, and whose orientation was self-education rather than the amelioration of psychopathology. Many techniques of the new group are not dissimilar from traditional psychotherapy, but the assumption made about the members is that they are *not* sick. This is true even when some or all group members are disturbed. But it is not necessary to feel that one "needs therapy" to join a group, for it appears that everyone can benefit from experimentation with new ways of behavior and new social arrangements, and the most effective groups are made up of "chronic undifferentiated people." These new groups are explosive because they concentrate on immediate behavior within the group, not on explanations of past behavior—that tempting search for a scapegoat. They are also unpredictable, because each participant is encouraged to scrutinize himself and his relationship to the world without the shackles of normal role expectations.

When a person is labeled—neurotic, psychotic, executive, teacher, salesman, psychologist—either by himself or by others, he restricts his behavior to the role and even may rely upon the role for security. This diminishes the kind of experience he is likely to have. Indeed, it is groups whose members have a shared label—be it schizophrenic or executive—that are hardest to help move into intimate contact.

The importance of avoiding labels is shown by the experience of a young bachelor, who was urged by myself and other group members to stop frittering away his time at the YMCA when he should be involved in the heterosexual world. By the last day of the marathon he walked like a tiger—his growth was impressive. Then I discovered he was a former mental patient. Had I known this earlier, I would have thought, "Your adjustment is pretty good, considering where you've been." I never would have responded to him so directly. And his marked behavioral change would have been blunted.

During group sessions, exclusive reliance on a narrow range of roles is broken down. The chronically hospitalized patient who helps another patient, or the juvenile delinquent who persuades a boy not to run away, sees himself in a new and liberating light. It is this opportunity to shift freely from the role of patient to that of therapist or observer that is the unique feature of group therapy.

Since the essence of the new group movement is flexibility and experimentation, new techniques and procedures constantly are being tried. Experiments with the length of sessions resulted in the marathon group; experiments with technological innovations resulted in the use of video tape to capture behavior; experiments with group makeup resulted in the family workshop.

The 300-Year Weekend

As its name implies, the marathon group, which grew out of my experiences in a sensitivity-training laboratory in 1963, is a continuous session. My first attempt to use the marathon—with a group of psychotics—was both rewarding and exciting. The model finally developed by George Bach, one of the pioneers in group psychotherapy, and myself lasts from twenty-four to thirty hours, often without a break for sleep—a distinct departure from the precisely scheduled "fifty-minute hour" of traditional psychotherapy. The marathon group represents a radical alteration in the quality of the psychotherapeutic experience. It assumes that people are capable of coping with undiluted, intense experience and do not require carefully measured exposure to therapy; it has been called a "pressure cooker" because of the tension it builds up. And like a pressure cooker, it also can compress the amount of time required to do its work. The development is infinitely more rapid than under conventional therapy and the progress can be startling. The marathon uniquely maximizes and legitimizes people's readiness for change.

The marathon group is more than an exercise in massive confrontation and involvement. It is an educational experience primarily useful for what *follows* the conflict—crisis, anxiety, and reaching out for contact.

And in order for what follows to be meaningful, it is essential that group members neither avoid nor dilute their discomfort. The tension must rise. Members of the group are asked to react to each other, immediately and spontaneously, at all times; these immediate reactions—the "feedback"—inform the recipient in un-

mistakable terms of just what impact he has on others in the group. Thus, ground rules for the marathon specify that the group remain together throughout the session; they outlaw psychological or psychiatric jargon of any school; and they call for authentic, honest, and direct reactions.

The group leader's role is quite different from his role in traditional therapy. He deliberately refrains from gathering case histories about the marathon group participants. The leader must build up his impression of participants exactly as other members of the group do, and he must share the impact of each participant. For, in a marathon group, being *understood* is not what is essential; the importance is in being *reacted* to.

The group leader sets the experience in motion so that the pressure gauge will begin to rise. His position is clear and unmistakable, but he does not remain the traditional, aloof clinician—he is also a group member, a distinct human being. For this reason, I frequently hold marathon groups in my home, and my wife participates.

Marathons run a fairly predictable course. In the first phase, participants tell their "stories." Basically, they present themselves as they wish the world to see them: they describe their frustrations or their life circumstances, with careful attention to the response they hope to evoke. They may anticipate solutions to their problems or look for support of their actions or attitudes. Inevitably they encounter static from the group—unexpected reactions that they find difficult to accept. Thus they meet their first crisis: feedback that is different from what they intended or wanted, or expected. And learning begins early. One man said that he felt—for the first time—that someone knew him well enough to tell him more about himself than he already knew.

Most people have learned that the best way to handle a crisis is to run away. However, the marathon does not offer that option. For one thing, retreat is against the rules. For another, each group member contributes to the crises of the other participants at the same time as he is experiencing his own, so that he is drawn closer to the very people with whom he is in conflict. A counterpoint between the urge to retreat and the necessity to become more involved characterizes the second phase of the marathon.

Tears and Threats

During this middle phase the group members, not surprisingly, learn a considerable amount about each other. They also learn to react more directly and honestly. Their ways of moving through the world become more and more apparent. They sense that their approach to others is limited and tentative, and so their awareness of other possibilities grows. No clear-cut solutions emerge, but the struggles at this point are intense. It is the most explosive period of the session. Dramatic, frightening, moving interchanges are likely to occur. Tears and threats are not uncommon.

It was at this point that I once had an extreme confrontation with a young man whose religious fanaticism made it impossible for him to have a relationship with anyone who did not share his feelings. As the marathon progressed, I found his insistent intrusion of religious dogma abrasive and, after making it clear that I did not operate within a religious framework, demanded that he specify his reactions to me. He was thrown into conflict between his usual stance and his feeling for me. Suddenly he cried and talked about his concern for hypocrisy he saw within his church.

Another young man, who had been observing quietly, also began to cry. He was so deeply moved by the religious man's struggle that tears coursed down his cheeks. He said it was the first time in his life that he had found himself touched by another human being. Now he realized how distantly he had conducted his life. And he wept. The change in this silent observer was as profound as that in the young man who was the temporary focus of the group. This "spectator therapy" is a group phenomenon that is accentuated by the marathon experience.

As the session nears its end, there is in any marathon group a new sense of intimacy among all the members, and positive feelings emerge in a spontaneous and deeply felt fashion. This phase has been called a "love feast," because participants reach out to one another with unguarded intimacy. They now permit themselves to experience more—more fear, more love, more empathy, and more excitement. A Negro youth, following a marathon experience, wrote: "It seemed to get me out of that fake shield that I had been hiding behind practically all of my life."

Solutions and alternatives begin to emerge, usually through the realization by the group member that he can reveal more of himself than he thought safe.

Taking part in a marathon is like watching oneself through the wrong end of a telescope: everything is sharp, concentrated, miniaturized. It becomes clear in this microcosm that one's life is, to a considerable degree, something one creates and something for which one is responsible. Gradually, the inhabitants of the small world learn to act upon their environment as well as to be acted upon. It becomes apparent that the larger world can be altered in similar fashion. This is my deep belief.

Mirror, Mirror on the Wall

One function of a group is to show its members the effect they have upon one another. Responding to other people develops one's ability to communicate perceptions directly and honestly; receiving responses increases one's self-knowledge. But it is hard to sit still and listen to information about one's self that may be unpleasant, and it is hard to assimilate what one is told in mere words. This is why I turned to a new medium, which some therapists since have adopted and which others question.

Video-tape equipment makes it possible for group members to see themselves in action, which they find highly informative as well as fascinating. In one group, a wife had spent considerable time complaining bitterly that her husband "behaved like a child" with her. On video tape, I was able to show her that she used many of the mannerisms of a scolding mother with him—she would glare, shake her finger, and, when pleased, pat his head. "I couldn't believe it," she said. "It was worth a thousand words."

Contrary to what one might expect, placing a television camera in the midst of a group does not seem to affect behavior. Television camera and video-tape machine become part of the group circle. The camera may be manned by a co-therapist or even by the group members themselves. This arrangement gives them a chance to observe the group from an unusual and therefore useful point of view. Their choice of what appears on the tape is in itself a commentary—on the action and on the cameraman as well.

Unless responses are observed soon after behavior, they have little value. So when Lee Myerhoff and I began to use video tape during marathons, I decided to interrupt the group from time to time and replay the tape. This did not break the continuity of group interaction. Instead, group members would react to themselves on the television monitor, and other members would react to this reaction. Consequently, the viewing usually was followed by fuller concentration than before on immediate group behavior and events.

Focused Feedback

Video tape shares one unfortunate characteristic with life: It contains too much information. It is necessary to select what relates to the goals of the group and to focus the attention of the group members on it. A rationale for focused feedback can be found in the works of George Herbert Mead, who preceded the technical reality of video tape by many decades. Essentially a social psychologist, Mead developed a theory of personality development that stressed the social environment within which man becomes human. Among Mead's speculations was the theory that preceding each act, people rehearse that act in their minds and anticipate the response others will give to it. On the basis of the anticipated response, the act is initiated; on the basis of the actual response, behavior is modified. An act consists of a range of gestures, some of which (such as speech) can be monitored by the initiator, and some of which (such as facial expressions) cannot.

Video tape shows the group member—sometimes all too clearly—the relationship between an anticipated and an actual response. Often the two correspond; at critical times they often do not. In either case, comparing them is extremely useful for the group member. Tape also makes clear the discrepancy between a person's inner state and what he communicates to others. Most people are surprised to discover how much effort they invest in hiding their true responses, as if life were a poker game.

The pictures on the video tape are added to the verbal pictures painted of each group member by himself and others. And on the screen, for the first time, the participant confronts himself instead of having to interpret information filtered through the mind of another individual. He also sees himself, on tape, in each of the three major group roles: the patient role, when he is the focus of attention; the therapist role, when he attempts to extend help to others; and the observer role, when he is an inactive witness to the struggles of others.

Recent studies by Margaret Robinson, conducted at Camarillo State Hospital for her doctoral research at the University of Southern California, tend to confirm my observation that after seeing himself on video tape, a group member often changes his behavior before incorporating the change into his self-concept. After four sessions of focused feedback, there was a marked drop in the incidence of specific behavior units that were the objects of the feedback, but the self-concept—as measured on self-rating tests—remained unchanged. When behavior first changes, there is a period of awkwardness, then an improved level of behavior. The changed behavior elicits new responses from other people, perhaps initiating a chain reaction.

Games Families Play

In our family workshops, developed in collaboration with Ann Dreyfuss, of Western Behavioral Sciences Institute, three or four families remain together for several days, generally for a weekend. At first, the scene is chaotic—children are everywhere, in constant motion. Because of their short attention span, young children sometimes are segregated from the main group from time to time during the weekend, but a rule of the family workshop is that *all* members participate, and no one is talked about when he is not present.

Parents are quite devious with their children, and they teach their children to be devious with them—beginning when the children still are at the preverbal level. And this is complicated by the fact that the family as a unit puts on an act before outsiders.

Families come to the workshop with ready-made relationships, but they have not learned to talk about them. As initial shyness and family chauvinism wear off, the interplay begins. Even very young children pick up the emotional tone of the workshop and seem to be aware that a struggle is taking place.

There are rules: Regardless of which family they belong to, group members are expected to respond to each other directly, and to express their perceptions as clearly as possible. As families get to know one another, they become aware of the implicit contractual arrangements that determine their behavior. The workshop, like the marathon, is a microcosm of the difficulties that families encounter at home; experimenting with new and more fruitful ways of dealing with these problems is a major goal of the session.

Early in our sessions, each family in turn is given a large piece of paper and pastels. The family is asked to draw a design together for five minutes, without speaking. Mothers are more likely to be uncomfortable in this situation than are fathers. Interestingly, most families will fight for space; each member will try to use the whole sheet and to invade others' territory.

After the picture is completed, the family members discuss their reactions, and then the rest of the group talks about how they perceived the family. During the discussion, family members tend to draw parallels between the ways they behaved in this situation and the ways they behave at home.

The picture exercise takes the workshop out of the realm of words and removes the advantage from the parent and gives it to the child. The art game actually helps teach youngsters to give feedback, and they soon warm to the task (see Figures 1 and 2).

On other occasions, a box is placed in the center of a family group. They are told that something terrible is inside the box and asked to imagine what it might be. Typical guesses range from "a little dinosaur" to "a creeping hand" or "something soft and gooey and icky." This game represents an attempt by the family to share their fears.

Sometimes we ask the chosen family to pass sticks in a circle according to a specified pattern, or to perform rhythmical handclapping "dances." The purpose of these games, which usually come late in the workshop, is to give the family a chance to have fun together, to cooperate under the easy conditions of play without the restrictions of the usual family roles. In other words, a mother is invited for a moment to stop functioning as a mother and to become instead a playmate with responsibilities no greater than her child's. Some mothers do this well and enjoy it, others do not—in either case, the results are informative.

If parents complain, as they often do, that their children never listen to them at home, the family may be asked to talk together for fifteen or twenty minutes, perhaps about their reasons for coming to the workshop. The rest of the group comments on this; their response is supplemented by a replay of video tape.

The family workshop has wider implications. The current American family is becoming increasingly unique in that it sees itself as an independent unit, operating without reliance on the extended family—grandparents, uncles, aunts, cousins. This is an impossible task. As families are brought up in isolation, social agencies move into the vacuum created by the dissolution of the extended family. And as the family influence diminishes, there is an accompanying growth in the strength of the adolescent culture.

The intimate relationships developed during the workshop can be the nucleus from which to explore and experiment with new social arrangements. An intimate network of families who had shared workshop experiences could be created. These families would provide the help and emotional support originally supplied by the clan or the extended family.

A powerful group experience permits the individual to explore his own resources, those of the people with whom he finds himself, and those of the world about him. Group experiments provide experiences, not intellectual exercises—and experiences have the power to reshape us. Perhaps we need to establish "colleges for growth." Just as a student is not stupid because he goes to college to learn, so a person is not sick because he seeks group therapy or encounter experience to help him grow.

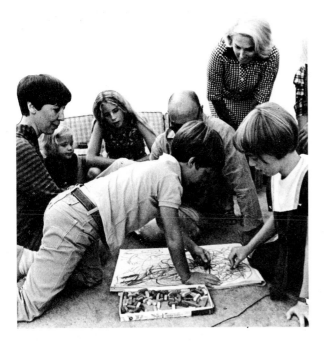

Figure 1. One family drawing. The mother tended to hang back, seemingly unhappy about the lack of structure inherent in the exercise. The father made more attempts to participate but these were largely toward the edge of the paper. The older girl worked in a neat fashion but the young boy began to fill the paper with his scribbling. Finally, there was an attempt on the part of the parents to involve the children in a tick-tack-toe game, which ultimately was scribbled over by the boy (including the tear in the paper). The mother complained that the boy inhibited her by his hyperactivity, but she could be seen as inviting him to fill space by her reluctance to act without structure.

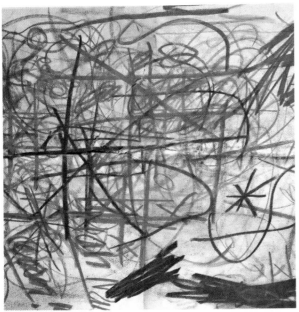

Figure 2. The family's product.

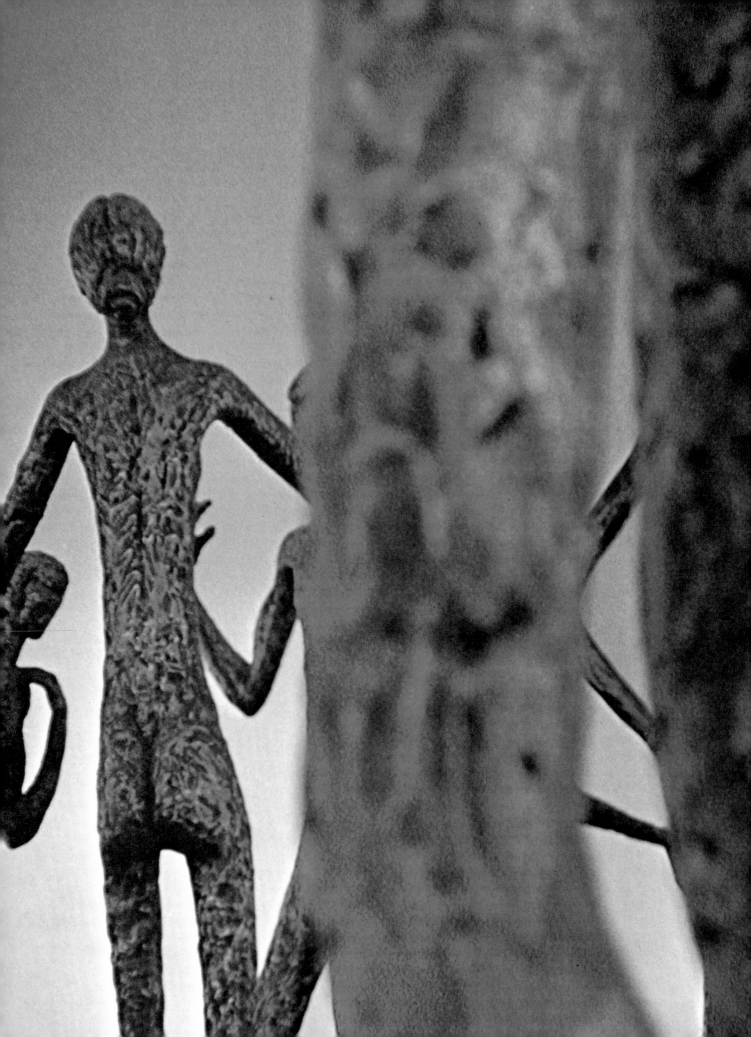

A Report on a Nude Marathon
Paul Bindrim

More than one selection in this series underscores the 1960s as a decade of innovation and exploration in modes of psychotherapy and ways of personal growth. An increased awareness of everyday events as well as a widened exposure to novelty have, for some, usurped the former goals of insight and adjustment.

Even a quiet revolution has its radicals, and this one in psychotherapy is no exception. Although few therapists or even leaderless groups resort to extremes, the trend toward experimentation and away from adherence to standard procedures is firmly set. Everywhere the seclusion schedule of the individual therapy hour is being supplemented or replaced by the weekend marathon, by deliberate exposure to stressful emotional experience, and by confrontation instead of privacy.

The new aims have brought with them new methods—or perhaps the methods have brought results that then turn into desirable goals. In either case, the current trend is best described by phrases such as total self-disclosure, sensory awareness, or complete openness. One logical extension of this trend is, naturally, the nude marathon. Is this merely the most daring of the new experiences being tracked by sensation-hungry Californians? Or is it a creative integration of techniques imbued with power to work marked personality change in a fairly short time? There is no longer a solid wedge between professional treatment and gimmickry, and there are no data that adequately describe the types of changes claimed by the "total experience" techniques. In fact, systematic data collection and scientific analysis are acts incompatible with the goal of becoming an emancipated, experientially guided being.

Ken: I think Lou said it much better . . . I was not so much inhibited as scared of my reaction to other people, and of course scared to death of having an erection.

MURRAY: I particularly enjoyed looking at the bodies of the women, at their genitals and breasts.

SANDRA: Normally I don't find that looking at a nude man is particularly exciting, but I thought you guys really looked great in the light show. It really brought out a lot of the strength, and I thought "that looks like what a man ought to look like."

LOUISE: I found myself thinking, "Do I look as good as her?" Comparing, and I didn't particularly like that reaction, and I felt like kicking myself for doing it, but I *was* doing it, and I thought, "I'm kind of fat here, and this and that, and do I want it to be out in the open

and out in the light and have someone looking at me and thinking the same things about me?" This kind of bothered me, especially when I was looking at Anita. She has such a lovely body.

LEO: I enjoyed the lovely female bodies last night. Many of your breasts—I wanted to touch them, feel them, put my face against them.

These remarks were made by participants at various times during a nude marathon. I've begun with them in order to get whatever sensationalism there might be about a nude encounter group not only out in the open but also out of the way.

The basic marathon is a period of no less than twenty hours of intimate, intensive, authentic human interaction, uninterrupted by subgrouping, eating, or sleeping. Such round-the-clock pressure leads the participants to take off their social masks, stop playing games, and start communicating openly and authentically. In theory, anyway, a marathon group moves from mistrust to trust, from polite acceptance to genuine critique, from peeping-Tomism to participation, from dependency to autonomy, from autocracy to democracy. During this trial by intimacy, one's roles, masks and pretenses tend to peel away layer by layer, revealing a more authentic self.

As emotional intimacy develops in clothed groups, marathon members have shown a spontaneous tendency to disrobe. On one occasion when a swimming pool was available, participants swam in the nude after the marathon. These spontaneous excursions into nudity seem to indicate that personal isolation and estrangement had been reduced.

Naturally enough, some of us wondered what would happen if marathon members first disrobed, and then interacted. Abraham Maslow, former president of the American Psychological Association, raised this question in *Eupsychian Management*. "I wonder what would happen if these encounter groups remained exactly as they are but only added a physical nudism." Later he defended nude marathons when they were attacked on ethical grounds, making possible the continuation of this research. Perhaps the whole process of becoming emotionally open and intimate would be hastened and intensified by nudity.

In addition most people in interacting groups—as well as in society—hesitate to touch each other. To touch is to be intimate, and to be intimate in that curious Henry Jamesian sense is to want or to have sexually. If full body contact between nude men and women were to be encouraged, and yet sexual expression prohibited, might this not lead more quickly to a sense of emotional intimacy and a sense of intensified personal identity that is the goal of all marathon groups?

(The wonderful Margaret Altmann has said of tourists throwing stones at her beloved wapiti elk that there is usually no malice or desire to hurt involved, but simply a thwarted desire to make contact with something elusive, strange, free, and beautiful. How many of us have not been in that position vis-à-vis other human beings?)

The results of the experimental marathon I'll be talking about in this article were good, and they thus help answer the question, why a *nude* marathon? Seventeen of the twenty participants felt that they had opened up to each other on more authentic and meaningful levels as a result of nudity; of the remaining three, none felt that nudity had hindered his ability to interact. Those clinical psychologists who participated felt that the group had integrated and become therapeutically functional more rapidly than participants had at clothed marathons they had attended. Five weeks after the marathon, fifteen of the participants gathered at Long Beach State College and reported beneficial changes in

their relationships with themselves, members of their families, colleagues, and the world in general. These changes were the result generally of increased self-confidence and self-expression, diminished fears of rejection, decreased anger or hostility toward one's own faults, and a readier and more level-headed overall acceptance of other persons.

But let me now fill in some of the details: how the marathon was set up, who the participants were, what they did, where they did it, and so on. My cosponsor of this experiment, Dr. William E. Hartman, professor of sociology at California State College at Long Beach, and I sent out announcements of the proposed nude marathon to psychologists, marriage counselors, participants in group and individual therapy, and persons who had attended typical marathons clothed.

Of the ten men and ten women who were selected for our marathon, there were three engineers, two schoolteachers, four clinical psychologists, one pharmacist, two magazine editors, two social workers, one artist, and five housewives. There was one married couple, and, although some married persons came without their mates, most of the participants were single.

We met at the Deer Park nudist camp near Escondido, California. Deer Park is large; it affords privacy in a beautiful natural setting. Its facilities include a swimming pool and a swirling hot Jacuzzi bath large enough for our entire group. Since the camp had just been closed to the public, the marathon had complete privacy.

The twenty participants agreed to:

1. Stay with the group for the entire session and avoid subgrouping;
2. Participate in all scheduled activities;
3. Remain in the presence of nude persons and feel free to remove one's clothes or not;
4. Use first names only, if they wished;
5. Abstain from alcoholic beverages and drugs throughout the session;
6. Refrain from overt sexual expression. Hugging and kissing would be permissible, but not the fondling of genitals or intercourse;
7. Take no photographs.

The group was in continuous session from 9 P.M. Friday until 3 P.M. Sunday, with six hours out each night for sleeping. Meals were served cafeteria style.

The participants were asked beforehand to bring with them the things they most enjoyed smelling, touching, tasting, looking at, and hearing, for use as stimuli in a sensory-saturation experience designed to induce a peak state perhaps best described as a mild turn-on.

It is probably simplest to describe the relevant events of the marathon in a straightforward, day-by-day narrative. By relevant events I mean those relating to the new factor or vector of nudity. Therapeutic interactions of the sort typical in clothed marathons took place as well, of course.

Friday

The group met on Friday evening with all members clothed. Everyone was asked to share with the group his anxieties, anticipations and fantasies about social nudity. Participants were again assured that they did not have to strip. This interaction took a little over an hour. The session then moved to the bath and members were told that they could bathe in the nude or otherwise, as they chose; everyone chose to bathe nude. The session in the bath was followed by an experience with colored lights in the main meeting room. Those who wished to participate actively stood in front, where colored patterns were thrown onto their bodies by a 35-mm slide projector; they could scrutinize the beautiful patterns and colors in a full-length mirror. Those who preferred to observe sat quietly in the darkened room. After the colored-light session, the group retired for the night.

Saturday

After an hour's walk around the grounds and then breakfast, members were asked at the day's opening session to share their impressions of Friday's activities. This session was held out of doors and was tape recorded. Members' responses may be summarized under the following headings.

A *sense of pleasure from the freedom to look at bodies of others and to be looked at in return.* The colored-light session permitted overt expression of voyeuristic and exhibitionist tendencies, of course. (As the marathon continued, the tendency to look excessively, or to experience self-consciousness when being looked at, declined almost to the point of disappearance.)

A *sense of personal comfort, exhilaration, and freedom.*

The desire to touch and a sense of being inhibited in this desire. There was little skin contact in the Friday session in the baths. Members were particularly aware of their reluctance to touch and repeatedly asked themselves why.

A *sense of group closeness.*

Relief and surprise among the men at their not having become unduly aroused sexually.

A *sense of guilty concern about one's body.* Members became, in retrospect, very aware of their negative feelings about their bodies—among the men there was concern whether their penises were large enough, and among both men and women there was a concern whether they were paunchy, or flabby, or wrinkled, whether they were as good-looking as certain other members, and so on. This concern about looks later dissolved or at least abated markedly; certain members commented that it seemed to come in part from movie

and magazine stereotypes. Members increasingly felt themselves to be right and beautiful, each in his own way, and forgot about *Playboy* and movie stars.

The experience of being high or at least unable to sleep for most of the night. The various exhilarations, worries, surprises, and so on seemed to give everyone something to think about and kindled a feeling of success exciting enough to keep him awake.

After lunch, another encounter was held in the Jacuzzi bath, followed by an hour of movement and sensory awareness, led by Sara McClure, a dance therapist. There was another brief bathing period in the evening. Full body contact became more spontaneous, particularly in the warm water of the pool, and less sexually centered. Dance therapy furthered this process.

Sunday

The Sunday morning session included an hour of meditation with sensory saturation. Each member, after prolonged periods of looking into the eyes of potential partners, selected as a partner a member of the opposite sex with whom eye contact was most comfortable and relaxing. Each member was then seated close to and facing the person of his choice. All were then asked to close their eyes and keep them closed. The prelude to Wagner's *Tristan und Isolde* was played. During this period, each member was asked to touch, taste and smell simultaneously the items he had selected for this experience. (One participant touched velvet, ate chocolate, and smelled a rose.) This sense-saturation led to a mild, drugless peak state, or high.

While he was in this state, each participant was asked to reexperience in fantasy the best moment of his life—a wonderful happening or experience in which he had felt joyous, free, close to the heart of his being, and at one with the world. When he had completed his fantasy recall and was turned on to his limit, each member was asked to touch fingertips with his partner's, and to gaze quietly into his partner's eyes. After twenty minutes of eye-centered meditation, members were asked to place their chairs in a circle and share their experiences.

Most of the participants felt that the periods of sensory-saturation, fantasy, and eye-centered meditation were the most profound experiences of the marathon. The general outlines of this experience are not unlike those of drug-induced, hypnotic, or Zen-meditational trips. Many members reported a sense of going out, a traveling through and beyond the boundaries of ordinary experience and an approach to something variously called "God," "warm, white light," "birth," "the beauty of the whole thing," "the stream of the universe," "a white nirvana," and so on. These experiences seemed to have a lasting effect on the postmarathon attitudes and behavior of many of the participants. An increased sense of inner worth, a sense of having com-

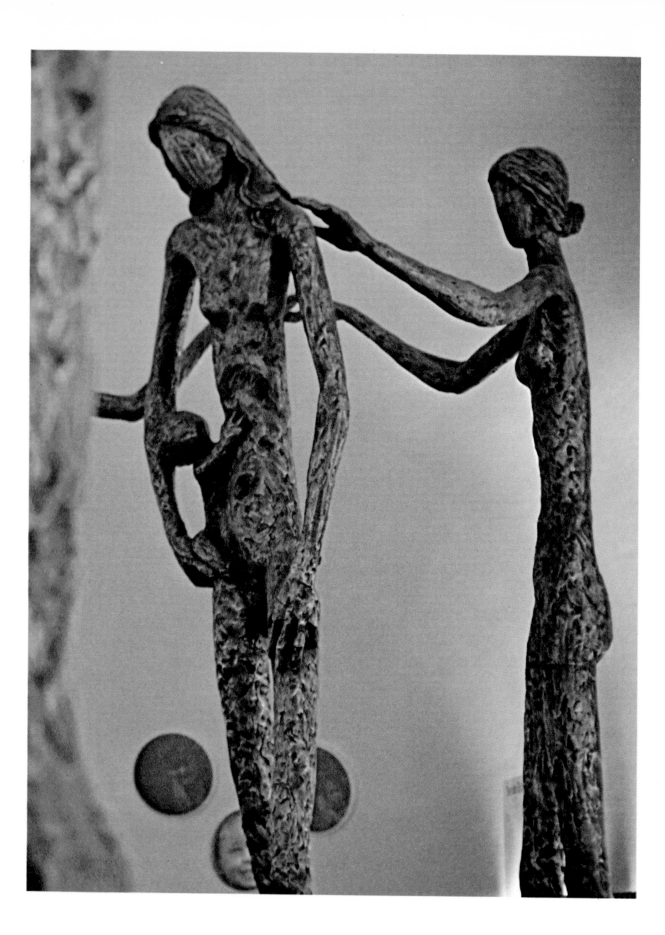

pleted a crucial psychic or spiritual cycle, helped some to a better understanding of their marriage partners. (In one case this expressed itself as an amicable divorce. In another, a remarkably beautiful woman whose husband had made childish and petulant fun of her body was able to get her husband to stop playing little boy and to move the entire relationship onto a much more stable, mature, and mutually satisfying level.) Several men and women reported that for the first time in years they had had friendly and adult relations with persons of the opposite sex.

The success of the peak experience encounter on Sunday was, I believe, strongly prepared for and mediated by the prior therapeutic experience of social nudity.

The tentative conclusions that I reached from this first nude marathon were encouraging. I reasoned that just as a lack of tender, tactile contact seems to be responsible in certain cases for infant deaths, the same deprivation may produce a nonlethal but chronic tension and anxiety among adults. That is, controlled skin contact might be therapeutic in and of itself. Perhaps the social world is such a jungle of polite estrangement that sensory isolation may create a famine in the heart that cannot be relieved by any *one* person, even one's mate. If purely physical contact (particularly between males who are most strongly inhibited in this respect) remains tenderly sensual yet takes place within an environment in which goals of a purely sexual nature have been deconditioned, then perhaps genuine mental and emotional exposure and acceptance can flower more naturally and more beautifully.

Self-acceptance, I reasoned, is often associated with one's body image. Open exposure to group reaction in the nude state might often remedy purely imaginary distortions, thereby increasing ego-strength and empowering men and women to make more honest and more salutary struggles with their core emotional problems.

Since sensual body contact is often a primary way of expressing one's self emotionally and of responding adequately to others, and since our culture defines sensuality and sexuality as bed-mates, perhaps we have blocked vital avenues of communication that might easily be reopened.

While such speculations are rather heady to have been based mainly on one experimental encounter involving twenty carefully selected participants, my initial conclusions continue to be verified. Since that first Deer Park marathon, I have held thirty-eight nude marathons. New techniques, drawn from my original theories, have increased the effectiveness of the sessions.

Sensitivity training has been criticized—and rightly—for the use of untrained and unsupervised leaders, for neither screening applicants nor providing follow-up, and for not testing its theories. None of these objections applies to the nude marathons I conduct. Half of the participants already have been prescreened in a sense, for they have been referred by other psychologists and psychiatrists. In addition, each participant is screened preliminarily by telephone and must agree to regard the first part of the marathon itself as a screening process, with the understanding that if I ask him to leave, he will go immediately. While this is not ideal, it serves as a compromise between the excessive costs of pretesting and the blind commitment to work with just anyone who shows up for a marathon. All participants attend a follow-up session, and I am always available for private consultation. Testing is underway.

Opposition to nude marathons continues from the uninformed and from those who are threatened by the thought of removing their own clothing. Accusations of gimmickry, manipulation, and publicity seeking have been made by some psychologists.

Conflicting viewpoints are common in the field of psychotherapy where few therapeutic techniques have been adequately tested. Only solid data can hope to settle these questions. Fortunately, academic psychologists have become interested in nude marathons as broad-spectrum learning experiences, and a number of research projects are being planned. One project at the Center for Behavior Therapy in Beverly Hills will attempt a more definitive behavioral analysis of nude marathons.

Qualified therapists who participate in nude sessions share my own optimism. The method has spread rapidly in spite of strong social pressures. Among the twenty-nine therapists now conducting nude marathons are the presidents of the Los Angeles Society of Clinical Psychologists and the American Association for Humanistic Psychology.

Examples of benefits from the nude encounter continue to multiply, though the nude marathon is still too new for long-term follow-up and evaluation. Frigid females, impotent males, and sexual exhibitionists have become at least temporarily symptom-free. Arthritics have been relieved of pain. Long-standing bachelors who could not commit themselves emotionally have married. Depressed individuals have been freed of suicidal tendencies. Psychotics in remission have lost their compulsive gestures and behaved normally by the end of a session. Swingers at one nude marathon found a new need for emotional relatedness in sexual expression. Marriages have been revitalized.

Is it any wonder that, both as therapist and as scientific reporter, I remain optimistic and thrilled about the possibilities of this new therapy?

IV
Abnormal Behavior and Public Concerns

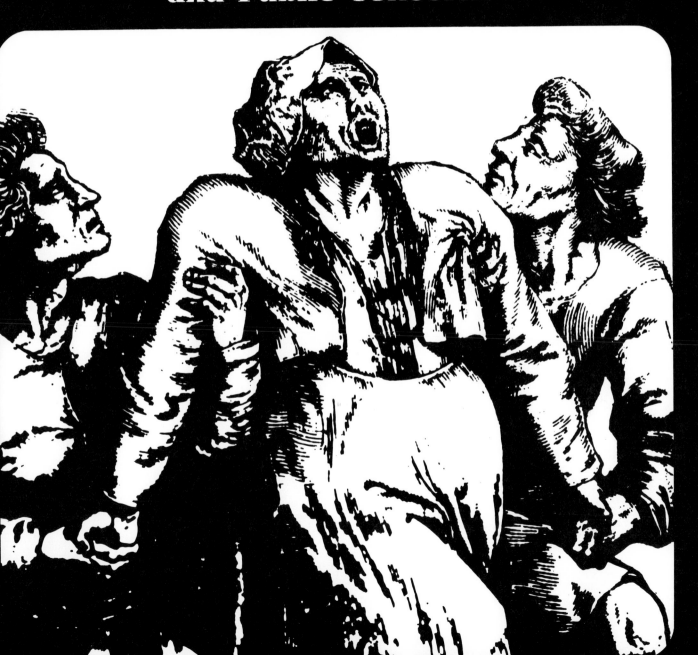

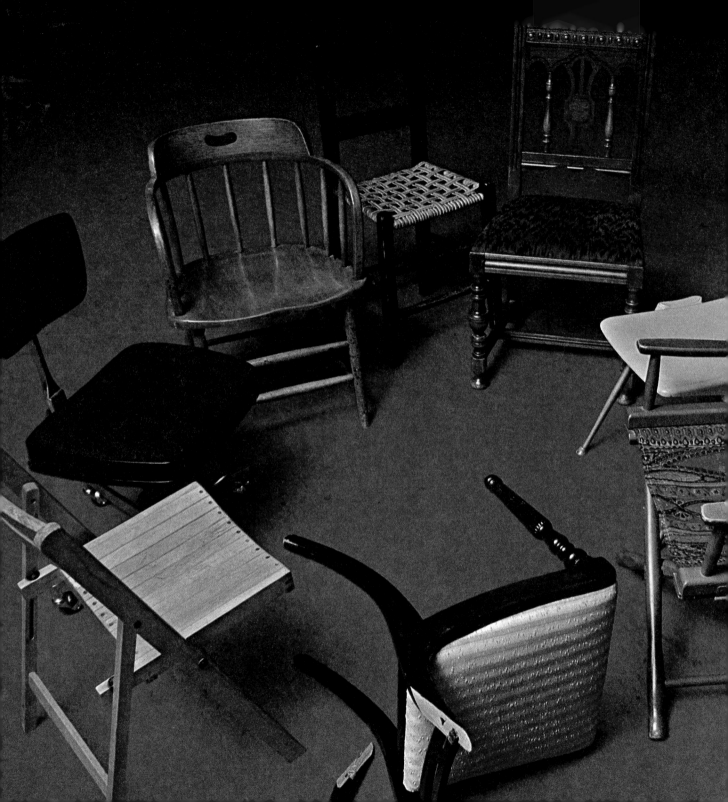

Group Therapy:
Let the Buyer Beware

Everett L. Shostrom

A shortage of professional manpower has resulted in programs to train students, housewives, grand-mothers, and even hospitalized patients to serve as therapists. These nonprofessional therapists have learned to use a variety of approaches, ranging from behavior modification to psychodynamic therapy. Such programs have had remarkable success; clearly, certain individuals can act as effective therapists with only a minimum of training and supervision. However, there is nothing to show that powerful con-frontation forms of therapy can be conducted successfully by persons with absolutely no training.

Despite this dearth of evidence, leaderless encounter groups and groups with untrained "facilitators" are becoming more and more popular. Perhaps this trend grows out of the attempt to discard the doctor-patient model and view the group leader as "one of the guys." The results of this approach have at times been humorous, at times disastrous. In his warning to the public, Everett Shostrom brings attention to the increasing problems of nonprofessional commercialism in the area of group therapy.

Joan was a fine scholar and teacher. She was fat and difficult, and had a grotesque limp, but true students loved her. She had made brilliant contributions to the High Minoan period, and her colleagues trembled as they waited to see what or whom she would demolish next. Joan was also pathologically sensitive about certain episodes of her adolescence. In a moment of dis-traction—she had been gleefully rebuked for a serious bibliographical error—Joan responded to an ad in the local underground paper; this ad promised an "en-counter" group, and Joan was eager to encounter some-thing. To her surprise, she found that two of the three other participants, including the leader, were university people whom she knew. Uncharacteristically, Joan said what the hell, and plunged into those interactions she had heard about. She found herself under cruel attack by the other participants, all of them therapeutically sophisticated; they quickly located and probed into the most painful segments of her life.

Initially, Joan felt herself rather better for the ex-perience. In the weeks that followed, however, she thought she heard allusions to her deeply classified torments, even at the most superficial of faculty gather-ings. Soon she began to suspect her most valued stu-dents of noninnocent, nonprofessional slyness—a quiz-zical smile here, a cool "Don't *you* think" there, a chuckle running through the lecture hall. . . . Three weeks later, on a bright afternoon, Joan drove her dusty and heretofore sluggish sedan into a bridge abutment.

They said she had been driving eighty miles an hour.

Doug worked in personnel, and his corporate star was rising. His people—applicants he had recommended—were turning out very well in the jobs he had selected them for. Doug was, however, bored and uneasy about his job—he felt that this "gift" his superiors were always talking about was overvalued. Doug went to an "attack-in" organized by his church; he was encouraged to give vent to his hostilities and critical scorn, and he did. It was great fun, and Doug carried the techniques back to his job. He got into a number of violent shout-ing matches with applicants and superiors, and was suddenly, and violently, fired.

Mr. and Mrs. Wassail had been married twenty-three years; they had done a commendable job of raising their children; they maintained respect for each other; and they had intelligent friends, eclectic but solid. On the advice of one of these close and trusted friends, they went to a sensory-awareness seminar. They arrived at a spectacular estate where very quickly they and some other persons very much like them abandoned them-selves to systematic depravity. Mr. and Mrs. Wassail enjoyed themselves for a while but found that they were literally unable to face each other or their children. After a few months, they separated, with a great deal of oblique bitterness.

Bill was a slender, handsome young man who had been fighting clearsightedly what he had identified—correctly, but on principle and without professional help—as homosexual panic. Bill read a newspaper ad that promised awareness and self-expansion. He signed up for sessions and was told—or rather shown—that everybody was really homosexual. Bill promptly, and with great relief, became a screaming queen. He alienated his parents and friends and found himself committed to a world in which he was by breeding, interests, and insight, truly and hopelessly alien.

Carl Rogers has said that the encounter group may be the most important social invention of the century, and he is probably right. The group experience has invaded every setting—industry, the church, universities, prisons, resorts. Corporation presidents have become group members, along with students, delinquents, married couples, dropouts, criminals, nurses, educators.

The demand for group experience—whether in the form of actualization groups, as I call them, or of T-groups, Synanon-like attack-ins, sensitivity-training groups, or marathons, nude and otherwise—has grown so tremendously that there are not now enough trained psychologists, psychiatrists, or social workers to meet it directly. As a result, groups organized by lay leaders have proliferated. While some of these lay groups have honestly and efficiently fulfilled their almost miraculous promises, others have been useless, stupid, dangerous, corrupt, and even fatal. I shall make it clear later that I am not arguing against lay leadership but rather for lay leadership that has been trained in such a way that the public will be protected. What I'd like to do at this point is suggest a few practical guidelines for choosing an encounter group, and then later take up a few general whys, maybes, and what-to-dos.

Each of the four examples with which I began this article contains elements that may be taken as fairly strict nos:

| 1. | Never respond to a newspaper ad. Groups run by trained professionals, or honestly supervised by them, are forbidden by ethical considerations to advertise directly. Modest and tasteful informational brochures are circulated among professionals in relevant disciplines, and referral by a reputable and well-informed counselor is one of the surest safeguards. Cheap mimeographed flyers promising marvels, especially erotic ones, are danger signals, as are donations or fees of less than $5.00. A good group is backed by a lot of labor and experience, which are today in very short supply.

| 2. | Never participate in a group of fewer than a half-dozen members. The necessary and valuable candor generated by an effective group cannot be dissipated, shared, and examined by too small a group, and scapegoating or purely vicious ganging-up can develop. Conversely, a group with more than sixteen members generally cannot effectively be monitored by anyone, however well trained or well assisted.

| 3. | Never join an encounter group on impulse—as a fling, binge, or surrender to the unplanned. Any important crisis in your life has been a long time in prepara-

tion and deserves reflection. If you are sanely suspicious of your grasp on reality, be doubly cautious. The intense, sometimes apocalyptic experience of the group can be most unsettling, particularly for persons who feel that they are close to what one layman calls "controlled schizophrenia." A trained person responsible for a meaningful session would not throw precariously balanced persons into a good encounter group. Nor would he allow persons who are diabolically experienced in the ways of group dynamics to form a group. If you find yourself in a group in which everybody talks jargon, simply walk out.

| 4. | Never participate in a group encounter with close associates, persons with whom you have professional or competitive social relations. Be worldly wise, or healthily paranoid, about this. As a corollary, never join a group that fails to make clear and insistent distinctions between the special environment of the group and the equally special environment of society. You should be told crisply that everything occurring within the group must be considered vitally privileged communication. You should always feel that the warm, vigorous disalienation that flowers in a good group is to a certain extent designed to suggest the richness of possibilities—in terms of self-knowing and other-knowing—and does not by any means imply a rigid code of behavior. In these matters, consult your common sense—it probably is one of the worst enemies you have, but it still is an entirely internalized enemy, hence deserving of notice.

| 5. | Never be overly impressed by beautiful or otherwise class-signaled surroundings or participants. Good group sessions can be held in ghetto classrooms, and all good sessions will include persons and life styles with which you do not identify intimately or on a day-to-day basis. Social or intellectual homogeneity in a group usually suggests an unimaginative, exploitative hostess mentality. A good group session should, I think, eventually unfold itself to every member as a kind of externalization or dramatization of himself—himself as fawner and snob, weakling and bully, villain and victim, poet and bureaucrat, critic and nice guy—himself as a small but complex galaxy of contraries. If you have a strong feeling that, as Huck Finn said, you've "been there before," you most probably have.

| 6. | Never stay with a group that has a behavioral ax to grind—a group that seems to insist that everybody be a Renaissance *mensch*, or a devotee of *cinéma vérité*—or a rightist or leftist, or a cultural, intellectual, or sexual specialist. This is narrow, destructive missionary zeal, or avocational education, and it has nothing to do with your self, your sweetest goals, or your fullest life as a self-knowing, self-integrating human being.

| 7. | Never participate in a group that lacks formal connection with a professional on whom you can check. Any reputable professional has a vital stake in any group he runs or in any group whose leader he has trained and continues to advise and consult. Such a professional

may be a psychiatrist (M.D.), a psychologist (M.A. or Ph.D. in psychology), a social worker (M.S.W.), or a marriage counselor (Ph.D.). One of the most significant questions to ask is, *Are you, or is your professional consultant, licensed to practice in this state?* If he has a Ph.D. and is not licensed, find out why not. Most reputable professionals are members of local, usually county, professional organizations; such organizations in many instances determine who may be listed where and how in your local Yellow Pages. If you can't find your group leader or the group's adviser in the Yellow Pages, check with the professional organization to find out why. It must be said at this point that all the training and accreditation in the world will not guarantee that every man in every place will be a good, efficient, worthy, or honest practitioner. Everyone knows that, but I am after all talking about rules of thumb, and rules and thumbs will take us just so far.

Any encounter group that uses the words *psychologist, psychiatrist, psychotherapy, psychotherapist, psychology,* or *therapy* in describing itself is usually subject to regulation by state laws and by the American Psychological Association, the American Psychiatric Association, or the National Association of Social Workers. In the past decade or so, however, humanistic psychology has explicitly and implicitly deemphasized therapy, at least in the sense of curing or treating people who are, on the analogy with physical medicine, mentally sick. Humanistic psychology, from whose passionate forehead the encounter group has sprung, tends to talk about *emotional growth, fulfillment of one's potential, feeling, contact,* and the participative *experiencing* of one's self and others with *honesty, awareness, freedom,* and *trust.* It has dealt usually with persons who are performing within socially acceptable parameters of legality, productivity, and success. It speaks usually to those who are not sick but rather normal—normally depressed, normally dissatisfied with the quality of their lives, normally tormented by irrelevance, meaninglessness, waste, loneliness, fear, and barrenness. Anyone can appropriate this humanistic vocabulary, set up shop as a lay encounter leader, and evade all professional and legal regulation by omitting psychological, psychiatric, and therapeutic terms from his descriptive catalogue or notice.

There are dangers in all group encounters—groups are crucibles of intense emotional and intellectual reaction, and one can never say exactly what will happen. It can be said generally, however, that well-trained people are equipped to recognize and deal with problems (and successes) before, while, and after they happen, and that ill-trained or untrained people often are not. Yet training—in the sense of specialized, formally accredited education—will not guarantee that a man or woman will be a helpful or successful group leader. Indeed, such researchers as Margaret Rioch have shown that natural group leaders with almost no training can

facilitate precisely the kind of ideal, joyful, alive, tender, and altogether marvelous self-learning that the most highly trained leaders strive for. Since there are not enough trained professionals to go around, the problem is to get good group leaders—to develop a set of standards that will allow us to enroll good people, teach them the necessary skills, and send them out with some formal approval that will give the public a fair chance to stay out of trouble.

Such well-selected, well-trained leaders should have a title and a certificate of some sort indicating that they have met certain nationally accepted standards. They would stand in some fairly well-defined relationship to professionals and to other licensed counselors. The analogy that most quickly, and perhaps most unhappily, comes to mind is the relationship of registered nurses to physicians.

A good model for the kind of nation-wide programmatic training I have in mind should be developed by such groups as the national psychological and psychiatric associations. (The California State Psychological Association is considering legislation that would permit nonlicensed persons to practice group leadership only when they are supervised by trained psychologists.) Research is badly needed to evaluate and measure competence and codify standards. In the meantime, there is a pilot program that can serve as an example at the National Center for the Exploration of the Human Potential in La Jolla, California, which sponsors a one-year course for adults who want to be encounter-group leaders. The center is advised by Abraham Maslow, Jack Gibb, Gardner Murphy, and Herbert Otto, among others.

Applicants for this training must have, among other things, a bachelor's degree. They must have some leadership experience (as a teacher or administrator, for example), and extensive encounter-group experience. They also must be evaluated by a psychologist or a psychiatrist. Then they are trained intensively and intelligently.

I'd like to propose that persons with such training call themselves facilitators and refer to their work in such a way that they distinguish themselves from certified counselors who work in institutional settings, and from licensed psychotherapists in professional practice. The National Center program is just an example, and it appears that many similar programs are developing. I think that the public is entitled to some ready means for distinguishing a rigorously selected and coached facilitator from, for instance, a member of Esalen Association. (Anyone may become a *member* of Esalen Association by paying annual dues; this indicates no other connection with Esalen Institute.)

Encounter groups in all their forms are far too valuable—and the demand for such groups is far too clamorous and desperate—for us to let ignorance, psychosocial greed, or false prophecy tarnish them.

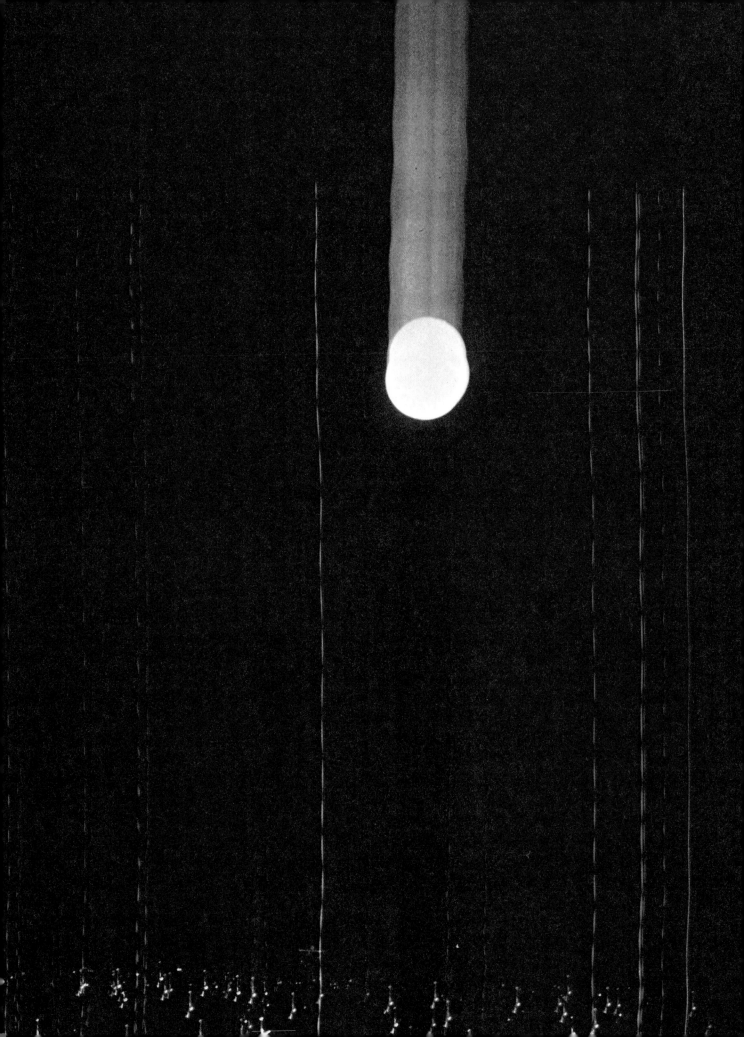

Chromosomes and Crime

Ashley Montagu

In the late nineteenth century, intelligence and personality were thought to be genetically determined. During the early twentieth century the emphasis shifted to environmental factors. Recent technological advances, such as refined methods for analyzing chromosomes, have swung the pendulum back toward the genetic side. The discovery of a chromosomal anomaly in one of the most common kinds of mental retardation, Mongolism (Down's syndrome), suggested that chromosomal anomalies might account for other atypical physiological and behavioral patterns.

Ashley Montagu reviews the presently accumulating evidence that some prisoners convicted of crimes of violence have an extra Y chromosome. Should further research confirm these findings, numerous issues will demand resolution. The results in both courtroom and laboratory during the next several years will have serious implications for the fields of child development, psychopathology, and forensic medicine.

Are some men "born criminals"? Is there a genetic basis for criminal behavior? The idea that criminals are degenerates because of "bad genes" has had wide appeal.

Johann Kaspar Spurzheim and Franz Joseph Gall, the inventors of phrenology early in the nineteenth century, associated crime with various bumps on the head, reflecting the alleged structure of the particular region of the brain within. Later in the last century, Cesare Lombroso, an Italian criminologist, listed physical stigmata by which criminals might be recognized. Lombroso's marks of degeneration included lobeless and small ears, receding chins, low foreheads and crooked noses. These traits supposedly foretold a biological predisposition to commit crimes.

In more recent years, Earnest A. Hooton of Harvard and William H. Sheldon of New York claimed to have found an association between body type and delinquent behavior. These claims, however, were shown to be quite unsound.

Of all the tales of "bad blood" and "bad genes," perhaps the two most famous are those of the Jukes and the Kallikaks. The tale of the Jukes was first published in 1875 by Richard L. Dugdale, a New York prison inspector. In his report, "The Jukes: A Study in Crime, Pauperism, Disease, and Heredity," Dugdale covers seven generations, 540 blood relatives and 169 related by marriage or cohabitation. Although Dugdale did not invent the Jukes, he often fell back upon his imagination to bolster his theory of the hereditary causes of crime when the facts failed. When information about individuals was hard to come by, Dugdale resorted to characterizations as "supposed to have attempted rape,"

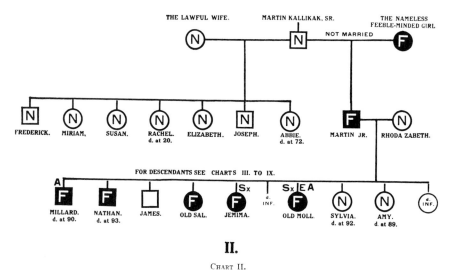

II.

Chart II.

N = Normal   F = Feeble-minded.   Sx = Sexually immoral   A = Alcoholic.   I = Insane.   Sy = Syphilitic.   C = Criminalistic.   D = Deaf.
d. inf. = died in infancy.   T = Tuberculous.

The good and the bad Kallikaks, from *The Kallikak Family* by Henry H. Goddard,
© Macmillan, 1912 (copyright renewed 1940 by Henry H. Goddard)

"reputed sheep-stealer, but never caught," "hardened character" and the like.

The Kallikaks were studied by Henry H. Goddard, director of a school for the mentally retarded in New Jersey. In his report, published in 1912, he followed the fortunes and misfortunes of two clans of Kallikaks. Both were descended from the same Revolutionary War soldier. The bad Kallikaks sprang from this soldier's union with a feeble-minded girl, who spawned a male so bad that he became known as "Old Horror."

"Old Horror" fathered ten other horrors, and they in turn became responsible for the hundreds of other horrible Kallikaks traced by Dr. Goddard. All of the good Kallikaks were descendants, of course, from the Revolutionary War soldier's marriage with a Quaker woman of good blood. Since none of the good Kallikaks seems to have inherited any "bad genes," something rather strange must have occurred in the lineage, for we know that a certain number of the good offspring should have shown some "degenerate" traits.

The Jukes and the Kallikaks are sometimes quoted as examples of what "good" and "bad" genes can do to human beings. While it is possible that a genetic defect may have been involved in some of these pedigrees, the disregard by the investigators of environmental effects renders their work valueless except for their quaint, anecdotal style of reporting.

Recently, the question of whether a man's genetic makeup may be responsible for his committing acts of violence has again come forward in the courts.

In France in 1968, Daniel Hugon was charged with the murder of a prostitute. Following his attempted suicide, he was found to be of XYY chromosomal constitution. Filled with remorse, Hugon had voluntarily surrendered to the police. His lawyers contended that

he was unfit to stand trial because of his abnormality.

The possible link between an XYY chromosomal constitution and criminals first came to light some years ago in a study of prison hospital inmates. In December 1965, Patricia A. Jacobs and her colleagues at Western General Hospital in Edinburgh published their findings on 197 mentally abnormal inmates undergoing treatment in a special security institution in Scotland. All had dangerous, violent, or criminal propensities.

Seven of these males were found to be of XYY chromosomal constitution, one was an XXYY, and another an XY/XXY mosaic. Since on theoretical grounds the occurrence of XYY males in the general population should be less frequent than the XXY type (the latter type occurs in some 1.3 out of 1,000 live births), the 3.5 percent incidence of XYY males in a prison population constituted a significant finding.

There is still too little information available concerning the frequency of XYY males among the newly born or adults, but there is little doubt that the frequency found by Jacobs and her colleagues is substantially higher than that in the general population. Few laboratories yet are able to do chromosome studies on a large scale, so information available is based on limited population samples from small areas. Current estimates of the frequency of XYY males at birth range from 0.5 to 3.5 per 1,000.

Jacobs also found that the XYY inmates were unusually tall, with a mean height of 6 feet 1.1 inches. Males in the institution with normal XY chromosomal constitution had a mean height of 5 feet 7 inches.

Since publication of the paper by Jacobs and her co-workers, about a dozen other reports have been published on XYY individuals, and all the reports confirm and enlarge upon the original findings (see Table 1).

TABLE 1

Summary of Published Reports on XYY Anomaly

No.	Population	Status	Height Inches	Intelligence	Traits	XYY	XXYY	XY/XXY	XXY	XYY/XYYY	XYYY	Investigator
10,725	Maternity	Newborn				—	1	5	12	—	—	Maclean, N. et al. *Lancet*, i: 286–290, 1964.
2,607	Ordinary			Subnormal		—	2	—	—	—	—	Maclean, N. et al. *Lancet*, i: 293, 1962.
197	Security	Criminal	73.1	Subnormal		7	1	1	—	—	—	Jacobs, P. et al. *Nature*, Vol. 208: 1351, 1352, 1965.
942	Institutional	Criminal		Subnormal		12	7	2	—	—	—	Casey, M. et al. *Nature*, Vol. 209: 641, 642, 1966.
50	Institutional Mentally ill	Non-criminal				4	—	—	—	—	—	Casey, M. et al. *Lancet*, i: 859, 860, 1966.
24	Institutional	Criminal				2	—	—	—	—	—	Casey, M. et al. *Lancet*, i: 859, 860, 1966.
315	Security	Criminal	6 over 72	8 Subnormal 1 Schizophrenic		9	—	—	—	—	—	Price, W. et al. *Lancet*, i: 565, 566, 1966.
464	Institutional	Delinquent		Subnormal	Aggressive Grand mal	1	—	—	—	—	—	Welch, J. et al. *Nature*, Vol. 214: 500, 501, 1967.
19	Detention center	Criminal Sex crimes	74.1	IQ 83	Negro Acne	1	—	—	—	—	—	Telfer, M. et al. *Lancet*, i: 95, 1968.
129	Institutional	Criminal	+72			5	—	—	7	—	—	Telfer, M. et al. *Science*, Vol. 159: 1249, 1250, 1968.
34	Prison	Criminal	69-82½	2 Subnormal	Psychopathic	3	—	—	—	1	—	Wiener, S. et al. *Lancet*, i: 159, 1968.
1,021	Institutional Boys	Delinquent	Tall	IQs 77, 78, 91	Property offenses	3	—	—	1	—	—	Hunter, H. *Lancet*, i: 816, 1968.
200	Institutional	Criminal	+72		Aggressive Sex offenders	9	—	—	—	—	—	Vanasek, F. et al., Atascadero State Hospital, Calif., 1968.
1	Ordinary	Embezzlement	78	IQ 118	Not overtly aggressive Depressed	1	—	—	—	—	—	Leff, J. and Scott, P. *Lancet*, i: 645, 1968.
1	Ordinary	8 yrs. 7 mo.	57	IQ 95	Aggressive	1	—	—	—	—	—	Cowie, J. and Kahn, J. *British Medical Journal*, Vol. 1: 748, 749, 1968.
1	Ordinary	5 yrs. 6 mo.		IQ 85	Undescended testes Simian creases	—	—	—	—	—	1	Townes, P. *Lancet*, i: 1041–1043, 1965.
1	Ordinary	44 yrs.	72	Average	Trouble keeping jobs	1	—	—	—	—	—	Hauschka, T. et al. *American Journal of Human Genetics*, Vol. 14: 22–30, 1962.
1	Ordinary	12 yrs.		Average	Undescended testes	1	—	—	—	—	—	Sandberg, A. et al. *New England Journal of Medicine*, Vol. 268: 585–589, 1963.

However, in many of these cases only inmates 6 feet or more in height were selected for study, so care must be taken in interpreting the findings.

In a sample of 3,395 prison and hospital inmates, 56 individuals were XYY, nine others had supernumerary Ys in one combination or another. Only eight of the inmates were XXY. Supernumerary Y chromosomes in any other combination are only one-fifth as frequent as the XYY—a significant fact that suggests it is the YY complement in the presence of a *single* X chromosome that constitutes the most frequent anomaly.

However, the presence of an extra Y chromosome, in any combination, appears to increase the chances of trouble. It also seems that the presence of an extra X chromosome, no matter what the number of extra Y chromosomes may be, in no way reduces the chance of trouble.

The Y chromosome, so to speak, seems to possess an elevated aggressiveness potential, whereas the X chromosome seems to possess a high gentleness component.

It appears probable that the ordinary quantum of aggressiveness of a normal XY male is derived from his Y chromosome, and that the addition of another Y chromosome presents a double dose of those potencies that may under certain conditions facilitate the development of aggressive behavior.

Of course, as with any chromosome, this does not

NORMAL MALE MEIOSIS
(Formation of the sperm)

Primary Spermatocyte

FIRST MEIOTIC DIVISION

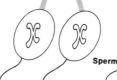

SECOND MEIOTIC DIVISION

Sperm

| SPERM | OVUM | NORMAL MALE | SPERM | OVUM | NORMAL FEMALE |

NONDISJUNCTION OF SEX CHROMOSOMES IN MALE MEIOSIS

Primary Spermatocyte   Primary Spermatocyte

NONDISJUNCTION AT FIRST MEIOTIC DIVISION   FIRST MEIOTIC DIVISION

SECOND MEIOTIC DIVISION   NONDISJUNCTION AT SECOND MEIOTIC DIVISION

Sperm

| SPERM | OVUM | MALE (Klinefelter's Syndrome) | SPERM | OVUM | MALE (XYY Syndrome) |

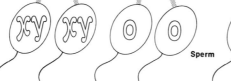   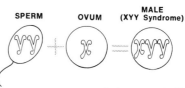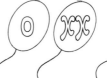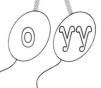

(autosomes omitted)

mean that the genes are directly responsible for the end effect. Rather, the genes on the sex chromosomes exercise their effects through a long chain of metabolic pathways. The final physiological or functional expression results from the interaction of the genes with their environments.

Genes do not determine anything. They simply influence the morphological and physiological expression of traits. Heredity, then, is the expression, not of what is given in one's genes at conception, but of the reciprocal interaction between the inherited genes and the environments to which they've been exposed.

Genes, chromosomes, or heredity are not to be interpreted, as so many people mistakenly do, as equivalent to fate or predestination. On the contrary, the genetic constitution, the genotype, is a labile system, capable of being influenced and changed to varying degrees.

Unchangeability and immutability are not characteristics of the genetic system. The genetic code for any trait contains a set of specific instructions. The manner in which those instructions will be carried out depends not only on those instructions but also upon the nature of their interaction with other sets of instructions as well as with their environments.

The phenotype, that is, the visible product of the joint action of genes and the environment, is variable. The idea of genetic or hereditary preformation is as incorrect and unsound as is the doctrine of hereditary predestination. In discussing the behavioral traits so frequently associated with the XYY type, these facts must be especially borne in mind.

How does the XYY chromosomal aberration originate? Most probably the double Y complement is produced during formation of the sperm. During the process of meiosis, in which chromosomes divide and duplicate themselves, normal separation of the sex chromosomes leads to two kinds of sperm—those with an X chromosome, and those with a Y chromosome. If an X sperm fertilizes a normal X ovum, an XX individual (normal female) will result. If the Y sperm fertilizes the ovum, a normal XY male will result.

Failure of the sex chromosomes to separate normally is called nondisjunction. There are two divisions during meiosis. If nondisjunction occurs during the first meiotic division in the production of sperm, this leads to two kinds of sperm cells—those with both the X and Y chromosomes, and those with no sex chromosomes. If an XY sperm fertilizes a normal ovum, an XXY individual will be the result. The XXY individual is a male (Klinefelter's Syndrome) but is usually sterile, lacking functional testes. About 80 percent of these males develop small breasts and at least 25 percent are of limited intelligence.

If nondisjunction occurs at the second meiotic division of the paternal germ cells, three types of sperm are produced: XX, YY, and those containing no sex chromosomes. Offspring resulting from fertilization of a normal ovum will be, respectively, XXX, XYY, and XO.

An XYY individual also could be produced if the sex chromosomes fail to separate normally in the early stages of division (mitosis) of a normal, fertilized XY ovum. However, in such an event, an individual with some type of mosaicism is more likely to occur.

Mosaicism refers to the existence of a different number of sex chromosomes in different tissues or parts of the body. For example, an individual may have only one X chromosome in some of his cells, and three chromosomes (XYY) in other cells. Such a mosaic would be designated XO/XYY. The O refers to the missing X or Y chromosome. If the single X chromosome is coupled with an isochromosome (I)—a chromosome with two identical arms—then the mosaic would be XI/XYY. Of course, other mosaics such as XY/XYY or XYY/XYYY occur.

Major physical abnormalities do not occur in XYY individuals for the reason that the Y chromosome carries relatively few genes. However, the physical abnormalities that do occur are interesting. As in most cases in which an extra sex chromosome is present, there is a high incidence of abnormal internal and external genitalia. Even in childhood, XYY individuals are usually strikingly tall, and as adults usually exceed six feet in height. Facial acne appears to be frequent in adolescence. Mentally, these individuals are usually rather dull, with IQs between 80 and 95. Abnormal electroencephalographic recordings, and a relatively high incidence of epileptic and epileptiform conditions, suggest a wide spectrum of brain dysfunction. Disorders of the teeth, such as discolored enamel, malocclusion and arrested development, also have been noted.

Allowing for the fact that in many cases tall prison inmates were selected for study of the XYY syndrome, and while a number of known XYY individuals fall several inches short of 6 feet, it is nonetheless clear that tallness usually characterizes the XYY individual.

This may be a significant factor in influencing the individual's behavioral development. Among children his own age, an XYY boy may be teased and taunted because of his height, and impelled either to withdrawal or aggression. As a juvenile, adolescent, or adult, he may find himself nurtured in environments that encourage physical aggression as a means of adaptation.

This should not be interpreted to mean that all tall men have an XYY constitution. Recently, Richard Goodman and his colleagues at Ohio State University examined the chromosomes of thirty-six basketball players ranging in height from 5 feet 11 inches to 6 feet 10 inches, and found no chromosomal abnormalities.

The resort to brawn rather than brain is not limited to individuals endowed with an extra Y chromosome. Most violent crimes are committed by chromosomally normal individuals. However, the high frequency with which individuals with XYY chromosomes commit crimes of violence leaves little doubt that in some cases the additional Y chromosome exerts a preponderantly powerful influence in the genesis of aggressive behavior.

In a maximum security prison in Melbourne, Australia, Saul Wiener and his colleagues found four XYY-type males in a study of thirty-four tall prisoners, all between 5 feet 9 inches and 6 feet 10.5 inches in height. A striking frequency of 11.8 percent! Of the three XYY inmates, one was charged with attempted murder, the second had committed murder, and the third, larceny. The fourth was an XYY/XYYY mosaic and had committed murder.

An interesting fact is that the tallest of the XYY murderers, 6 feet 10.5 inches tall, had a sister who was even taller. The tallness of the sister indicates that even though the X chromosome is not usually associated with excessive height in families where the males are extremely tall, a trait for tallness may be also carried in the X chromosome.

As a consequence of the discovery of what may be called the XYY syndrome, there now can be very little doubt that genes do influence, to some extent, the development of behavior.

It also appears clear, that, with all other factors constant, genes of the same kind situated at the same locus on the chromosomes of different people may vary greatly both in their penetrance and their expressivity.

Penetrance refers to the regularity with which a gene produces its effect. When a gene regularly produces the same effect, it is said to have complete penetrance. When the trait is not manifested in some cases, the gene is said to have reduced penetrance.

Expressivity refers to the manifestation of a trait produced by a gene. When the manifestation differs from individual to individual, the gene is said to have variable expressivity. For example, the dominant gene for allergy may express itself as asthma, eczema, hay fever, urticarial rash, or angioneurotic edema.

Hence, it would be an error to identify the XYY constitution as *predisposed* to aggressive behavior. Whatever genes are involved, they often fail to produce aggressive behavior, and even more often may be expressed in many different ways. In fact, the XYY phenotype, the product of the joint action of genes and environment, does vary from normal to various degrees of abnormality.

Some individuals, however, seem to be driven to their aggressive behavior as if they are possessed by a demon. The demon, it would seem, lies in the peculiar nature of the double Y chromosome complement. That the combined power of several Y chromosomes can be so great, in some cases, as to cause a man to become unrestrainedly aggressive is dramatically borne out by a case reported by John Cowie and Jacob Kahn of East Ham Child Clinic, London, in March 1968.

The first-born, wanted child of a mother aged twenty-three and a father aged twenty-five was referred at the age of four and a half years to a psychiatrist because he was unmanageable at home, destructive, mischievous,

and defiant. He would smash his toys, rip the curtains, set fire to the room in his mother's absence, kick the cat, and hit his eight-month-old brother. He was over-adventurous and without fear. At two years of age, he began wandering away from home and was brought back by the police on five occasions. He started school at five years and at once developed an interest in sharp-pointed objects. He would shoot drawing compasses across the schoolroom from an elastic band and injured several children. In one incident, he rammed a screwdriver into a little girl's stomach.

At the age of eight years, seven months, he was 4 feet 9 inches tall, handsome, athletically proportioned, and of normal appearance. He is of average intelligence and often considerate and happy. His electroencephalogram is mildly abnormal. Both his parents and his brother have normal chromosomal complements, but the boy is of XYY constitution. His brother is a normally behaving child, and the parents are concerned, loving people.

As illustrated by this case, there is now an increasing amount of evidence that XYY individuals commence their aggressive and social behavior in early prepubertal years. In many cases, the offenses committed are against property rather than against persons. The XYY anomaly, therefore, should not be associated with one particular behavioral trait but rather regarded as an aberration characterized by a wide spectrum of behavioral possibilities ranging from totally normal to persistent antisocial behavior. The degree of aggressiveness varies and constitutes only one component of the highly variable spectrum of behavioral contingencies.

We have shown how the XYY chromosomal aberration can originate in nondisjunction during meiosis or during mitosis. But does an XYY male transmit the abnormality to his offspring? To this question the answer is: probably not. One report on an Oregon XYY man indicates the double Y chromosome complement may not be transmitted. The man has six sons, and all are of normal XY chromosomal constitution.

On the other hand, T. S. Hauschka of Roswell Park Memorial Institute and the Medical Foundation of Buffalo, and his colleagues, who discovered one of the first XYY individuals in 1961, suggest that there may be a hereditary predisposition to nondisjunction. The XYY individual they identified was a normal male who came to their attention because he had a daughter who suffered from Down's syndrome (mongolism). Since Down's syndrome, in most cases, also arises as a result of nondisjunction, this, coupled with other abnormalities in his offspring, suggested that he might be transmitting a hereditary tendency to nondisjunction.

The fact that the XYY complement is now known to be associated with persistent antisocial behavior in a large number of individuals raises a number of questions that the reasonable society, if not the Great Society, must consider seriously.

A first question, if not a first priority, is whether it would not now be desirable to type chromosomally all infants at birth or shortly after. At least 1 percent of all babies born have a chromosomal abnormality of some sort, and about one-quarter of these involve sex chromosome abnormalities. Some of these will be XYY. Forearmed with such information, it might be possible to institute the proper preventive and other measures at an early age. These measures would be designed to help the individuals with the XYY chromosomal constitution to follow a less stormy development than they otherwise might.

A second question is how society should deal with individuals known to be of XYY constitution. Such individuals are genetically abnormal. They are not normal and, therefore, should not be treated as if they were.

If the individual has the misfortune to have been endowed with an extra chromosome Number 21, he would have suffered from Down's syndrome (mongolism). He would not have been expected to behave as a normal individual. And why should the XYY individual be held any more responsible for his behavior than a mongoloid? Mongoloids are usually likeable, unaggressive individuals, and most sociable. The aggressive XYY individual is often the very opposite. Yet the unaggressive behavior of mongoloids is as much due to their genetic constitution as is, at least in part, the aggressive and antisocial behavior of the XYY individual.

Recognizing this fact, it becomes very necessary for us to consider how society and the law should deal with such individuals. We have learned how to identify and treat the hereditary defect of PKU (phenylketonuria), which can result in idiocy if not treated. Cannot we also develop measures to treat the XYY? Surgical intervention, such as sterilization, is totally inappropriate since it will not "cure" or alleviate the condition, nor will it reduce the frequency of XYY individuals in the general population. The XYY aberration, as far as we know, is not directly inherited and quite probably arises primarily from nondisjunction of the sex chromosomes in completely normal parents.

Although we are in no position to control the genetic inheritance of an individual, we can do a great deal to change certain environmental conditions that may encourage the XYY individual to commit criminal acts.

A society does not properly acquit itself of its responsibilities if it places the entire burden of caring for abnormal individuals upon the parents. What we are talking about here is not a program of eugenic control but a program of social therapy. There is every reason to believe that if we can successfully develop effective methods to help the aggressive XYY individual, then we will be moving in the right direction to control those social conditions that drive men to crime—regardless of their genotype.

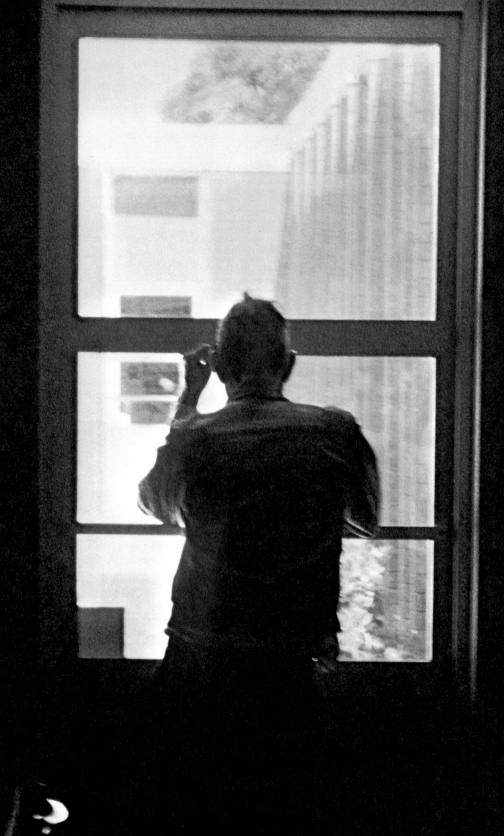

The Psychiatrist's Power in Civil Commitment

Alan M. Dershowitz

This article is concerned with civil commitments, those proceedings in which a court commits a person to a mental hospital for a period of evaluation and treatment. In such hearings, psychiatric testimony is weighed very heavily and almost always determines the outcome. Yet, the psychiatrist's decision regarding commitment is based solely on what he thinks is best. There are no tests and no diagnostic procedures that predict how dangerous a person may be to others, let alone how much he will benefit from hospitalization.

The medical model is brought into the courtroom in the cause of individual protection and social justice. Yet we must ask how well that cause is being served. How often do hospitals function as jails for persons whose behavior is socially but not legally offensive? We must also consider how psychiatrists and psychologists can offer testimony uncolored by their personal values.

These problems would be of less gravity if hospital commitments, in either civil or criminal cases, actually brought help to those committed. But, as Thomas Szasz forcefully states in the following article, in many of our hospitals this is simply not the case.

In the trial scene from *Brothers Karamazov*, Dostoevsky, speaking through the lips of the defense attorney, issued a stern warning to the legal profession:

Profound as psychology is, it's a knife that cuts both ways. . . . You can prove anything by it. I am speaking of the abuse of psychology, gentlemen.

I will speak here about another knife that cuts two ways: psychiatry in the legal process. Much has been written about one cutting edge: the contributions made by psychiatry. I will focus on the other side of the blade: the social costs incurred by the increasing involvement of the psychiatrist in the administration of justice. An important—if subtle—consequence of psychiatric involvement has been the gradual introduction of a medical model in the place of the law's efforts to articulate legally relevant criteria. These costs may be illustrated by reference to the process known as civil commitment of the mentally ill, whereby almost one

million persons are today confined behind the locked doors of state mental hospitals, though never convicted of crime.

Not in every society and not in every age were the insane confined by the state. The building of asylums on a wide scale did not begin until the seventeenth century. Such confinement was originally designed to further vaguely articulated legal goals. In the eighteenth and early nineteenth century these laws were part of a larger tapestry, which included "suppression of rogues, vagabonds, common beggars and other idle, disorderly and lewd persons." The legislative purpose seems clear: to isolate those persons who—for whatever reason—were regarded as intolerably obnoxious to the community. Medical testimony had little to offer in making this judgment: the people knew whom they regarded as obnoxious. By the middle of the nineteenth century madness was becoming widely regarded as a disease that should be treated by physicians with little, or no, interference by courts. The present situation comes close to reflecting that view: the criteria for confinement are so vague that courts sit—when they sit at all—merely to review decisions made by psychiatrists. Indeed, the typical criteria are so meaningless as even to preclude effective review.

In Connecticut, for example, the court is supposed to commit any person who a doctor reasonably finds is "mentally ill and a fit subject for treatment in a hospital for mental illness, or that he ought to be confined." This circularity is typical of the criteria—or lack thereof—in about half of our states. Even in those jurisdictions with legal-sounding criteria—such as the District of Columbia, where the committed person must be mentally ill and likely to injure himself or others—the operative phrases are so vague that courts rarely upset psychiatric determinations.

The distorting effect of this medical model of confinement may be illustrated by comparing two recent cases from the District of Columbia. One involved Bong Yol Yang, an American of Korean origin who appeared at the White House gate asking to see the President about people who were following him and "revealing his subconscious thoughts." The gate officer had him committed to a mental hospital. Yang demanded a jury trial, at which a psychiatrist testified that he was mentally ill—a paranoid schizophrenic—and that although there was no "evidence of his ever attacking anyone so far," there is always a possibility that "if his frustrations . . . became great enough, he may potentially attack someone. . . ." On the basis of this diagnosis and prediction, the judge permitted a jury to commit Yang until he is no longer mentally ill and likely to cause injury.

The other case involved a man named Dallas Williams, who at age thirty-nine had spent half his life in jail for seven convictions of assault with a deadly weapon and one conviction of manslaughter. Just before his scheduled release from jail, the government petitioned for his civil commitment. Two psychiatrists testified that although "at the present time [he] shows no evidence of active mental illness . . . he is potentially dangerous to others and if released is likely to repeat his patterns of criminal behavior, and might commit homicide." The judge, in denying the government's petition and ordering Williams' release, observed that: "the courts have no legal basis for ordering confinement on mere apprehension of future unlawful acts. They must wait until another crime is committed or the person is found insane." Within months of his release, Williams lived up to the prediction of the psychiatrists and shot two men to death in an unprovoked attack.

Are there any distinctions between the Williams and Yang cases that justify the release of the former and the incarceration of the latter? There was no evidence that Yang was more dangerous, more amenable to treatment, or less competent than Williams. But Yang was diagnosed mentally ill and thus within the medical model, whereas Williams was not so diagnosed. Although there was nothing about Yang's mental illness that made him a more appropriate subject for involuntary confinement than Williams, the law attributed conclusive significance to its existence vel non. The outcomes in these cases—which make little sense when evaluated against any rational criteria for confinement—are typical under the present civil commitment process. And this will continue, so long as the law continues to ask the dispositive questions in medical rather than legally functional terms, because the medical model does not ask the proper questions, or asks them in meaningless, vague terms: Is the person mentally ill? Is he dangerous to himself or others or in need of care or treatment?

Nor is this the only way to ask questions to which the civil commitment process is responsive. It will be instructive to restate the problem of civil commitment without employing medical terms and to see whether the answers suggested differ from those now given.

What Is Risk? What Is Harm?

There are, in every society, people who may cause trouble if not confined. The trouble may be serious (such as homicide); trival (making offensive remarks); or somewhere in between (forging checks). The trouble may be directed at others, at the person himself, or at both. It may be very likely that he will cause trouble, or fairly likely, or fairly unlikely. In some instances this likelihood may be considerably reduced by a relatively short period of involuntary confinement; in others, a longer period may be required with no assurances of reduced risk; while in still others, the likelihood can never be significantly reduced. Some people will have fairly good insight into the risks they pose and the costs entailed by an effort to reduce those risks; others will have poor insight into these factors.

When the issues are put this way, there begins to emerge a series of meaningful questions capable of traditional legal analyses:

What sorts of anticipated harm warrant involuntary confinement?

How likely must it be that the harm will occur? Must there be a significant component of harm to others, or may it be to self alone?

If harm to self is sufficient, must the person also be incapable, because he lacks insight, of weighing the risks to himself against the costs of confinement?

How long a period of involuntary confinement is justified to prevent what sorts of harms? Must the likelihood of the harm increase as its severity decreases? Or as the component of harm to others decreases?

These questions are complex, but this is as it should be, for the business of balancing the liberty of the individual against the risks a free society must tolerate is very complex. That is the business of the law, and these

PSYCHIATRIST'S POWER IN CIVIL COMMITMENT

are the questions that need asking and answering before liberty is denied, but they are obscured when the issue is phrased in medical terms that frighten—or bore—lawyers away. Nor have I simply manufactured these questions. They are the very questions that are being implicitly answered every day by psychiatrists, but they are not being openly asked, and many psychiatrists do not realize that they are, in fact, answering them.

Let us consider two of these questions and compare how they are being dealt with—or not dealt with—under the present system with how they might be handled under functional nonmedical criteria.

The initial and fundamental question that must be asked by any system authorizing incarceration is: which harms are sufficiently serious to justify resort to this rather severe sanction? This question is asked and answered in the criminal law by the substantive definitions of crime. Thus, homicide is a harm that justifies the sanction of imprisonment; miscegenation is not; and adultery is a close case about which reasonable people may, and do, disagree. It is difficult to conceive of a criminal process that did not make some effort at articulating these distinctions. Imagine, for example, a penal code that simply made it an imprisonable crime to cause injury to self or others, without defining injury. It is also difficult to conceive of a criminal process—at least in jurisdictions with an Anglo-American tradition —in which these distinctions were not drawn by the legislature or courts. The question of which harms do, and which do not, justify incarceration is a legal—indeed a political—decision, to be made by the constitutionally authorized agents of the people. Again, try to imagine a penal code that authorized incarceration for anyone who performed an act regarded as injurious by a designated expert, say a psychiatrist or penologist.

Yet this is precisely the situation that prevails with civil commitment. The statutes authorize preventive incarceration of mentally ill persons who are likely to injure themselves or others. Generally, "injure" is not further defined in the statutes or in the case law, and the critical decision—whether a predicted pattern of behavior is sufficiently injurious to warrant incarceration—is relegated to the psychiatrist's unarticulated judgments.

Some psychiatrists are perfectly willing to provide their own personal opinions—often falsely disguised as expert opinions—about what harms are sufficiently serious. One psychiatrist recently told a meeting of the American Psychiatric Association that "you"—the psychiatrist—"have to define for yourself the word danger, and then having decided that in your mind . . . look for it with every conceivable means. . . ."

On Liberty

As one would expect, some psychiatrists are political conservatives while others are liberals; some place a greater premium on safety, others on liberty. Their opinions about the harms that do and those that do not justify confinement probably cover the range of opinions one would expect to encounter in any educated segment of the public. But they are opinions about matters that each of us is as qualified to form as they are. Thus, this most fundamental decision is almost never made by the legislature or the courts; often it is never explicitly made by anybody; and when it is explicitly made, it is by an unelected and unappointed expert operating outside the area of his expertise.

Consider, for example, the age-old philosophical dispute about the government's authority to incarcerate someone for his own good. The classic statement denying such authority was made by John Stuart Mill in *On Liberty*. He deemed it fundamental:

That the only purpose for which power can be rightfully exercised against any member of a civilized community, against his will, is to prevent harm to others. He cannot rightfully be compelled to do or forbear because it will be better for him to do so, because it will make him happier, because . . . to do so would be wise or even right. . . .

The most eloquent presentation of the other view was made by the poet John Donne in a famous passage from his *Devotions*:

No man is an island, entire of itself; every man is a piece of the continent, a part of the main; if a clod be washed away from the sea, Europe is the less . . . any man's death diminishes me, because I am involved in mankind; and therefore never send to know for whom the bell tolls; it tolls for thee.

In our complex and interdependent society, there is hardly a harm to one man that does not have radiations beyond the island of his person. But this observation does not, in itself, destroy the thrust of Mill's argument. Compare, for example, a recent case that arose under the civil commitment process with a similar fact situation that produced no real case at all. Mrs. Lake, a sixty-two-year-old woman, suffers from arteriosclerosis that causes periods of relative irrationality. One day she was found wandering around downtown Washington looking confused but bothering no one, whereupon she was committed to a mental hospital. She petitioned for release and at her trial testified, during a period of apparent rationality, that she was aware of her problem, that she knew that her periods of confusion endangered her health and even her life, but that she had experienced the mental hospital and preferred to assume the risk of living—and perhaps dying—outside its walls. Her petition was denied, and despite continued litigation, she is still involuntarily confined in the closed ward of the mental hospital.

Compare Mrs. Lake's decision to one made by Supreme Court Justice Robert H. Jackson who, at the same age of sixty-two, suffered a severe heart attack while serving on the Supreme Court. As Solicitor General Simon E. Sobeloff recalled in his memorial tribute, Jackson's "doctors gave him the choice between years of comparative inactivity or a continuation of his normal activity at the risk of death at any time." Characteristically, Jackson chose the second alternative and suffered a fatal heart attack shortly thereafter. No court interfered with his decision. A similar decision, though in a lighter vein, is described in a limerick entitled "The Lament of a Coronary Patient":

My doctor has made a prognosis
That intercourse fosters thrombosis
But I'd rather expire
Fulfilling desire
Than abstain, and develop neurosis.

Few courts, I suspect, would interfere with that decision. Why then do courts respond so differently to what appear to be essentially similar decisions by Mrs. Lake, Justice Jackson, and the coronary patient? Because these similarities are obscured by the medical model imposed upon Mrs. Lake's case but not upon the other two. Most courts would distinguish the cases by simply saying that Mrs. Lake is mentally ill, while Jackson and the coronary patient are not, without pausing to ask whether there is anything about her "mental illness" that makes her case functionally different from the others. To be sure, there are some mentally ill people whose decisions are different from those made by Justice Jackson and the coronary patient. Some mentally ill people have little insight into their condition, the risks it poses, and the possibility of change. Their capacity for choosing between the risks of liberty and the security of incarceration may be substantially impaired. In some cases, perhaps the state ought to act in *parens patriae* and make the decision for them. But not all persons so diagnosed are incapable of weighing risks and making important decisions.

Defining Likelihood

There is another important question that rarely gets asked in the civil commitment process: how likely should the predicted event have to be to justify preventive incarceration? Even if it is agreed, for example, that preventing a serious physical assault would justify incarceration, an important question still remains; how likely should it have to be that the person will assault before incarceration is justified? If the likelihood is very high—say 90 percent—then a strong argument can be made for some incarceration. If the likelihood is very small—say 5 percent—then it would be hard to justify confinement. Here, unlike the process of defining harm, little guidance can be obtained from the criminal law, for there are only a few occasions where the criminal law is explicitly predictive, and no judicial or legislative guidelines have been developed for determining the degree of likelihood required.

But someone is deciding what degree of likelihood should be required in every case. Today the psychiatrist makes that important decision; he is asked whether a given harm is likely, and he generally answers yes or no. He may—in his own mind—be defining "likely" to mean anything from virtual certainty to slightly above chance. And his definition will not be a reflection of any expertise but again of his own personal preference for safety or liberty.

Not only do psychiatrists determine the degree of likelihood that should be required for incarceration; they also decide whether that degree of likelihood exists in any particular case.

Overprediction

Now this, you may be thinking, is surely an appropriate role for the expert psychiatrist. But just how expert are psychiatrists in making the sort of predictions upon which incarceration is presently based? Considering the heavy—indeed exclusive—reliance the law places on psychiatric predictions, one would expect there to be numerous follow-up studies establishing their accuracy. Over this past year, with the help of two researchers, I conducted a thorough survey of all the published literature on the prediction of antisocial conduct. We read and summarized many hundreds of articles, monographs, and books. Surprisingly enough, we were able to discover fewer than a dozen studies that followed up psychiatric predictions of antisocial conduct. And even more surprisingly, these few studies strongly suggest that psychiatrists are rather inaccurate predictors—inaccurate in an absolute sense—and even less accurate when compared with other professionals, such as psychologists, social workers, and correctional officials, and when compared to actuarial devices, such as prediction or experience tables. Even more significant for legal purposes, it seems that psychiatrists are particularly prone to one type of error—overprediction. They tend to predict antisocial conduct in many instances where it would not, in fact, occur. Indeed, our research suggests that for every correct psychiatric prediction of violence, there are numerous erroneous predictions. That is, among every group of inmates presently confined on the basis of psychiatric predictions of violence, there are only a few who would, and many more who would not, actually engage in such conduct if released.

One reason for this overprediction is that a psychiatrist almost never learns about his erroneous predictions of violence—for predicted assailants are generally incarcerated and have little opportunity to prove or disprove the prediction; but he always learns about his erroneous predictions of nonviolence—often from newspaper headlines announcing the crime. This higher visibility of erroneous predictions of nonviolence inclines him, whether consciously or unconsciously, to overpredict violent behavior.

What, then, have been the effects of virtually turning over to the psychiatrists the civil commitment process? We have accepted a legal policy—never approved by an authorized decision maker—that permits significant overprediction, in effect a rule that it is better to confine ten men who would not assault than to let free one man who would. We have defined danger to include all sorts of minor social disruptions. We have equated harm to self with harm to others without recognizing that question's debatable nature.

Now it may well be that if we substitute functional legal criteria for the medical model, we would still accept many of the answers we accept today. Perhaps our society is willing to tolerate significant overprediction. Perhaps we do want incarceration to prevent minor social harms. Perhaps we do want to protect people from themselves as much as from others. But we will never learn the answers to these questions unless they are exposed and debated. Such open debate is discouraged—indeed made impossible—when the questions are disguised in medical jargon against which the lawyer—and the citizen—feels helpless.

The lesson of this experience is that no legal rule should ever be phrased in medical terms; that no legal decision should ever be turned over to the psychiatrist; that there is no such thing as a legal problem that cannot—and should not—be phrased in terms familiar to lawyers. And civil commitment of the mentally ill is a legal problem; whenever compulsion is used or freedom denied—whether by the state, the church, the union, the university, or the psychiatrist—the issue becomes a legal one; and lawyers must be quick to immerse themselves in it. The words of Louis Brandeis ring as true today as they did in 1927, and are as applicable to the psychiatrist as to the wiretapper:

Experience should teach us to be most on our guard to protect liberty when the Government's purposes are beneficent. Men born to freedom are naturally alert to repel invasion of their liberty by evil-minded rulers. The greatest dangers to liberty lurk in insidious encroachment by men of zeal, well-meaning but without understanding.

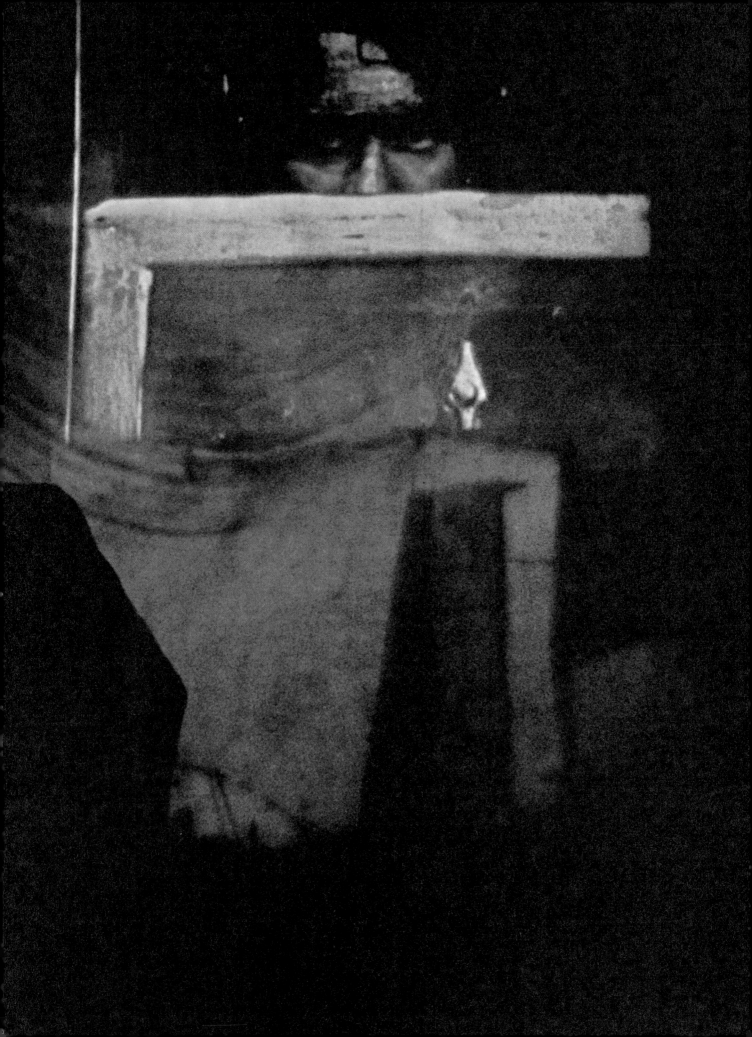

The Crime of Commitment

Thomas Szasz

What are we doing when we call a person "mentally ill" and put him into a hospital for treatment? Drawing an analogy between the relationship of a slave master to his slave and that of a psychiatrist to an unwilling patient he commits to an institution, Szasz provokes a reconsideration of the trust placed in the disease model of mental disorder. Should a person who is unable to cope with life's problems be called ill and thus be thought of as a patient? When such persons are placed in a hospital, do we help them into health or mold them into the role of the good patient?

Reason underpins Szasz's dramatic overstatement, but his argument must be countered by the question "What alternative to the mental hospital—beside prison—do we have?" Or, more pointedly, what alternative do we want? The question is idle without some crucial information. We must learn more about and from society's needs and values: Is a person who has offended society to be punished or treated sympathetically? Above all, we must uncover the kinds of treatment that have the highest efficacy in the shortest time, whether they be for the people who act against society or for those who act against themselves.

Physicians and laymen alike generally believe persons are involuntarily confined in mental hospitals because they are mentally ill but don't know they are sick and need medical treatment. This view, to put it charitably, is nonsense. In my opinion, mental illness is a myth. People we label "mentally ill" are not sick, and involuntary mental hospitalization is not treatment. It is punishment.

Involuntary confinement for "mental illness" is a deprivation of liberty that violates basic human rights, as well as the moral principles of the Declaration of Independence and the United States Constitution. In short, I consider commitment a crime against humanity.

Any psychiatrist who accepts as his client a person who does not wish to be his client, who defines him as "mentally ill," who then incarcerates his client in an institution, who bars his client's escape from the institution and from the role of mental patient, and who proceeds to "treat" him against his will—such a psychiatrist, I maintain, creates "mental illness" and "mental patients." He does so in exactly the same way as the white man created slavery by capturing the black man, bringing him to America in shackles, and then selling and using the black man as if he were an animal.

Illness Versus the Sick Role

To understand the injustice of commitment it is necessary to distinguish between *disease* as a *biological condition* and the *sick role* as a *social status*. Though a simple one, this distinction is rarely made in articles on mental illness, and there is a good reason for this: Once this distinction is made, psychiatry ceases to be what it is officially proclaimed, namely, a medical specialty, and becomes instead social engineering.

Strictly speaking, *illness* is a biological (physicochemical) abnormality of the body or its functioning. A person is sick if he has diabetes, a stroke, or cancer.

The *sick role*, on the other hand, refers to the social status of claiming illness or assuming the role of patient. Like husband, father, or citizen, the *sick role* denotes a certain relationship to others in the society.

A person may be ill but may prefer not to assume the sick role, as when we have a severe cold but go about our business. Conversely, a person may be healthy but choose to assume the sick role, as when we feel perfectly well but offer illness as an excuse for avoiding an obligation to go to the office or a party. Soldiers often assume the sick role—called "malingering"—to avoid the dangers of combat.

Where does the distinction between illness and sick role leave the alleged mental patient? He is said to be "very sick" by his relatives and the psychiatrists retained by them, but the patient maintains he is perfectly well and rejects medical or psychiatric help. Society then uses the police power of the state to force such a person into the sick role: this is done by calling the person a "mental patient," by incarcerating him in a "mental hospital," and by "treating" him for his "mental illness" whether he likes it or not. The underlying issue, however, is whether or not an individual has the right to refuse to be cast into the role of mental patient.

To answer this question, it is necessary to consider the problem of what mental illness is. Mental illness is not a physicochemical abnormality of the body, that is, an organic illness. If it were, we would simply call it illness and have no need for the qualifying adjective "mental." Actually, what we call "functional" mental diseases are not diseases at all. Persons said to be suffering from such disorders are socially deviant or inept, or in conflict with individuals, groups, or institutions.

Not only does mental illness differ fundamentally from physical illness, but mental hospitalization differs from medical hospitalization. Mental hospitalization is typically involuntary, whereas medical hospitalization is typically voluntary. In a free society, a person cannot be committed and treated against his will for cancer or heart disease, but he can be committed for depression or schizophrenia.

Should future research establish that certain so-called functional mental illnesses are actual physical disorders, they would then be treated like other organic disorders, and the question of involuntary hospitalization for them would become irrelevant.

If schizophrenia, for example, turns out to have a biochemical cause and cure, schizophrenia would no longer be one of the diseases for which a person would be involuntarily committed. Pellagra once sent many persons to mental hospitals with symptoms resembling schizophrenia until its cause was found to be a vitamin deficiency.

Mental Illness or Undesirable Behavior?

A person is said to be mentally ill if he behaves in certain "abnormal" ways. Since what is abnormal to one person is normal to another, mental illness is a kind of loose-fitting, quasi-medical synonym for bad or undesirable behavior. To a Christian Scientist, going to a doctor is abnormal. To a hypochondriac, *not* going is. To a Roman Catholic, using artificial birth control is abnormal. To a non-Catholic eager to avoid pregnancy, *not* using it is abnormal. The fact that mental illness designates a deviation from an ethical rule of conduct, and that such rules vary widely, explains why upper-middle-class psychiatrists can so easily find evidence of "mental illness" in lower-class individuals; and why so many prominent persons in the past fifty years or so have been diagnosed by their enemies as suffering from some type of insanity. Barry Goldwater was called a "paranoid schizophrenic"; Whittaker Chambers, a "psychopathic personality"; Woodrow Wilson, a "neurotic," frequently "very close to psychosis" (by no less a psychiatrist than Sigmund Freud!). Jesus himself, according to two psychiatrists quoted by Dr. Albert

Schweitzer in his doctoral thesis, was a "born degenerate" with a "fixed delusional system," manifesting a "paranoid clinical picture [so typical] it is hardly conceivable people can even question the accuracy of the diagnosis."

My argument that commitment is a crime against humanity is opposed on the grounds that commitment is necessary for the protection of the healthy members of society. To be sure, commitment does protect the community from certain threats. But the question should not be *whether* the community is protected, but precisely *from what*, and *how*.

Commitment shields nonhospitalized members of society from having to accommodate to the annoying or idiosyncratic demands of persons who have *not* violated any criminal statutes. The commitment procedure has already been used against General Edwin Walker and Ezra Pound. Conceivably it could be used against a Stokely Carmichael or an Eldridge Cleaver.

But what about those persons who are actually violent? Society could, if it were willing, protect itself from violence and threats of violence through our system of criminal laws, which provides for the imprisonment of violators in correctional institutions.

What about so-called emotionally disturbed persons who have not violated any statute but are believed to be violence-prone? Everything possible should be done to give them help, but is it just to hospitalize them or treat them involuntarily for being "potentially dangerous"?

To be judged potentially violent, a patient must be interviewed by a psychiatrist, which in effect violates the patient's right under the Fifth Amendment to refuse to incriminate himself. Few "mental patients" receive legal advice prior to being committed, but if they refused to be seen or interviewed by a physician, commitment would be impossible.

Psychiatrists cannot predict whether a person will be violent. Many "mental patients" who lose their liberty never have been and never will be violent.

Being "potentially dangerous" is not a crime. Most of us equate emotional disturbance with being violence-prone. Studies show, however, that "mental" patients are no more violence-prone than "normals."

Psychiatrist as Slave Master

To further clarify the political dimensions and implications of commitment practices, let us note some of the fundamental parallels between master and slave on the one hand and the institutional psychiatrist and involuntarily hospitalized mental patient on the other. In each instance the former member of the pair defines the social role of the latter and casts the latter in that role by force. The committed patient must accept the view that he is "sick," that his captors are "well"; that the patient's own view of himself is false and his captors' view of him is true; and that to effect any change in his social situation, the patient must relinquish his "sick" views and adopt the "healthy" views of those who have power over him. By accepting himself as "sick" and the institutional environment and the various manipulations imposed by the staff as "treatment," the patient is compelled to authenticate the psychiatrist's role as that of benevolent physician curing mental illness. The patient who maintains the forbidden image of reality—that the psychiatrist is a jailer—is considered paranoid. Since most patients (like oppressed people generally) eventually accept the ideas imposed on them by their superiors, hospital psychiatrists are constantly immersed in an environment in which their identity as "doctor" is affirmed. The moral superiority of white men over black was similarly authenticated and affirmed.

Suppose a person wishes to study slavery. He might start by studying slaves—and he would then find that slaves are, in general, brutish, poor, and uneducated. The student of slavery might then conclude that slavery is the slave's natural or appropriate social state. Such, indeed, have been the methods and conclusions of innumerable men through the ages. For example, Aristotle held that slaves were naturally inferior and hence justly subdued.

Another student, biased by contempt for slavery, might proceed differently. He would maintain there can be no slave without a master holding the slave in bondage. This student would accordingly consider slavery a type of human relationship, a social institution supported by custom, law, religion, and force. From this perspective, the study of masters is at least as relevant to the study of slavery as is the study of slaves. I hold that the study of institutional psychiatrists is as relevant to the study of involuntary hospitalization as is the study of mental patients.

Mental illness has been investigated for centuries and continues to be investigated today, in much the same way slaves were studied in the antebellum South and before. Men took for granted the existence of slaves. Scientists duly noted and classified the biological and social characteristics of the slaves. In the same way, we take for granted the existence of mental patients. Indeed, many Americans believe the number of such patients is steadily increasing. And it is generally believed that the psychiatrist's task is to observe and classify the biological, psychological, and social characteristics of mental patients.

The defenders of slavery claimed the Negro was happier as a slave than as a free man because of the "peculiarities of his character." As historian S. M. Elkins has said, "The failure of any free workers to present themselves for enslavement can serve as one test of how much the analysis of the happy slave may have added to Americans' understanding of themselves." The failure of most persons with so-called mental illness to present themselves for hospitalization is a test of how much current analysis of mental health problems may have added to our understanding of ourselves.

Today, of course, involuntary mental hospitalization is a universally accepted method of social control, much as slavery was in the past. Our unwillingness to look searchingly at this problem may be compared to the unwillingness of the South to look at slavery. "A democratic people," wrote Elkins, "no longer reasons with itself when it is all of the same mind." Today the Supreme Court of Iowa can say: "Such loss of liberty [as is entailed in commitment of the insane] is not such liberty as is within the meaning of the constitutional provision that 'no person shall be deprived of life, liberty or property without due process of law.'" I submit, however, that just as slavery is an evil, so is hospitalizing anyone without his consent, whether that person is depressed or paranoid, hysterical or schizophrenic.

Punishment Without Crime

Commitment practices flourished long before there were mental or psychiatric "treatments" for "mental diseases." Indeed madness, or mental illness, was not always a requirement for commitment. The Illinois commitment laws of 1851 specified that, "Married women . . . may be entered or detained in the hospital on the request of the husband of the woman . . . *without* the evidence of insanity required in other cases." Regulations for the Bicêtre and Salpêtrière, the two Parisian "mental hospitals" that became world famous, made it possible in 1680 to lock up children (of artisans and poor people) who "refused to work or who used their parents badly." Girls "debauched or in evident danger of becoming so," and prostitutes or "women who ran bawdy houses" were also considered fit subjects for incarceration.

Today, commitment laws usually specify that, for involuntary hospitalization, a person not only must be mentally ill but must also be dangerous to himself or to others. But even if a mental patient has expert legal advice, what facts can *he* offer to prove that he is not dangerous when a psychiatrist claims he is? Clearly, it is impossible to *prove* that a person is not dangerous.

Involuntary mental hospitalization remains today what it has been ever since its inception in the seventeenth century: an extra-legal, quasi-medical form of social control for persons who annoy or disturb others and whose nonconformity cannot be controlled through the criminal law. To be sure, the rhetoric has changed. Formerly, a housewife's commitment could be justified by her husband's disaffection and his unsupported complaints. Today, commitment must be justified by calling the housewife "mentally ill." The locus of confinement has changed. The Bedlams of old have been replaced by state mental hospitals and community mental-health centers. But the social reality remains the same: commitment is still punishment without trial, imprisonment without time limit, and stigmatization without hope of redress.

Biographies

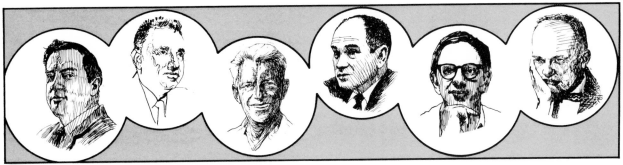

BARRON   BASSIN   BESDINE   BINDRIM   BRAMS   CLARK

FRANK BARRON ("The Dream of Art and Poetry") is professor of psychology at the University of California, Santa Cruz, and is also a staff member of the Institute of Personality Assessment and Research on the Berkeley campus. It was at Berkeley that he received his Ph.D. after earlier graduate work at both the University of Minnesota and Cambridge University. He is a graduate of LaSalle College.

For a number of years Barron has been studying creativity. His 1963 study, *Creativity and Psychological Health* (Van Nostrand), won the Outstanding Research Award of the American Personnel and Guidance Association. A revised and expanded second edition of it was published in 1968 in paperback under the title *Creativity and Personal Freedom*. His most recent book is *Creative Person and Creative Process* (Holt, Rinehart and Winston).

Dr. Barron is a past president of the International Child Art Center and has been a member of the Board of Directors of the International Council of Psychologists.

ALEXANDER BASSIN ("Daytop Village") was a member of the study team whose report led to the founding of the Daytop experiment, and later, as director of research for the New York Supreme Court Probation Department, he was in an excellent position to observe the progress of Daytop.

Dr. Bassin, an associate professor of criminology and corrections at Florida State University, taught courses in group therapy, group dynamics, and counseling methods at the Yeshiva University Graduate School. He remains a consultant to Daytop's Board of Directors and is a member of its Board of Governors. For the past few years, Dr. Bassin has been associated with Dr. William Glasser in promoting the use of Reality therapy through workshops and institutes in all parts of the United States. Dr. Bassin received his B.A. from Brooklyn College and his M.A. and Ph.D. in social psychology from New York University.

MATTHEW BESDINE ("Mrs. Oedipus") considers himself basically a Freudian psychoanalyst in private practice. Having taken on teaching duties as a clinical professor at Adelphi University's postdoctoral program in psychotherapy and psychoanalysis, at the National Psychological Association for Psychoanalysis, and at the Institute for Practicing Psychotherapists, Dr. Besdine has in a sense come full cycle, since he started out as a graduate of the City College of New York in 1926, prepared to teach history in the New York City schools.

The late Clara Thompson invited him to study at the William Alanson White Institute, and he was among a group of students who later arranged a series of private seminars with Theodore Reik to complete their training. This nucleus became the charter membership of the NPAP in 1948. At about the same time, Dr. Besdine completed his residence credits in the doctoral program in clinical psychology at New York University.

Dr. Besdine has been president of NPAP, co-chairman of the Joint Council for Mental Health Services and a fellow of the Center of Human Development at the Hebrew University in Jerusalem, among other things. He is presently doing a psychoanalytic study of Isadora Duncan and other female geniuses.

PAUL BINDRIM ("A Report on a Nude Marathon") has been a licensed clinical psychologist for more than twenty years, and has a private practice at 2000 Can- tata Drive, Hollywood, California. He did his undergraduate work at Columbia University and received his M.A. from Duke University, where he studied with J. B. Rhine. After leaving Duke in 1947, he joined the faculty of El Camino Junior College in California and also began private practice.

In June 1967, he conducted the first nude group-therapy marathon. He has since run more than three dozen sessions and a series of nude sensitivity training workshops.

JEROME BRAMS ("From Freud to Fromm") completed his doctoral studies at the University of Missouri and for two years was a postdoctoral fellow at New York University. From 1965 to 1967 he was in Cuernavaca, Mexico, as Erich Fromm's research associate. He is currently associate professor of psychology, Florida State University.

Brams writes: "Since my return from Mexico, I've been impressed by the political and social activism of some college students. But at the same time, there seems to be a paradoxical sense of alienation from self among many of these and other students."

WALTER HOUSTON CLARK ("The Psychology of Religious Experience") retired from the faculty of the Andover Newton Theological School in 1968. In the early 1940s, he did postgraduate work at Harvard, the university of William James. Currently, he is fascinated by the possibilities for the study of religious consciousness afforded by the psychedelics, if properly handled. He has guided about 150 LSD "trips" under experimental conditions, most of them in cooperation with the Worcester Foundation for Experimental Biology.

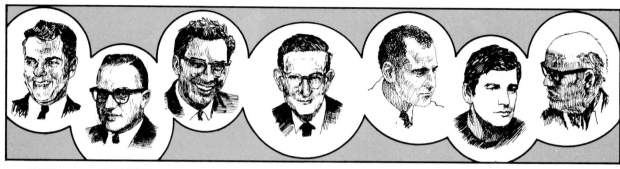

COYNE DERSHOWITZ DOMHOFF EYSENCK FERSTER FRANKEL HALL

JOHN M. COYNE ("Hypnotherapeutic Conditioning") divides his time between the Loma Psychological Center, where he is clinical director, and the University Hospital of San Diego County, where he is a clinical psychologist. After receiving his Ph.D. from Stanford University, he spent two years studying clinical neurology in the National Aeronautics and Space Administration School of Aviation Medicine. For four years he was a research neuropsychologist with the Life Sciences Branch of NASA's Manned Space Program Division. He is the author of *Clinical Neuropsychology* (Harper & Row).

ALAN M. DERSHOWITZ ("The Psychiatrist's Power in Civil Commitment: A Knife That Cuts Both Ways"), currently professor of law at Harvard University Law School, received his A.B. from Brooklyn College and his LL.B. from Yale Law School, where he was editor in chief of the *Yale Law Journal*. Following law school he served as law clerk to then-Justice Arthur Goldberg of the U.S. Supreme Court and Chief Justice David Bazelon, U.S. Circuit Court of Appeals, District of Columbia Circuit.

A frequent contributor to law journals, he—with Jay Katz and Joseph Goldstein—published *Psychoanalysis, Psychiatry and the Law*.

BILL DOMHOFF (coauthor, "Dreams of Freud and Jung") is a cofounder, with Calvin S. Hall, of the Institute of Dream Research, established in Miami and located since 1966 in Santa Cruz, California. He also teaches psychology at the University of California, Santa Cruz.

Domhoff's doctorate is from the University of Miami, where he and Hall met. Before joining the psychology depart-

ment at Santa Cruz in 1965, Domhoff taught psychology at California State College, Los Angeles, for several years. He is coeditor of *C. Wright Mills and the Power Elite* and author of *Who Rules America?* as well as several research articles on dreams.

HANS J. EYSENCK (New Ways in Psychotherapy") is a professor of psychology at the University of London and director of the Psychological Department at the Institute of Psychiatry, Maudsley and Bethlem Royal Hospitals. His experimental research in the field of personality has earned him international recognition. He has published more than 100 articles as well as eight books, including *The Structure of Human Personality*, *The Uses and Abuses of Psychology*, and *The Psychology of Politics*. He takes this in stride but is proud of the fact he also has been published in *Punch* magazine.

Born in Berlin in 1916, Eysenck left Germany in 1934 to study French and English history and literature at the Universities of Dijon and Exeter, and received his Ph.D. in psychology in 1940 from the University of London.

C. B. FERSTER ("The Autistic Child") is a professor of psychology at Georgetown University in Washington, D.C. For several years before joining the Georgetown faculty, he served as a director and as senior research associate at the Institute for Behavioral Research in Silver Spring, Maryland, working under a research career development award from the National Institutes of Health.

Dr. Ferster did his undergraduate work at Rutgers University and received his M.A. and Ph.D. from Columbia. After leaving Columbia, he spent five years as a research fellow at Harvard, and then moved on for more research and teaching

at the Yerkes Laboratory of Primate Biology in Florida, the Institute of Psychiatric Research at Indiana University, and the University of Maryland.

He is coauthor of *Behavior Principles* (with M. C. Perrott, 1968) and of *Schedules of Reinforcement* (with B. F. Skinner, 1957) and has written more than 50 articles for professional journals.

MARVIN FRANKEL ("Morality in Psychotherapy") is an assistant professor of psychology at the University of Chicago. Frankel's Ph.D. thesis was on child-rearing practices, the need for achievement, and risk-taking behavior in the Brahmin and Vaisha castes of northern India. He did his research during 1962 and 1963 while on a Murphy Fellowship in India. His psychotherapy internship was at the University of Chicago's counseling center.

CALVIN S. HALL ("Dreams of Freud and Jung") is a cofounder, with Bill Domhoff, of the Institute of Dream Research in Santa Cruz, California. Dr. Hall is director of the institute, which has one of the largest collections of dream reports in the world; and he also teaches psychology at the University of California, Santa Cruz.

Hall received his B.A. and Ph.D. in psychology from the University of California, Berkeley. A member of the faculty of Western Reserve University for twenty years, he has also taught at Berkeley, the University of Oregon, Syracuse University and the University of Miami, and has served as a Fulbright Professor in the Netherlands. He is coauthor of *The Content Analysis of Dreams* and author of *The Primer of Freudian Psychology*, *The Meaning of Dreams*, and (with G. Lindzey) *Theories of Personality*.

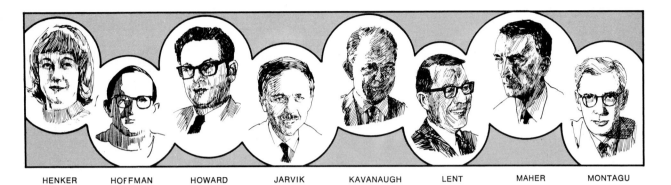

HENKER   HOFFMAN   HOWARD   JARVIK   KAVANAUGH   LENT   MAHER   MONTAGU

BARBARA A. HENKER, contributing editor, received her A.B. from San Francisco State College and her Ph.D. in clinical psychology from Ohio State University; she did postgraduate studies under a fellowship from the U.S. Public Health Service at Harvard, working with Jerome Kagan.

Currently teaching at the University of California, Los Angeles, Dr. Henker has two research interests with which she is actively involved. The first is the study of attentional processes and observational learning in very young children; one goal of the study is the early identification of children with atypical cognitive development, and the other is the development of new therapeutic and remedial techniques for the very young child.

The second research project, of which she is director and Carol K. Whalen codirector, is the Therapeutic Pyramid Project, conducted at Fairview State Hospital, Costa Mesa, California. Here modeling procedures and operant techniques are being used to teach a basic social repertoire to young (6–10) severely retarded inmates; the "therapists" are themselves retarded inpatients, either adolescents or adults. The results of the project so far show that both the children and their tutors make dramatic gains in this situation with these techniques.

MARTIN HOFFMAN ("Homosexuality and Social Evil"), a University of Illinois M.D., has been a psychiatric resident at the State University of New York at Syracuse and at Mount Zion Hospital and Medical Center in San Francisco. Dr. Hoffman, the author of *The Gay World* (Basic Books, 1968), serves as consultant to the Gender Identity Research and Treatment Clinic at the UCLA School of Medicine. He is also staff psychiatrist at the San Francisco Health Department's Center for Special Problems.

KENNETH I. HOWARD (coauthor, "Inside Psychotherapy") is a staff therapist at the Katharine Wright Mental Health Clinic in Chicago. He did his undergraduate work at the University of California, Berkeley, and received his Ph.D. from the University of Chicago. He has spent several years as research associate for the University of Chicago and for the Loyola University School of Medicine. At present he is with the Institute for Juvenile Research and is a professor of psychology at Northwestern University.

MURRAY E. JARVIK ("The Psychopharmacological Revolution") is a professor of pharmacology at the Albert Einstein College of Medicine in New York City. He received his M.D. and his Ph.D. from the University of California, Berkeley. Dr. Jarvik's chief professional interests are the actions of drugs on behavior and the physiological basis of memory.

ROBERT E. KAVANAUGH ("The Grim Generation") is Revelle College Counselor, University of California, San Diego. In his work with students, he concentrates on the solution of problems that interfere with academic achievement or personal growth. Kavanaugh has been a management consultant, a child-welfare worker, and a member of the faculty at Michigan State University. He has been involved in marriage, family- and sex-education clinics and programs. His fields are both philosophy and the social sciences.

JAMES R. LENT ("Mimosa Cottage: Experiment in Hope") specializes in applying the principles of operant conditioning to the problems of handicapped children. He is particularly interested in programs that allow the placement of mentally retarded children in the community.

After receiving his doctorate in special education from Syracuse University, Lent worked with handicapped children in several states. He joined the staff of the Parsons Research Center in 1964. The Mimosa Cottage Project, financed by a National Institute of Mental Health grant, is conducted by the Research Center under the joint auspices of Parsons State Hospital and Training Center and the Bureau of Child Research at the University of Kansas.

BRENDAN MAHER ("The Shattered Language of Schizophrenia") was born in England, and did his undergraduate work at the University of Manchester. A Fulbright Scholarship brought him to Ohio State University, from which he received his Ph.D. in 1954.

After serving briefly as psychologist in Her Majesty's prison, Wakefield, England, Maher then taught at Northwestern University, Louisiana State University, Harvard, and Wisconsin; currently, he is Riklis Professor of Behavioral Science at Brandeis.

ASHLEY MONTAGU ("Chromosomes and Crime"), noted anthropologist and social biologist, was born in England and came to the United States in 1930. He received his Ph.D. from Columbia University in 1937. He has written extensively on race, genetics, and human evolution and was responsible for drafting the UNESCO statement on race. Among his 31 books are *The Human Revolution*, *Human Heredity*, and *The Natural Superiority of Women*.

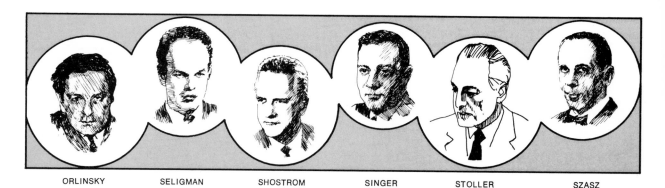

ORLINSKY   SELIGMAN   SHOSTROM   SINGER   STOLLER   SZASZ

DAVID E. ORLINSKY (coauthor, "Inside Psychotherapy") is a staff therapist at the Katharine Wright Mental Health Clinic in Chicago. He also serves as senior research associate at the Institute for Juvenile Research in Chicago and teaches at the University of Chicago, where he received his bachelor's degree and his doctorate as well.

MARTIN E. P. SELIGMAN ("For Helplessness: Can We Immunize the Weak?") is an assistant professor of psychology at Cornell University. He took his B.A. in philosophy at Princeton and his Ph.D. at the University of Pennsylvania.

Dr. Seligman's major research interest is the psychology of learning and motivation, in particular the effect of unpredictable and uncontrollable trauma.

EVERETT L. SHOSTROM ("Group Therapy: Let the Buyer Beware") is a member of the training staff of the Institute of Industrial Relations at the University of California, Los Angeles. He holds his Ph.D. from Stanford University and has taught at Stanford and Oregon State University and at Pepperdine College, where he was head of the Psychology Department.

He is coauthor of, among other books, *Therapeutic Psychology, Fundamentals of Actualization Counseling and Therapy*, which is used in 200 universities, and is author of *Man, the Manipulator*, published in 1967. He is also the author of two tests, the Personal Orientation Inventory and the Caring Relationship Inventory, and has produced and directed six psychological films.

JEROME L. SINGER ("The Importance of Daydreaming") has directed research programs on the psychology of daydreams and related fantasy processes for over ten years. He obtained his doctorate at the University of Pennsylvania, and later attended the William Alanson White Institute, where he received his certificate as a psychoanalyst.

Dr. Singer is professor of psychology and director of the Clinical Psychology Training Program, City College of the City University of New York. He also has a private practice in psychoanalysis.

He is the author of *Daydreaming: An Introduction to the Experimental Study of Inner Experience*.

FREDERICK H. STOLLER ("The Long Weekend"), after receiving his doctorate from UCLA, where he was trained in classical clinical psychology, served as a senior psychologist at Camarillo State Hospital. There he "obtained first-hand experience with people in trouble and learned not to be frightened of them—an important asset." He is now senior research associate at the Public Systems Research Institute and associate professor in the School of Public Administration, University of Southern California. The center is operated under the auspices of the School of Public Administration, and Dr. Stoller finds his contact with an interdisciplinary group studying broader social structures a valuable supplement to his primary work on research and training in group methods.

THOMAS SZASZ ("The Crime of Commitment"), born in Budapest, Hungary, is a professor of psychiatry at the State University of New York Upstate Medical Center in Syracuse. He obtained his M.D. degree from the University of Cincinnati where his top-of-the-class rank won him the Stella Feiss Hofheimer Award. After that he worked as an intern, resident, and training-research fellow at several clinics and universities before earning a certificate from Chicago's Institute for Psychoanalysis.

He is a member of the board of consultants of *The Psychoanalytic Review* and of the editorial boards of *The Journal of Nervous and Mental Disease*, and *Journal of Drug Addiction*. He serves as a consultant to the committee on Mental Hygiene of the New York State Bar Association.

Bibliographies

I. Psychopathology and Personality Dynamics

The Dreams of Freud and Jung

AGGRESSION IN DREAMS. C. S. Hall, B. Domhoff in *International Journal of Social Psychiatry*, Vol. 9, pp. 259–267, 1963.

THE CONTENT ANALYSIS OF DREAMS. C. S. Hall, R. L. Van de Castle. Appleton-Century-Crofts, 1966.

FRIENDLINESS IN DREAMS. C. S. Hall, B. Domhoff in *Journal of Social Psychology*, Vol. 62, pp. 309–314, 1964.

THE INTERPRETATION OF DREAMS. S. Freud. Hogarth Press, 1953. Vols. IV and V, Standard Edition.

THE LIFE AND WORK OF SIGMUND FREUD. E. Jones. Basic Books, 1955.

MEMORIES, DREAMS, REFLECTIONS. C. G. Jung. Pantheon, 1963.

ON DREAMS. S. Freud. Hogarth Press, 1953. Vol. V, Standard Edition.

The Importance of Daydreaming

DAYDREAMING: AN INTRODUCTION TO THE EXPERIMENTAL STUDY OF INNER EXPERIENCE. J. Singer. Random House, 1966.

DAYDREAMING PATTERNS OF AMERICAN SUBCULTURAL GROUPS. J. Singer, V. McCraven in *International Journal of Social Psychiatry*, Vol. 8, pp. 272–282, 1962.

EYE MOVEMENTS ACCOMPANYING DAYDREAMING, VISUAL IMAGERY AND THOUGHT SUPPRESSION. J. Antrobus, J. S. Antrobus, J. Singer in *Journal of Abnormal and Social Psychology*, Vol. 69, pp. 244–252, 1964.

A FACTOR-ANALYTIC STUDY OF DAYDREAMING AND RELATED COGNITIVE AND PERSONALITY VARIABLES. J. Singer in *Perceptual and Motor Skills*, Monograph Supplement, Vol. 3, No. 17, 1963.

STUDIES IN THE STREAM OF CONSCIOUSNESS: EXPERIMENTAL ENHANCEMENT AND SUPPRESSION OF SPONTANEOUS COGNITIVE PROCESSES. J. S. Antrobus, J. Singer, S. Greenberg in *Perceptual and Motor Skills*, Vol. 23, pp. 399–417, 1966.

The Dream of Art and Poetry

CREATIVITY AND PERSONAL FREEDOM. F. Barron. Van Nostrand, 1968.

THE EARLY MENTAL TRAITS OF 300 GENIUSES. C. Cox. Stanford University Press, 1936.

FORMS OF THINGS UNKNOWN. H. Read. Meridian, 1963.

GENETIC STUDIES OF GENIUS. L. Terman, *et al.*, eds. Stanford University Press.

SCIENTIFIC CREATIVITY. F. Barron, C. Taylor, eds. Wiley, 1963.

Mrs. Oedipus

THE CREATIVE IMAGINATION. H. M. Ruitenbeek, ed. Quadrangle, 1965.

THE DEVELOPMENTAL PSYCHOLOGY OF JEAN PIAGET. J. H. Flavell. Van Nostrand, 1963.

THE FIRST YEAR OF LIFE. R. A. Spitz. International Universities Press, 1965.

JOCASTA AND OEDIPUS: ANOTHER LOOK. M. Besdine in *Pathways in Child Guidance*. Bureau of Child Guidance, New York City Board of Education, March 1968.

THE JOCASTA COMPLEX, MOTHERING AND GENIUS. M. Besdine in *The Psychoanalytic Review*, Vol. 55, No. 2, 1968.

THE MAN BEHIND THE ARTIST: A PSYCHOANALYTIC STUDY OF MICHELANGELO BUONARROTTI. M. Besdine (in press).

The Grim Generation

THE AMERICAN COLLEGE. N. Sanford. Wiley, 1962.

NO TIME FOR YOUTH: GROWTH AND CONSTRAINT IN COLLEGE STUDENTS. J. Katz, *et al.* Jossey-Bass, 1968.

THE STUDENT AND HIS STUDIES. E. Raushenbush. Wesleyan University Press, 1964.

THE STUDENT IN HIGHER EDUCATION. J. Kaufmann, *et al.* Hazen Foundation, 1968.

THE UNCOMMITTED. K. Keniston. Harcourt, Brace & World, 1965.

YOUNG RADICALS: NOTES ON COMMITTED YOUTH. K. Keniston. Harcourt, Brace & World, 1968.

The Psychology of Religious Experience

THE EXPLORATION OF THE INNER WORLD. A. T. Boisen. Harper & Row, 1936.

THE FUTURE OF AN ILLUSION. S. Freud. Liveright, 1932.

THE INDIVIDUAL AND HIS RELIGION. G. W. Allport. Macmillan, 1950.

LSD: THE PROBLEM-SOLVING DRUG. P. G. Stafford, B. H. Golightly. Award, 1967.

MODERN MAN IN SEARCH OF A SOUL. C. G. Jung. Harcourt, Brace and World, 1933.

THE PSYCHOLOGY OF RELIGION. W. H. Clark. Macmillan, 1958.

THE VARIETIES OF RELIGIOUS EXPERIENCE. W. James. Mentor, 1958.

Homosexuality and Social Evil

CITY OF NIGHT. J. Rechy. Grove Press, 1963.

THE GAY WORLD: MALE HOMOSEXUALITY AND THE SOCIAL CREATION OF EVIL. M. Hoffman. Basic Books, 1968.

GIOVANNI'S ROOM. J. Baldwin. Dial Press, 1956.

THE PROBLEM OF HOMOSEXUALITY IN MODERN SOCIETY. H. Ruitenbeek, ed. Dutton, 1963.

SEXUAL INVERSION: THE MULTIPLE ROOTS OF HOMOSEXUALITY. J. Marmor, ed. Basic Books, 1965.

The Shattered Language of Schizophrenia

THE NEUROLOGY OF PSYCHOTIC SPEECH. M. Critchley in *British Journal of Psychiatry*, Vol. 110, pp. 353–364, 1964.

PATHOLOGICAL AND NORMAL LANGUAGE. J. Laffal. Atherton Press, 1965.

SCHIZOPHRENIA: LANGUAGE AND THOUGHT. B. Maher in *Principles of Psychopathology*, Chapter 15. McGraw-Hill, 1966.

STUDIES IN PSYCHOTIC LANGUAGE. B. Maher, K. O. McKean, and B. McLaughlin in *The General Inquirer: A Computer Approach to Content Analysis* (P. J. Stone, D. C. Dunphy, M. S. Smith and D. M. Ogilvie, eds.). M.I.T. Press, 1966.

A THEORY OF VERBAL BEHAVIOR IN SCHIZOPHRENIA. L. J. Chapman, L. Chapman, and G. A. Miller in *Progress in Experimental Personality Research*, Vol. 1. Academic Press, 1964.

II. Psychotherapy and Behavioral Change— Research and Theories

From Freud to Fromm

AN AUTOBIOGRAPHICAL STUDY. S. Freud. Norton, 1963.

ESCAPE FROM FREEDOM. E. Fromm. Holt, Rinehart, and Winston, 1941.

THE FUTURE OF AN ILLUSION. S. Freud. Liveright, 1955.

THE HEART OF MAN. E. Fromm. Harper & Row, 1964.

MAN FOR HIMSELF. E. Fromm. Holt, Rinehart and Winston, 1947.

NEW INTRODUCTORY LECTURES ON PSYCHOANALYSIS. S. Freud. Norton, 1933.

AN OUTLINE OF PSYCHOANALYSIS. S. Freud. Norton, 1949.

THE SANE SOCIETY. E. Fromm. Holt, Rinehart and Winston, 1955.

New Ways in Psychotherapy

CAUSES AND CURES OF NEUROSIS. H. J. Eysenck, S. Rachman. Robert Knapp, 1965.

CASE STUDIES IN BEHAVIOR MODIFICATION. L. P. Ullman, L. Krasner. Holt, Rinehart and Winston, 1965.
CONDITIONING TECHNIQUES IN CLINICAL PRACTICE AND RESEARCH. C. Frank. Springer, 1964.
EXPERIMENTS IN BEHAVIOR THERAPY. H. J. Eysenck. Pergamon Press, 1963.
PSYCHOTHERAPY BY RECIPROCAL INHIBITION. J. Wolpe. Stanford University Press, 1958.

For Helplessness: Can We Immunize the Weak?

ALLEVIATION OF LEARNED HELPLESSNESS IN THE DOG. M. Seligman, S. F. Maier, J. H. Geer in *Journal of Experimental Psychology*, Vol. 73, pp. 256–262, 1968.
CHRONIC FEAR PRODUCED BY UNPREDICTABLE ELECTRIC SHOCK. M. Seligman in *Journal of Comparative and Physiological Psychology*, Vol. 66, pp. 402–411, 1968.
FAILURE TO ESCAPE TRAUMATIC SHOCK. M. Seligman, S. F. Maier in *Journal of Experimental Psychology*, Vol. 74, pp. 1–9, 1967.
INTERNAL VS. EXTERNAL CONTROL OF REINFORCEMENT; A REVIEW. H. M. Lefcourt in *Psychological Bulletin*, Vol. 65, pp. 206–221, 1966.
ON THE PHENOMENON OF SUDDEN DEATH IN ANIMALS AND MAN. C. P. Richter in *Psychosomatic Medicine*, Vol. 19, pp. 191–198, 1967.
UNPREDICTABLE AND UNCONTROLLABLE AVERSIVE EVENTS. M. Seligman, S. F. Maier, R. L. Solomon in *Aversive Conditioning and Learning*. F. R. Brush, ed. Academic Press, 1969.

Morality in Psychotherapy

ANALYSIS OF A PHOBIA IN A FIVE-YEAR-OLD BOY. S. Freud in *The Complete Psychological Works of Sigmund Freud*. Hogarth Press, 1955. Vol. XIV.
AN APPETITIONAL THEORY OF SEXUAL MOTIVATION. K. R. Hardy in *Psychological Review*, pp. 1–18 and 71, 1964.
BEHAVIOR THERAPY TECHNIQUES. A. A. Lazarus, J. Wolpe. Pergamon Press, 1966.
THE CONCEPT OF MOTIVATION. R. S. Peters. Routledge & Kegan Paul, 1958.
A GENERAL INTRODUCTION TO PSYCHOANALYSIS. S. Freud. Liveright, 1920.
THE NEW GROUP THERAPY. O. H. Mowrer. Van Nostrand, 1964.
THE ORDEAL OF CHANGE. E. Hoffer. Harper & Row, 1964.

THE PSYCHOANALYTIC TECHNIQUE. A. Bernstein in *Handbook of Clinical Psychology*. McGraw-Hill, 1965.
THE PSYCHOPATHOLOGY OF EVERYDAY LIFE. S. Freud. Ernest Benn, 1904.
A STORY OF THREE DAYS. M. Wertheimer in *Documents of Gestalt Psychology*. University of California Press, 1961.
VALUE: BEHAVIORAL DECISION THEORY. G. M. Becker, C. G. McClintock in *Annual Review of Psychology*. Annual Reviews, 1967.

Inside Psychotherapy

COMMUNICATION RAPPORT AND PATIENT PROGRESS. D. E. Orlinsky, K. I. Howard in *Psychotherapy: Theory, Research and Practice*, 1968.
DIMENSIONS OF CONJOINT EXPERIENTIAL PROCESS IN PSYCHOTHERAPY RELATIONSHIPS. D. E. Orlinsky, K. I. Howard in *Proceedings, 75th Annual Meeting*, American Psychological Association, pp. 251–252, 1967.
THE GOOD THERAPY HOUR: EXPERIENTIAL CORRELATES OF PATIENTS' AND THERAPISTS' EVALUATIONS OF THERAPY SESSIONS. D. E. Orlinsky, K. I. Howard in *Archives of General Psychiatry*, Vol. 16, pp. 621–632, 1967.
THE PATIENT'S EXPERIENCE OF PSYCHOTHERAPY: SOME DIMENSIONS AND DETERMINANTS. K. I. Howard, D. E. Orlinsky, J. A. Hill in *Multivariate Behavioral Research*, 1968.
THE THERAPIST'S FEELINGS IN THE THERAPEUTIC PROCESS. K. I. Howard, D. E. Orlinsky, J. A. Hill in *Journal of Clinical Psychology*, 1968.

The Psychopharmacological Revolution

DRUGS AND ANIMAL BEHAVIOUR. H. Steinberg in *British Medical Bulletin*, Vol. 20, pp. 75–80, 1964.
DRUGS USED IN THE TREATMENT OF PSYCHIATRIC DISORDERS. M. E. Jarvik in *The Pharmacological Basis of Therapeutics*, L. S. Goodman, A. Gilman, eds. Macmillan, 3rd ed., pp. 159–214, 1965.
THE HALLUCINOGENIC DRUGS. F. Barron, M. E. Jarvik, S. Bunnell, Jr. in *Scientific American*, Vol. 210, pp. 3–11, April, 1964.
THE INFLUENCE OF DRUGS UPON MEMORY. M. E. Jarvik in *Animal Behaviour and Drug Action*. Hannah Steinberg, A. V. S. de Reuck, Julie Knight, eds. Churchill, 1964.
THE RELATION OF PSYCHIATRY TO PHARMACOLOGY. A. Wikler. Williams & Wilkins, 1957.

III. Psychotherapy and Behavioral Change—Approaches

The Autistic Child

ARBITRARY AND NATURAL REINFORCEMENT. C. B. Ferster in *The Psychological Record*, Vol. 17, No. 3, pp. 341–347, 1967.
AN EVALUATION OF BEHAVIOR THERAPY WITH CHILDREN. C. B. Ferster, J. Simons in *The Psychological Record*, Vol. 16, No. 1, pp. 65–71, 1966.
INFANTILE AUTISM. B. Rimland. Appleton-Century-Crofts, 1964.
OPERANT REINFORCEMENT OF INFANTILE AUTISM. C. B. Ferster in *An Evaluation of the Results of the Psychotherapies*. S. Lesse, ed. Charles C Thomas, 1968.
PERSPECTIVES IN PSYCHOLOGY: XXV, TRANSITION FROM ANIMAL LABORATORY TO CLINIC. C. B. Ferster in *The Psychological Record*, Vol. 17, No. 2, pp. 145–150, 1967.
POSITIVE REINFORCEMENT AND BEHAVIORAL DEFICITS OF AUTISTIC CHILDREN. C. B. Ferster in *Child Development*, Vol. 32, No. 3, pp. 437–456, 1961.

Hypnotherapeutic Conditioning

BASIC READINGS IN NEUROPSYCHOLOGY. R. L. Isaacson, ed. Harper & Row, 1964.
THE HUMAN BODY and THE HUMAN BRAIN. I. Asimov. Houghton Mifflin, 1963.
HYPNOTISM. A. M. Weitzenhoffer. Wiley, 1953.
NEURO-ENGINEERING: THE "NEW FRONTIER" FOR LIFE SCIENCES RESEARCH. J. M. Coyne in *Proceedings, San Diego Symposium for Biomedical Engineering*, 1963.
PSYCHOSOMATIC MEDICINE. J. H. Nodine, J. H. Moyer. Lea & Febiger, 1962.
THE STRESS OF LIFE. H. Selye. McGraw-Hill, 1956.

Mimosa Cottage: Experiment in Hope

THE EFFECT OF AN INSTITUTION ENVIRONMENT UPON THE VERBAL DEVELOPMENT OF IMBECILE CHILDREN. J. G. Lyle in *Journal of Mental Deficiency Research*, Vol. 3, pp. 122–128, 1959.
ENVIRONMENTAL INFLUENCE ON VERBAL OUTPUT OF MENTALLY RETARDED CHILDREN. B. B. Schlanger in *Journal of Speech and Hearing Disorders*, Vol. 19, pp. 339–345, 1954.
PROGRAMMED INSTRUCTION AS AN APPROACH TO TEACHING OF READING,

Tell us what you think

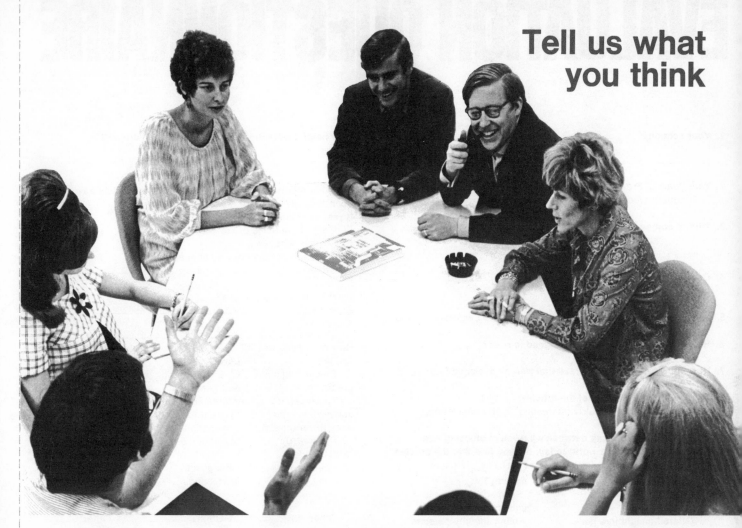

All over the country today students are taking an active role in the quality of their education. They're telling administrators what they like and what they don't like about their campus communities. They're telling teachers what they like and what they don't like about their courses.

This response card offers you a unique opportunity as a student to tell a publisher what you like and what you don't like about his book.

EVALUATION QUESTIONNAIRE

1. Your school:_____

_____

2. Your year: ☐ Freshman ☐ Sophomore ☐ Junior ☐ Senior
   ☐ Graduate student

3. Title of course in which READINGS was assigned:_____

_____

4. Course level: ☐ First year ☐ Second year ☐ Third year
   ☐ Fourth year ☐ Graduate

5. Length of course: ☐ Quarter ☐ Trimester ☐ Semester ☐ Year

6. How many articles were you assigned to read?_____

7. How many articles did you read that weren't assigned?_____

8. Did you find the majority of the articles:
   ☐ Very interesting ☐ Fairly interesting ☐ Not interesting

9. If you think there's a gap between what you're studying and
   what's going on in the world today, did you find that the articles
   in READINGS helped bridge that gap? ☐ Yes ☐ No

   If yes, how?
   ☐ Shed light on events in the news.
   ☐ Offered insight into personal problems and gave me ideas about solving them.
   ☐ Discussed the problems of individuals in ways that helped explain people I know.
   ☐ Offered insight into social problems and gave me ideas about solving them.
   ☐ Gave me information and arguments for attacking ideas I disagree with.
   ☐ Presented information and arguments that changed my own ideas.
   ☐ Other:_____

   _____

   If no, why?
   ☐ Seemed irrelevant to events in the news.
   ☐ Didn't identify personal problems important to me or suggest ways to solve them.
   ☐ Didn't make discussion of individual problems relevant to people I know.
   ☐ Didn't identify social problems important to me or suggest ways to solve them.
   ☐ Discussed individual and social problems but didn't make them important to me personally or show ways to deal with them.
   ☐ Didn't cause me to change my ideas about any important topic.
   ☐ Other:_____

10. How interesting were the materials used in your course?
    How do you rate them?
    Rating: 1 = Most interesting   7 = Least interesting
    Materials used:

	1	2	3	4	5	6	7
☐ **READINGS**	☐ 1	☐ 2	☐ 3	☐ 4	☐ 5	☐ 6	☐ 7
☐ Textbook	☐ 1	☐ 2	☐ 3	☐ 4	☐ 5	☐ 6	☐ 7
☐ Lectures	☐ 1	☐ 2	☐ 3	☐ 4	☐ 5	☐ 6	☐ 7
☐ Films	☐ 1	☐ 2	☐ 3	☐ 4	☐ 5	☐ 6	☐ 7
☐ Laboratory work	☐ 1	☐ 2	☐ 3	☐ 4	☐ 5	☐ 6	☐ 7
☐ Paperbacks	☐ 1	☐ 2	☐ 3	☐ 4	☐ 5	☐ 6	☐ 7
☐ Other_____	☐ 1	☐ 2	☐ 3	☐ 4	☐ 5	☐ 6	☐ 7

11. How helpful were the introductions to each article?
    ☐ Very helpful   ☐ Sometimes helpful
    ☐ Not helpful   ☐ Did not read them

12. Would additional materials printed with each article have
    been helpful? ☐ Yes ☐ No
    If yes, what kind?
    ☐ Marginal outlines of key points.
    ☐ Review questions.
    ☐ Glossaries of themes and concepts.
    ☐ Other:_____

13. What textbook did you use?
    Author(s):_____

    Title:_____

    How would you rate it?

Content:	Level:	Illustrations:
☐ Covered each area fully.	☐ Easy to read and generally interesting.	☐ Easy to understand, attractive, informative.
☐ Too much on some topics, not enough on others.	☐ Hard to read: explanations too complicated.	☐ Inadequate: hard to understand.
☐ Seemed up to date.	☐ Quality of writing not interesting.	☐ Unclear, unattractive.
☐ Seemed out of date.		☐ Didn't help in understanding.
☐ Other:_____	☐ Other:_____	☐ Other:_____

14. Are laboratory experiments part of your course work?
    ☐ Yes ☐ No
    If no, would you have liked to have had the equipment and
    opportunity to do psychological experiments as part of your
    course work? ☐ Yes ☐ No

15. Comments on course, text materials, etc.: _____

    _____

    _____

    _____

    _____

16. What do you think of this questionnaire?_____

    _____

    _____

    _____

    _____

WRITING, AND ARITHMETIC TO RE-
TARDED CHILDREN. S. W. Bijou *et al.*
in *Psychological Record*, Vol. 16, pp.
505–552, 1966.
RESIDENTIAL CARE OF MENTALLY HANDI-
CAPPED CHILDREN. J. Tizzard in *Brit-
ish Medical Journal*, Vol. 1, pp.
1041–1046, 1960.
SHIFTING STIMULUS CONTROL OF ARTICU-
LATION RESPONSES BY OPERANT TECH-
NIQUES. J. McLean. Unpublished
doctoral dissertation, University of
Kansas, 1965.
A STUDY OF THE EFFECTS OF COMMUNITY
AND INSTITUTIONAL SCHOOL CLASSES
FOR TRAINABLE MENTALLY RETARDED
CHILDREN. L. F. Cain, S. Levine. San
Francisco State College, 1961.

Daytop Village

DAYTOP LODGE—A NEW TREATMENT AP-
PROACH FOR DRUG ADDICTS. J. A.
Shelly, A. Bassin in *Corrective Psy-
chiatry*, Vol. 11, No. 4, pp. 186–195,
1965.
THE NEW GROUP THERAPY. O. H.
Mowrer. Van Nostrand, 1964.
REALITY THERAPY: A NEW APPROACH TO
PSYCHIATRY. W. Glasser. Harper &
Row, 1965.
SO FAIR A HOUSE: THE STORY OF SYNA-
NON. D. Casriel. Prentice-Hall, 1963.
THE PROCESS OF THE BASIC ENCOUNTER
GROUP. J. Bugental in *Challenges of
Humanistic Psychology*. McGraw-
Hill, 1967.
THERAPEUTIC PSYCHOLOGY: FUNDAMEN-
TALS OF ACTUALIZATION COUNSELING
AND THERAPY. 2nd ed. L. Brammer,
E. Shostrom. Prentice-Hall, 1968.

The Long Weekend

FACE TO FACE WITH THE DRUG ADDICT:
AN ACCOUNT OF AN INTENSIVE GROUP
EXPERIENCE. D. Kruschke, F. H.
Stoller in *Federal Probation*, Vol. 31,
No. 2, pp. 47–52, 1967.
FOCUSED FEEDBACK: EXTENDING GROUP
FUNCTIONS WITH VIDEO TAPE and
MARATHON GROUP THERAPY. F. H.
Stoller in *Innovations in Group Ther-
apy*. G. M. Gazda, ed. Charles C
Thomas, 1967.
GROUP PSYCHOTHERAPY ON TELEVISION:
AN INNOVATION WITH HOSPITALIZED
PATIENTS. F. H. Stoller in *American
Psychologist*, Vol. 22, pp. 158–162,
1967.

THE LEMON EATERS. J. Sohl. Simon and
Schuster, 1967.
THE MARATHON GROUP: INTENSIVE PRAC-
TICE OF INTIMATE INTERACTION.
G. R. Bach in *Psychological Reports*,
Vol. 18, pp. 995–1002, 1966.
THE USE OF FOCUSED FEEDBACK VIA
VIDEO TAPE IN SMALL GROUPS. F. H.
Stoller in *Explorations in Human Re-
lations Training and Research*, No. 1,
National Training Laboratories, Na-
tional Educational Association, 1966.

A Report on a Nude Marathon

CULTIVATING PEAK EXPERIENCE. P. Bin-
drim in *Ways of Growth*. H. Otto,
J. Mann, eds. Grossman, 1968.
EUPSYCHIAN MANAGEMENT: A JOURNAL.
A. Maslow. Irwin, 1965.
THE MARATHON GROUP: INTENSIVE PRAC-
TICE OF INTIMATE INTERACTION. G.
R. Bach in *Psychological Reports*,
Vol. 18, pp. 995–1002, 1966.
NUDISM IN AMERICA: A SOCIAL PSYCHO-
LOGICAL STUDY. W. E. Hartman, M.
Fithian. Crown (in press).
PEAK-ORIENTED PSYCHOTHERAPY: AN AP-
PROACH TO SELF-ACTUALIZATION
THROUGH THE CULTIVATION OF PEAK
EXPERIENCES. P. Bindrim. Mimeo-
graphed report, 1966.
PEAK-ORIENTED PSYCHOTHERAPY: CASE
HISTORIES AND TAPED TRANSCRIPTIONS
OF THERAPY SESSIONS. P. Bindrim.
Mimeographed report, 1966.
A REPORT ON A NUDE MARATHON. P. Bin-
drim in *Psychotherapy: Theory, Re-
search and Practice*, Vol. 5, No. 3,
pp. 180–188, September, 1968.
TIME-EXTENDED MARATHON GROUPS. E.
E. Minz in *Psychotherapy: Theory,
Research, and Practice*, Vol. 4, No.
2, pp. 65–70, May, 1967.

IV. Abnormal Behavior and Public Concerns

Group Therapy: Let the Buyer Beware

THE INCREASING INVOLVEMENT OF THE
PSYCHOLOGIST IN SOCIAL PROBLEMS.
C. Rogers in *The California State
Psychologist*, Vol. 9, No. 7, p. 29,
1968.

MAN, THE MANIPULATOR. E. Shostrom.
Abingdon, 1967.
THE MANIPULATOR AND THE CHURCH. M.
Dunnam, G. Herbertson, E. Sho-
strom. Abingdon, 1968.

Chromosomes and Crime

HUMAN HEREDITY. A. Montagu. World
Publishing, 1964.
THE GENETIC CODE. I. Asimov. Grossman,
1963 (in paperback, Signet).
GENETICS. *Biology and Behavior Series*.
David C. Glass, ed. Rockefeller Uni-
versity Press and Sage Foundation,
1968.
HUMAN POPULATION CYTOGENETICS.
W. M. C. Brown. Wiley, 1967.
THE YY SYNDROME. *Lancet*, March 12,
1966.

The Psychiatrist's Power in Civil Commitment

CRIME AND INSANITY IN ENGLAND. N.
Walker. Edinburgh University Press,
1968.
THE DEFENSE OF INSANITY. A. Goldstein.
Yale University Press, 1968.
PSYCHOANALYSIS, PSYCHIATRY AND LAW.
J. Katz, J. Goldstein, A. M. Dersho-
witz. Free Press, 1967.
VARIOUS JUDICIAL OPINIONS OF CHIEF
JUDGE DAVID BAZELON, U.S. COURT
OF APPEALS, DISTRICT OF COLUMBIA.

The Crime of Commitment

ASYLUMS: Essays on the Social Situation
of Mental Patients and Other In-
mates. E. Goffman. Doubleday-
Anchor, 1961.
THE MENTALLY DISABLED AND THE LAW:
The Report of the American Bar
Foundation on the Rights of the
Mentally Ill. F. T. Lindman, D. M.
McIntyre, Jr. University of Chicago
Press, 1961.
ONE FLEW OVER THE CUCKOO'S NEST. K.
Kesey. Viking, 1962.
PSYCHIATRY AND THE LAW. M. S. Gutt-
macher, H. Weihofen. Norton, 1952.
WARD NO. 6 [1892]. A. P. Chekhov in
Seven Short Stories by Chekhov.
Bantam, 1963. Pp. 106–157.

Index

Picture Credits

Cover photograph by William G. MacDonald

Photographs by
Raimondo R. Borea: pages 131, 132
Steve McCarroll: pages 22, 32, 76, 86, 92, 104, 126, 134
    152, 160
John Oldenkamp: pages 25, 52, 118, 123, 138, 139
Tom Suzuki: pages 2, 8, 16, 28, 34, 46, 56, 64, 74, 110, 140,
    144, 166
Steve Wells: page 148

Illustrations by
Philip Kirkland: pages 62, 80, 116
Karl Nicholason: page 40
George Price: pages 42, 43, 44, 171–174

CRM BOOKS
David A. Dushkin, *President and Publisher*, CRM BOOKS

Richard L. Roe, *Vice-President*, CRM BOOKS, *and Director, College Department*
Richard M. Connelly, *Sales Manager, College Department*
Nancy Le Clere, *Fulfillment Manager, College Department*
College Department Staff: Elaine Kleiss, Carol Walnum, La Delle M. Willett

Jean Smith, *Vice-President and Managing Editor*, CRM BOOKS
Editors: Arlyne Lazerson, Gloria Joyce, Cecie Starr, Betsy H. Wyckoff
Editorial Assistants: Jacquelyn Estrada, Cynthia MacDonald, Johanna Price, Ann Scales
Rights and Permissions: Donna L. Taylor

Jo Ann Gilberg, *Vice-President*, CRM BOOKS, *and Director, Manufacturing and Production*
Production Manager: Eugene G. Schwartz
Production Supervisors: Barbara Blum, E. Cecile Mayer, P. Douglas Armstrong
Production Assistants: Georgene Martina, Patricia Perkins, Toini Jaffe
Production Staff: Mona F. Drury, Margaret M. Mesec

Tom Suzuki, *Vice-President*, CRM BOOKS, *and Director of Design*
Art Director: Leon Bolognese
Designer: George Price
Associate Designers: Catherine Flanders, Reynold Hernandez
Assistant Designers: Robert Fountain, Pamela Morehouse
Art Staff: Jacqueline McLoughlin

Paul Lapolla, *Vice-President*, CRM BOOKS, *and Director, Psychology Today Book Club*
Assistant: Karen De Laria

Controller: Robert Geiserman
Assistant: Maryann Errichetti

Office Manager: Lynn D. Crosby
Assistant: Janie Fredericks

Officers of Communications/Research/Machines, Inc.
John J. Veronis, *President;* Nicolas H. Charney, *Chairman of the Board;*
David A. Dushkin, *Vice-President;* James B. Horton, *Vice-President*

This book was composed by American Book–Stratford Press, Inc., New York, New York
The book was printed and bound by The Kingsport Press, Inc., Kingsport, Tennessee